SPEECH AND LANGUAGE DISORDERS IN CHILDREN

Implications for the Social Security Administration's Supplemental Security Income Program

Committee on the Evaluation of the
Supplemental Security Income (SSI) Disability Program
for Children with
Speech Disorders and Language Disorders

Sara Rosenbaum and Patti Simon, *Editors*

Board on the Health of Select Populations

Board on Children, Youth, and Families

Institute of Medicine

Division of Behavioral and Social Sciences and Education

The National Academies of
SCIENCES · ENGINEERING · MEDICINE

THE NATIONAL ACADEMIES PRESS
Washington, DC
www.nap.edu

THE NATIONAL ACADEMIES PRESS 500 Fifth Street, NW Washington, DC 20001

This study was supported by Contract/Grant No. SS00-13-60048/0004 between the National Academy of Sciences and the Social Security Administration. Any opinions, findings, conclusions, or recommendations expressed in this publication do not necessarily reflect the views of any organization or agency that provided support for the project.

International Standard Book Number-13: 978-0-309-38875-7
International Standard Book Number-10: 0-309-38875-9
Library of Congress Control Number: 2016933601
Digital Object Identifier: 10.17226/21872

Additional copies of this report are available for sale from the National Academies Press, 500 Fifth Street, NW, Keck 360, Washington, DC 20001; (800) 624-6242 or (202) 334-3313; http://www.nap.edu.

Printed in the United States of America

Suggested citation: National Academies of Sciences, Engineering, and Medicine. 2016. *Speech and language disorders in children: Implications for the Social Security Administration's Supplemental Security Income Program.* Washington, DC: The National Academies Press. doi: 10.17226/21872.

The National Academies of
SCIENCES · ENGINEERING · MEDICINE

The **National Academy of Sciences** was established in 1863 by an Act of Congress, signed by President Lincoln, as a private, nongovernmental institution to advise the nation on issues related to science and technology. Members are elected by their peers for outstanding contributions to research. Dr. Ralph J. Cicerone is president.

The **National Academy of Engineering** was established in 1964 under the charter of the National Academy of Sciences to bring the practices of engineering to advising the nation. Members are elected by their peers for extraordinary contributions to engineering. Dr. C. D. Mote, Jr., is president.

The **National Academy of Medicine** (formerly the Institute of Medicine) was established in 1970 under the charter of the National Academy of Sciences to advise the nation on medical and health issues. Members are elected by their peers for distinguished contributions to medicine and health. Dr. Victor J. Dzau is president.

The three Academies work together as the **National Academies of Sciences, Engineering, and Medicine** to provide independent, objective analysis and advice to the nation and conduct other activities to solve complex problems and inform public policy decisions. The Academies also encourage education and research, recognize outstanding contributions to knowledge, and increase public understanding in matters of science, engineering, and medicine.

Learn more about the National Academies of Sciences, Engineering, and Medicine at **www.national-academies.org**.

COMMITTEE ON THE EVALUATION OF THE SUPPLEMENTAL SECURITY INCOME (SSI) DISABILITY PROGRAM FOR CHILDREN WITH SPEECH DISORDERS AND LANGUAGE DISORDERS

SARA ROSENBAUM (*Chair*), Harold and Jane Hirsh Professor of Health Law and Policy, Milken Institute School of Public Health, The George Washington University

WILLIAM J. BARBARESI, Associate Chief, Division of Developmental Medicine, Director, Developmental Medicine Center, Wade Family Foundation Chair in Developmental Medicine, Boston Children's Hospital; Associate Professor of Pediatrics, Harvard Medical School

STEPHEN M. CAMARATA, Professor of Hearing and Speech Sciences, Vanderbilt University School of Medicine

CHRISTINE DOLLAGHAN, Associate Dean and Professor, School of Behavioral and Brain Sciences, The University of Texas at Dallas

SIDNEY M. GOSPE, JR., Herman and Faye Sarkowsky Endowed Chair, Head, Division of Pediatric Neurology and Professor of Neurology and Pediatrics, University of Washington

GLORIA L. KRAHN, Barbara Emily Knudson Endowed Chair in Family Policy Studies, Oregon State University

ELYSA MARCO, Associate Professor of Neurology, University of California, San Francisco, School of Medicine

MARY PAT MOELLER, Director, Center for Childhood Deafness, Director, Language Development Laboratory, Boys Town National Research Hospital

SUSAN L. PARISH, Nancy Lurie Marks Professor of Disability Policy; Director, Lurie Institute for Disability Policy, and Associate Dean for Research, The Heller School for Social Policy and Management, Brandeis University

RAMESH RAGHAVAN, Professor and Associate Dean for Research, School of Social Work, Rutgers, The State University of New Jersey

AUDREY M. SORRELLS, Associate Dean of Students for Research and Associate Professor, The University of Texas at Austin, The College of Education & The Office of the Dean of Students, Division of Student Affairs

J. BRUCE TOMBLIN, Emeritus Professor, University of Iowa

KARL R. WHITE, Professor of Psychology and Director, National Center for Hearing Assessment and Management, Utah State University

Consultants

HOWARD H. GOLDMAN, Professor of Psychiatry, University of Maryland School of Medicine, Baltimore
MICHAEL McGEARY, Former Study Director, Institute of Medicine, The National Academies of Sciences, Engineering, and Medicine, Washington, DC
BARBARA C. SONIES, Research Professor, Department of Hearing and Speech Sciences, University of Maryland, College Park

Study Staff

PATTI SIMON, Study Director, Senior Program Officer
GUY CARMELI, Senior Program Assistant[1]
JENNIFER FLAUBERT, Associate Program Officer
ROHIT MUKHERJEE, Senior Program Assistant[2]
SARA THARAKAN, Research Associate[3]
FREDERICK "RICK" ERDTMANN, Director, Board on the Health of Select Populations
KIMBER BOGARD, Director, Board on Children, Youth, and Families[4]

---

[1] Starting June 2015.
[2] Through June 2015.
[3] Starting March 2015.
[4] Through July 2015.

Acknowledgments

Beyond the work of the study committee and the Institute of Medicine (IOM) project staff, this report reflects contributions from numerous other individuals and groups. The committee takes this opportunity to recognize those who so generously gave their time and expertise to inform its deliberations.

This study was sponsored by the Social Security Administration. We wish to thank Gina Clemons, Robin Doyle, Joanna Firmin, Marianna LaCanfora, Scott Marko, Natalie Scannell, Melissa Spencer, Marquita Sullivan, and Jim Twist for their guidance and support. In addition, the committee would like to thank the following individuals for their help: Terrance Flannery, Susan Guberman, Angela Harper, Gene Jerry, Chere Johnson, Joseph Karevy, Frances Mardesich, Dana Mercer, Stephanie Myers, Mary Beth Rochowiak, Cheryl A. Williams, Jessica Wisner, and Amanda Wulf.

The committee greatly benefited from the opportunity for discussion with the individuals who made presentations at and attended the committee's workshops and meetings: Kathy Bainbridge, Stephen J. Blumberg, Paul S. Davies, Jeffrey Hemmeter, Howard J. Hoffman, Ann P. Kaiser, Michelle M. Macias, Lemmietta G. McNeilly, Cheryl K. Messick, Meredith Miceli, Rhea Paul, Kalman Rupp, Steven F. Warren, Nora Wells, and Larry Wexler. The committee is thankful for the useful contributions of these many individuals. We extend special thanks to the following individuals who were essential sources of information, generously giving their time and knowledge to further the committee's efforts: Ilhom Akobirshoev, Esther Son, and Rajan Sonik.

Many staff within the IOM provided support in various ways to this project. The committee would like to thank Lorraine Bell, Laura DeStefano, Chelsea Frakes, Greta Gorman, Karen Helsing, Linda Kilroy, Fariha Mahmud, Maureen Mellody, Bettina Ritter, Julie Wiltshire, and Joel Wu. The committee gratefully acknowledges Rick Erdtmann, director of the Board on the Health of Select Populations, for his guidance on this study. Finally, Rona Briere and Alisa Decatur are to be credited for the superb editorial assistance they provided in preparing the final report.

Reviewers

This report has been reviewed in draft form by individuals chosen for their diverse perspectives and technical expertise. The purpose of this independent review is to provide candid and critical comments that will assist the institution in making its published report as sound as possible and to ensure that the report meets institutional standards for objectivity, evidence, and responsiveness to the study charge. The review comments and draft manuscript remain confidential to protect the integrity of the deliberative process. We wish to thank the following individuals for their review of this report:

Kathy Bainbridge, National Institutes of Health National Institute on Deafness and Other Communication Disorders
Heidi M. Feldman, Stanford University School of Medicine
Lisa Goffman, Purdue University
George Howard, University of Alabama at Birmingham
Catherine Lord, Weill Cornell Medical College
Susan Nittrouer, University of Florida
Patricia M. Owens, Patricia M. Owens Consultations in Disability Programs and Policy
Doris Trauner, University of California, San Diego, School of Medicine
David K. Urion, Boston Children's Hospital
Steven F. Warren, University of Kansas

Although the reviewers listed above provided many constructive comments and suggestions, they were not asked to endorse the report's overall conclusions, nor did they see the final draft of the report before its release. The review of this report was overseen by **Bradford H. Gray,** Urban Institute, and **Rosemary A. Chalk,** independent consultant. They were responsible for making certain that an independent examination of this report was carried out in accordance with institutional procedures and that all review comments were carefully considered. Responsibility for the final content of this report rests entirely with the authoring committee and the institution.

Preface

For low-income children who experience a severe disability, the Supplemental Security Income (SSI) program offers a vital source of financial support. Indeed, so important is the assistance made available through the SSI children's program that its scope and reach were the focus of a landmark 1990 decision by the U.S. Supreme Court, *Sullivan v. Zebley.* Under its targeted standards, most recently updated by Congress in 1996, the SSI program reaches more than 1.3 million children annually.

Most people think of speech and language as skills that children automatically acquire as they grow, and for the vast majority of children, this is the case. But the development of speech and language is an extraordinarily complex process, and for a small proportion of children, appropriate development can be interrupted or can cease altogether. Up to 16 percent of children have such disorders; for a fraction of these children, the disorder can involve an unusual level of severity.

In their severest form, speech and language disorders can have a devastating impact on children's health and development. These disorders can profoundly affect children's ability to communicate; learn; and establish and maintain strong family, peer, and community relationships. They elevate risk for a wide variety of adverse outcomes, including social isolation and mental health disorders, learning disabilities, behavior disorders, poor academic achievement, long-term placement in special education, and lifetime unemployment. Children with the severest forms of speech and language disorders who live in low-income families may be able to qualify for SSI benefits as well as Medicaid, which is essential to their ability to gain access to appropriate medical treatment.

With support from the Social Security Administration (SSA), the

National Academies of Sciences, Engineering, and Medicine formed the Committee on the Evaluation of the SSI Disability Program for Children with Speech Disorders and Language Disorders. The committee's charge was to identify past and current trends in the prevalence and persistence of these disorders among the general population of children under 18 and to compare these trends with trends among the SSI child population. The committee also was asked to provide an overview of the current status of diagnosis and treatment of speech and language disorders and the levels of impairment due to these disorders among children under 18.

To carry out its charge, the committee engaged in extensive study over the course of nearly 1 year, holding five formal meetings and participating in numerous telephone and email exchanges. As part of its work, the committee held two invitational workshops to gain insight from more than 16 experts in research on and measurement of speech and language disorders among children, as well as in the treatment of such disorders and the administration of educational and social programs and services for affected children.

It is the committee's hope that the findings and conclusions presented in this report will have impacts both practical and educational. On the practical side, the committee anticipates that its work will help inform the SSA's policy and program administration activities. On the educational side, the committee hopes that the report will convey to a broader audience the enormous personal, familial, and social consequences of severe speech and language disorders in childhood, and thus the vital importance of effective programs for affected children and their families.

This committee was especially fortunate to have a membership that not only possessed the full range of expertise needed to produce this report but also was uncommonly dedicated to its work and to the highest level of collaboration. The committee was extremely fortunate to be supported throughout its work by talented and gracious staff of the Institute of Medicine: Patti Simon, study director; Sara Tharakan and Jennifer Flaubert, research staff; Guy Carmeli and Rohit Mukherjee, who provided logistical and administrative support; and Dr. Rick Erdtmann, Director of the Academies Board on the Health of Select Populations. The committee also wishes to thank Dr. Howard Goldman for his expertise, guidance, and support throughout the study process.

The committee hopes that this report will further a greater understanding of the challenges faced by the children whose health conditions were the subject of its work, as well as of the central importance of programs such as SSI to the lives of these children.

Sara Rosenbaum, *Chair*
Committee on the Evaluation of the
Supplemental Security Income (SSI) Disability Program
for Children with Speech Disorders and Language Disorders

Contents

Summary

Speech and language are central to the human experience, and their acquisition is a seemingly automatic process that continues from birth through adolescence. The identification of speech and language disorders often occurs when a child does not achieve expected or normative developmental milestones. Such disorders impair a child's functioning, and when they are severe enough to disrupt a child's ability to communicate, they have especially serious consequences. In their most severe forms, moreover, such conditions can be expected to persist over a lifetime. When combined with other risks, such as poverty, severe speech and language disorders can increase risk for a wide variety of adverse outcomes, including social isolation and mental health disorders, learning disabilities, behavior disorders, poor academic achievement, and chronic underemployment. These outcomes—some of which can be mitigated through early identification and intervention—point to the array of needs children with speech and language disorders are likely to have and to the kinds of ongoing support they may require.

The Supplemental Security Income (SSI) program for children provides financial assistance to children from low-income, resource-limited families who have been determined to have conditions that meet the disability standard required under law. When sufficiently severe, speech and language disorders can qualify children for SSI disability assistance. Over the past several decades, the number of children receiving SSI has risen overall, and the number receiving SSI on the basis of speech and language disorders also has risen. A 2010 report issued by the U.S. Government Accountability Office (GAO) found an increase between 2000 and 2010 in both applications and allowances (applicants determined to meet the disability criteria) for children with speech and language impairments. During this period, the number of applications for speech and language impairments increased from 21,615 to 49,664, while the number of children found to meet the disability criteria increased from 11,565 to 29,147.

Based on the GAO's findings, the Social Security Administration (SSA) determined that additional research was needed to understand the increases in the number of children applying for and receiving SSI benefits on the basis of speech and language disorders. It is in the context of the changes observed in the SSI program for children that the SSA requested this study.

STUDY CHARGE

In 2014, the SSA Office of Disability Policy requested that the Institute of Medicine of the National Academies of Sciences, Engineering, and Medicine convene a consensus committee to identify past and current trends in the prevalence and persistence of speech and language disorders among the general U.S. population under age 18 and compare those trends with trends among the SSI childhood disability population, and to provide an overview of the current status of the diagnosis and treatment of speech and language disorders and the levels of impairment due to these disorders in the U.S. population under age 18. (See Box S-1 for the committee's full statement of task.)

OVERALL CONCLUSIONS

The committee reviewed a range of sources to respond to its charge, including published research on the etiology, epidemiology, and treatment of childhood speech and language disorders; expert testimony; data from clinical studies; data from nationally representative surveys; and data from federal programs. Collectively, the findings and conclusions presented in this report represent the committee's responses to the objectives, goals, and activities specified in its statement of task. The findings are statements of the evidence; the conclusions are inferences, interpretations, or generalizations drawn from the evidence and supported by the committee's findings.

After reviewing the evidence, the committee arrived at seven overall conclusions. Each of these is described in detail in the sections that follow.

Impact of Severe Speech and Language Disorders

Severe speech and language disorders in children are associated with significant impairment in functioning. Children with severe speech and language disorders—those whose functioning is considered to be two or more

BOX S-1
Statement of Task

An ad hoc committee will conduct a study to address the following task order objectives:

- Identify past and current trends in the prevalence and persistence of speech disorders and language disorders for the general U.S. population under age 18 and compare those trends to trends in the Supplemental Security Income (SSI) childhood disability population; and
- Provide an overview of the current status of the diagnosis and treatment of speech disorders and language disorders, and the levels of impairment in the U.S. population under age 18.

To accomplish this goal, the committee will:

- Compare the national trends in the number of children with speech disorders and language disorders under age 18 with the trends in the number of children receiving SSI on the basis of speech disorders and language disorders; and describe the possible factors that may contribute to any differences between the two groups; and
- Identify current professional standards of pediatric and adolescent health care for speech disorders and language disorders and identify the kinds of care documented or reported to be received by children in the SSI childhood disability population.

To perform the above activities, the committee shall do the following with respect to the two child populations:

- Identify national trends in the prevalence of speech disorders and language disorders in children and assess factors that influence these trends.
- Identify the causes of speech disorders and language disorders and determine how often these disorders are the result of known causes.
- Identify the average age of onset and the gender distribution and assess the levels of impairment within age groups.
- Assess how age, development, and gender may play a role in the progression of some speech disorders and language disorders.
- Identify common comorbidities among pediatric speech disorders and language disorders.
- Identify which speech disorders and language disorders are most amenable to treatment and assess typical or average time required for improvement in disorder to manifest following diagnosis and treatment.
- Identify professionally accepted standards of care (such as diagnostic evaluation and assessment, treatment planning and protocols, and educational interventions) for children with speech disorders and with language disorders.

standard deviations from the norm—may lack the ability to communicate effectively. The committee found that these disorders can have a lasting and profound impact on the children and families they affect. Specifically, the committee concluded that

1. **Severe speech and language disorders in children are conditions that interfere with communication and learning and represent serious lifelong threats to social, emotional, educational, and employment outcomes.**

The functional requirements for language and communication increase continually throughout childhood. For children with moderate to severe speech and language disorders, these requirements often outpace their development. Thus, even if a child with such a disorder is able to make at least some developmental progress through treatment, the gap between his or her abilities and functional expectations may nonetheless continue to widen.

Prevalence and Comorbidity

The committee was asked to identify past and current trends in the prevalence of speech and language disorders in the general population under age 18. As a first step to this end, the committee sought to arrive at a current estimate of the overall prevalence of speech and language disorders in children. In addition, the committee was asked to identify common comorbidities (or co-occurring conditions) of childhood speech and language disorders. To do so, the committee consulted numerous sources of data, including clinical data from small treatment studies, population-based data from large national surveys, and administrative data from large federal programs. From this review, the committee concluded that

2. **Speech and language disorders affect between 3 and 16 percent of U.S. children. Approximately 40 percent of children with speech and language disorders in nationally representative studies have serious comorbidities such as intellectual disabilities, autism spectrum disorder, and other neurodevelopmental and behavioral disorders.**

This range is based on the best evidence available: prevalence estimates of speech and language disorders from peer-reviewed studies of U.S. children (between 3.8 and 15.6 percent) and prevalence estimates of speech and language disorders from three national surveys (between 3.2 and 7.7 percent). However, the available data regarding the prevalence of childhood speech and language disorders within the general population are limited in several ways. Specifically, the sources of data considered by the committee vary markedly in how speech and language impairments are defined and identified, the degree to which the level of severity is documented, the reporting sources, and the characteristics of the populations within each dataset. For example, many of the sources of data include information reported by a parent or a caregiver but include no corroborating information from clinical assessment.

The few but varied data collection strategies used to estimate the prevalence of speech and language disorders in children leave room for both undercounts and overcounts. For example, conditions that commonly co-occur with speech and language disorders, such as autism spectrum disorder and attention deficit hyperactivity disorder, may initially be identified as speech and language disorders, thereby inflating the number of speech and language disorders reported. Conversely, speech and language disorders may be included in other reported categories, such as "development delays" or "multiple disabilities," or reported as impairments secondary to primary conditions such as autism spectrum disorder or primary disorders of hearing, thereby effectively deflating the number of speech and language disorders reported.

Although the committee encountered challenges, it found sufficient evidence to estimate that 3 to 16 percent of the general population of children from birth through age 21 experience problems with speech or language.[1] For example, studies on childhood speech sound disorders show overall prevalence rates ranging from 3 to 16 percent. Research on childhood language disorders shows overall prevalence rates of 6 to 15 percent. And one population-based study of specific language impairment found a prevalence rate of 7.4 percent among children in kindergarten. In addition, data from the National Survey of Children with Special Health Care Needs and the National Survey of Children's Health show reported prevalence of speech and language disorders between 3 and 5 percent. And one recent national survey on voice, swallowing, speech, and language problems in children found that 7.7 percent had such problems according to parent or guardian reports. Finally, National Health Interview Survey data from 2000 to 2012 indicate that more than 40 percent of children with speech and language problems experienced comorbidities such as developmental delay (estimated at 32 percent), autism (estimated at 12 percent), and intellectual disability (estimated at 10 percent).

Within the population of all children with speech and language disorders, a small group will have disorders severe enough to meet the standard of disability for the SSI program. Within that latter population, even fewer children will both meet the SSI financial eligibility standard and actually enroll in the program (see Figure S-1).

---

[1] While the primary population of focus for this study is children under age 18, the committee reviewed and has included here relevant Individuals with Disabilities Education Act (IDEA) data (which include children from birth to age 21).

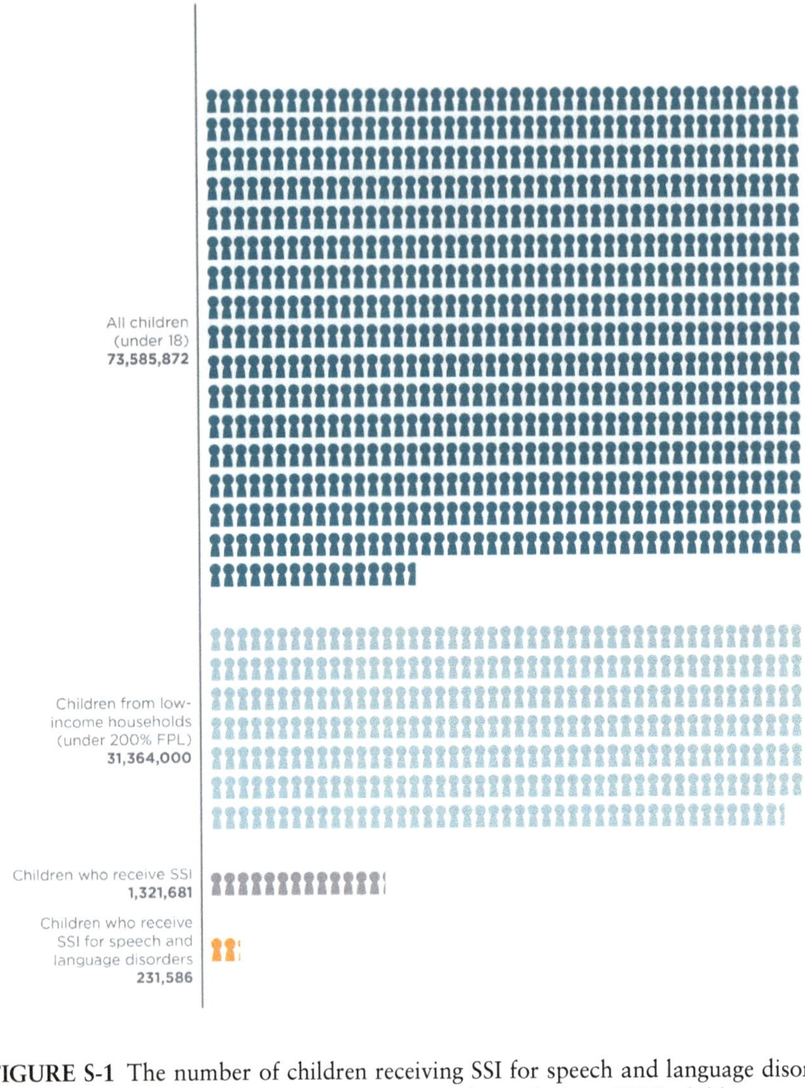

FIGURE S-1 The number of children receiving SSI for speech and language disorders is a small subpopulation among the general population of U.S. children.
NOTES: FPL = federal poverty level; SSI = Supplemental Security Income. All data are from 2013. Scale = 1 symbol to 100,000 children. The Current Population Survey table creator was used to generate numbers of children below 200 percent of the federal poverty level. Parameters used to generate the numbers include get count of: persons in poverty universe (everyone except unrelated individuals under 15); years: 2004 to 2013; census 2010 weights; row variable: age; column variable: income-to-poverty ratio; and customized formatting: income-to-poverty ratio percent cutoff of 200 percent. These populations are not mutually exclusive.

Supplemental Security Income

Childhood poverty and the accompanying deprivations have significant adverse implications for children with disabilities. Research has established that childhood poverty can exacerbate disabilities and their effects and lead to deleterious outcomes across a range of indicators, including emotional, social, and mental development; academic achievement; and employment during adulthood. The converse is true as well: the consequences of poverty are likely to be especially serious for children with disabilities because of their heightened vulnerabilities, elevated needs for health care, and overall poor health.

The SSI program for children was established to address the needs of children with disabilities living in low-income households because they were determined to be "among the most disadvantaged of all Americans and are deserving of special assistance." SSI recipients include children whose health conditions or disabilities are severe enough to meet the program's disability eligibility criteria and whose family income and assets are within limits specified by the SSA. The committee concluded that

3. **Children of families with low incomes are more likely than the general population to have disabilities, including speech and language disorders. The Supplemental Security Income (SSI) program is designed to award benefits to the most severely impaired children from low-income, resource-limited families. Currently, 0.31 percent of U.S. children receive SSI benefits for speech and language disorders.**

In December 2014, 213,688 children were receiving SSI benefits as the result of a primary speech or language impairment (16 percent of all children receiving SSI benefits). Figure S-1 shows that these children represent a small subpopulation among the general population of U.S. children. The majority of children who receive SSI benefits are from families with a household income less than 200 percent of the federal poverty level (FPL). The number of families with incomes less than 200 percent of the FPL changes over time. That is, as economic conditions deteriorate, more families join the ranks of those with incomes at or below a defined poverty level. This occurred most recently following the 2008-2009 recession in the United States. As a result, more children would have met the financial eligibility criteria for SSI benefits. This means that an increase in the number of children with speech and language disorders receiving SSI may not reflect an increase in these disorders, but instead may arise from an increased number of children with these disorders who meet the poverty threshold for SSI eligibility

(NASEM, 2015). However, there are no reliable estimates of the number of children living in poverty who also have speech and language disorders.

Assessment, Evaluation, and Standards of Care

The committee reviewed standards of care, including diagnostic evaluation and assessment, treatments and protocols, and educational interventions, for children with speech and language disorders. The committee reviewed the literature and invited speech, language, and special education experts to provide additional insights into current standards of care and practices for children with speech and language disorders, including evidence on the efficacy of treatments and interventions, when available.

In addition, the committee was asked to identify the kinds of care documented or reported to be received by children in the SSI disability program. The committee requested a review of a random sample of case files of children who receive SSI benefits for speech and language disorders. The results of this review helped demonstrate the kinds of evidence the SSA considers when making a disability determination for a child. Based on its review of professional standards of care and the documentation included in a random sample of case files, the committee concluded that

4. **To determine the severity of speech and language disorders in children, the Social Security Administration employs the results of professionally administered assessments and also takes into account other clinical evidence that would be consistent with severe speech and language disorders.**

To qualify for SSI benefits, children must meet a complex and detailed set of eligibility criteria that are income- and resource-related, work-related, and disability-related. The evidence required to document severity of disability is extensive and includes both medical evidence—such as formal testing to provide developmental and functional information, signs, symptoms, and laboratory findings—and parental and teacher reports. Under the SSA's standards, observations and information from a single source—such as a parent or caregiver are an insufficient basis for a finding of disability. For example, the majority of the cases in the random sample included evidence of standardized testing (143 of 152 files), and virtually all of the case files included information from speech-language pathologists regarding the child's speech and language status (150 of 152 files). While these findings cannot be considered representative of the entire SSI child population with speech and language disorders, the review offered valuable information that is consistent with other sources of evidence considered by the committee.

Trends in the General U.S. Population Compared with Trends in the Supplemental Security Income Program

One of the committee's primary objectives was to consider past and current trends in the prevalence of speech and language disorders among the general U.S. population under age 18 and to compare those trends with trends observed among participants in the SSI childhood disability program. To this end, the committee analyzed clinical studies, nationally representative survey data, and administrative or service data from a range of sources. These data, however, are primarily serial cross-sections as opposed to longitudinal data. Thus, these data reflect changes in the prevalence of speech and language disorders observed within populations of respondents (in the case of survey data) or beneficiaries (in the case of SSI data) over successive years and do not follow individual children over time. Without longitudinal data, it is not possible to describe the natural course of these disorders. Moreover, because children observed in one year may not be the same as those observed in another, the composition of the populations reflected in the data changes from year to year. Not only may changes in population composition over time affect rates of observed occurrence; changes in programs that provide supports for children with severe disabilities also will affect the size and characteristics of the population of children who receive benefits based on a severe disability in any given year. Thus, over time, SSI eligibility standards and the eligibility determination process itself, along with broader economic factors such as the recession of 2008-2009, may influence the rate at which speech and language disorders are observed among any given population of children at any given point in time.

Despite the above limitations, the committee was able to draw conclusions from the evidence regarding the extent to which speech and language disorders are documented in specific populations of children over time.

Trends in the General U.S. Population

The committee used the best evidence available to assess trends in the prevalence of speech and language disorders in the general U.S. child population. Several sources that collect data on speech and language disorders in children suggest that over the past decade, the prevalence of these conditions has increased. Although there have been no studies describing why the prevalence of speech and language disorders has increased over time, available epidemiologic literature related to children with autism spectrum disorder and attention deficit hyperactivity disorder may provide insight. Factors identified as causes for these increases include increased awareness of developmental disorders, increased availability of early intervention and special education services, and changes in the definition of certain conditions (e.g., autism spectrum disorder). The two nationally representative surveys that include measures of speech and language disorders in children at multiple points in time are the National Survey of Children's Health and the National Survey of Children with Special Health Care Needs. The National Survey of Children's Health showed an increase in prevalence of speech and language disorders from 3.8 percent in 2007 to 4.8 percent in 2011, a 26 percent increase. The National Survey of Children with Special Health Care Needs showed an increase in prevalence from 3.2 percent in 2005-2006 to 5.0 percent in 2009-2010, an increase of 56 percent. Although not a direct comparison, the committee reviewed data on initial SSI allowances for speech and language disorders for two points in time to determine the percent increase in those initial allowances.[2] The number of initial allowances for speech and language disorders increased by nearly 40 percent between 2007 and 2011 (from 21,135 to 29,309). Therefore, the committee concluded that

5. **The best available evidence shows an increase in the prevalence of speech and language disorders over the past decade in the U.S. child population. Trends in annual Supplemental Security Income initial allowances parallel this overall increase.**

Causes, Treatment, and Persistence

The committee was asked to identify causes of speech and language disorders and to determine how often those causes are known. The evidence shows a variety of known etiologies (e.g., cleft palate, congenital brain tumors, and genetic disorders) and potential risk factors (e.g., toxic exposures, nutritional deficiencies, and injuries), as well as the common comorbidities noted earlier (e.g., autism spectrum disorder and attention deficit hyperactivity disorder). In some cases, the cause may not be known.

A range of strategies are used to treat mild, moderate, and severe speech and language disorders in children. In its review of the evidence, the committee found that with treatment, mild speech and language disorders may completely resolve or be limited to relatively minor impairments; moderate speech and language disorders may substantially diminish, with residual impairments in an associated domain, such as reading and literacy. In the most severe cases, however—even with treatment—core speech and language deficits will likely continue into adolescence and may be lifelong. Therefore, the committee concluded that

[2] Initial allowances are the total number of new cases within any given period of time of children found to be eligible for disability benefits based on both the financial and the disability criteria.

6. **Children with mild to moderate speech and language disorders will benefit from a variety of treatments. For children with severe speech and language disorders, treatment improves function; with few exceptions, however, substantial functional limitations will persist.**

An implication of this conclusion is that a severe disorder will persist over time, thereby necessitating ongoing educational, social, and health supports and, in the case of children from low-income families, continuing eligibility for financial assistance through the SSI program.

Trends Among Participants in the Supplemental Security Income Program

To identify trends among participants in the SSI program, the committee reviewed administrative data collected by the SSA on initial allowances and recipients[3] for primary speech and language impairments. Between 2004 and 2014, the total number of children receiving benefits for speech and language disorders increased from 90,281 to 315,523, a 249 percent increase. The committee reviewed older data to help explain this substantial growth in the total number of recipients. At the committee's request, the SSA provided supplemental data for review beginning in 1994, the year in which the primary impairment code for speech and language impairments (3153) was introduced. From this review, the committee concluded that

7. **The total number of children receiving Supplemental Security Income for speech and language disorders more than tripled in the past decade. In addition to an increase in prevalence of these disorders in the general U.S. child population, this growth is explained primarily by two factors:**
    - **the introduction of a new impairment code for speech and language disorders in 1994, and**
    - **the continuing eligibility of children whose severe speech and language disorders persist throughout childhood.**

Prior to 1994, there were zero initial allowances for the impairment code for speech and language disorders in children (3153). The current total number of recipients reflects both the accumulation over time of new individuals in this impairment category and the very low attrition from the program due to the persistence of severe speech and language disorders. Thus, the increase in the number of annual initial *allowances* leads to a much larger percent increase in the total number of *recipients* over time,

[3] Recipients refer to the current number of children receiving SSI benefits.

because once qualified for SSI, few children with severe speech and language disorders subsequently become ineligible for the program.

Several additional factors contribute to the changes observed in the number of children receiving SSI benefits for speech and language disorders. For example, the total number of child SSI recipients fluctuates depending on the number of initial allowances, terminations, suspensions, and reentries from suspension. When the number of allowances exceeds the number of terminations and suspensions in 1 year, the total number of recipients increases for that year. Overall growth in the population of children would be expected to contribute some growth in the program as well. In addition to severity, a statutory condition of eligibility for SSI is either duration or death. Therefore, children with speech and language disorders who qualify for SSI will continue to have a severe speech and language disorder, and unless their eligibility changes for some other reason, they will not exit the program before they reach 18 years of age. Finally, allowances are affected by macroeconomic conditions. During a period of economic expansion, as family income increases and joblessness decreases, fewer children are likely to meet the SSA's financial eligibility criteria. By contrast, during periods of economic downturn—for example, during the recent recession—more children will meet the financial eligibility criteria of the program because of relatively higher unemployment.

CONCLUSION

The evidence presented in this report underscores the long-term and profound impact of severe speech and language disorders on children and their families. It also helps explain the degree to which children with such disorders can be expected to be a significant presence in a program such as SSI, whose purpose is to provide financial assistance to families of children with the severest disabilities. It is the committee's hope that this report will make a substantial contribution to understanding the nature of severe speech and language disorders in children and provide a strong foundation for future efforts in policy, practice, and research.

The committee's findings and conclusions characterize the current state of knowledge. Its findings also highlight the challenges that arise in undertaking a close examination of children's health status in the area of speech and language because of deficiencies in the evidence both across the general population and, in this case, the specific population of children enrolled in the SSI program. Despite its limitations, the evidence presented in this report offers valuable insight into the relationship between children with speech and language disorders in the general population and those participating in the SSI program. Furthermore, the evidence presented here can assist policy makers, health and education professionals, and SSI program administrators in understanding the extent to which the SSI program's basic design and administrative process operate together to connect the nation's most severely impaired and disadvantaged children with speech and language disorders to the benefits that program offers.

REFERENCE

NASEM (National Academies of Sciences, Engineering, and Medicine). 2015. *Mental disorders and disabilities among low-income children.* Washington, DC: The National Academies Press.

1

Introduction

Speech and language are central to the human experience; they are the vital means by which people convey and receive knowledge, thoughts, feelings, and other internal experiences. Acquisition of communication skills begins early in childhood and is foundational to the ability to gain access to culturally transmitted knowledge, to organize and share thoughts and feelings, and to participate in social interactions and relationships. Speech and language skills allow a child to engage in exchanges that lead to the acquisition of knowledge in his or her community and the educational arena. Communication skills are crucial to the development of thinking ability, a sense of self, and full participation in society.

Speech and language disorders—disruptions in communication development—can have wide-ranging and adverse impacts on the ability not only to communicate but also to acquire new knowledge and participate fully in society. Most children acquire speech and language by a seemingly automatic process that begins at birth and continues through adolescence. Typically, basic communication skills are developed (although not complete) by the time a child enters kindergarten, enabling the child to begin learning from teachers and interacting fluently with peers and caregivers (Oller et al., 2006). Severe disruptions in speech or language acquisition thus have both direct and indirect consequences for child and adolescent development, not only in communication but also in associated abilities such as reading and academic achievement that depend on speech and language skills. When combined with other developmental risks, such as poverty (Williams, 2013), severe speech and language disabilities can become high-impact, adverse conditions with long-term cognitive, social, and academic sequelae and high social and economic costs.

STUDY CONTEXT

Like other entitlement programs, the Supplemental Security Income (SSI) program has generated considerable and recurring interest in its growth, effectiveness, accuracy, and sustainability. Questions have arisen in both the media and policy-making settings regarding the appropriateness of SSI benefits for children with speech and language disorders.

As an example, the *Boston Globe* published a series of articles in December 2010 describing the experiences and challenges of families who either were currently receiving or had sought to become eligible to receive SSI benefits for their children. These articles focused on the growing number of children enrolled in SSI on the basis of speech and language disorders. In response to issues raised in these articles, members of Congress directed the U.S. Government Accountability Office (GAO) to conduct an assessment of the SSI program for children. This assessment was designed to examine decade-long trends in the rate of children receiving SSI benefits based on mental impairments;[1] the role played by medical and nonmedical information, such as medication use and school records, in the initial eligibility determination; and steps taken by the Social Security Administration (SSA) to monitor children's continued eligibility based on disability.

The GAO assessment was conducted between February 2011 and June 2012. Midway through the assessment, on October 27, 2011, the Subcommittee on Human Resources of the House Ways and Means Committee convened a hearing on SSI for children, including an interim report by the GAO on its findings regarding the SSI program for children. In that report, the GAO found that between 2000 and 2011, the annual number of children applying for SSI benefits had increased from 187,052 to 315,832. Of these applications, 54 percent had been denied.

The GAO also found that mental impairments constituted approximately 65 percent of all child SSI allowances. The three most prevalent primary mental impairments[2] for children found eligible were attention deficit hyperactivity disorder (ADHD), speech and language impairments,[3]

[1] The SSI program categorizes "speech and language impairments" as mental disorders.

[2] See the report *Mental Disorders and Disabilities Among Low-Income Children* for trends in prevalence for mental disorders (NASEM, 2015).

[3] Impairment code 3153 was changed from "speech and language delays" to "speech and language impairments" in August 2015.

and autism/developmental delays.[4] From December 2000 to December 2011, the total number of children receiving SSI benefits for mental impairments had increased annually, from approximately 543,000 in 2000 to approximately 861,000 in 2011, an almost 60 percent increase. Secondary impairments were present for many of those found medically eligible. In addition, the GAO estimated that in 2010, 55 percent of children with speech and language impairments who received SSI benefits had an accompanying secondary impairment recorded; 94 percent of those recorded secondary impairments were other mental disorders.

In its final report, the GAO suggested that several factors may have contributed to the observed changes in the size of the SSI program for children, including

- long-term receipt of assistance, with fewer children leaving the disability program prior to age 18;
- increased numbers of children living in poverty in the United States;
- increased awareness and improved diagnosis of certain mental impairments;
- a focus on identifying children with disabilities through public school special education services; and
- increased health insurance coverage of previously uninsured children.

The GAO found an increase between 2000 and 2010 in both applications and allowances (applicants determined to meet the disability criteria) for children with speech and language impairments (GAO, 2012). During this period, the number of applications for speech and language impairments increased from 21,615 to 49,664, while the number of children found to meet the disability criteria increased from 11,565 to 29,147 (GAO, 2012). The cumulative number of allowances for children with speech and language impairments has continued to increase. In December 2014, 213,688 children were receiving benefits as the result of a primary speech or language impairment (16 percent of all children receiving SSI benefits) (SSA, 2015). The factors that contributed to these changes are a primary focus of this report and are discussed at length in Chapters 4, 5, and 6.

Based on the GAO findings, the SSA determined that additional study was needed to understand the increases in the total number of children

[4] "Autism/developmental delays" is language drawn directly from the GAO report. However, autism spectrum disorder is a distinct neurodevelopmental disorder with distinct clinical characteristics. For further reading on autism spectrum disorder, see *Mental Disorders and Disabilities Among Low-Income Children* (NASEM, 2015).

receiving SSI benefits as a result of speech and language disorders. This study was requested to meet that need.

STUDY CHARGE AND SCOPE

In 2014, the SSA's Office of Disability Policy requested that the Institute of Medicine (IOM) of the National Academies of Sciences, Engineering, and Medicine convene a consensus committee to (1) identify past and current trends in the prevalence and persistence of speech and language disorders among the general U.S. population under age 18 and compare those trends with trends among the SSI childhood disability population; and (2) provide an overview of the current status of the diagnosis and treatment of speech and language disorders and the levels of impairment due to these disorders in the U.S. population under age 18. (See Box 1-1 for the committee's full statement of task.)

This report addresses the charge defined in the committee's statement of task. It should be noted that this report is not intended to provide a comprehensive discussion of speech and language disorders in children, but to provide the SSA with information directly related to the administration of the SSI program for children with these disorders. In addition, this committee was not charged with providing an evaluation of the SSI program or addressing any other questions related to policy or rulemaking.

Finally, it is important to note that this study was conducted at the same time that the Committee on the Evaluation of the Supplemental Security Income (SSI) Disability Program for Children with Mental Disorders study was under way. Although the two studies have related statements of task and were both sponsored by the SSA, the work was conducted by two distinct committees, which held separate meetings and underwent independent report review processes. The report *Mental Disorders and Disabilities Among Low-Income Children* was released in September 2015 (NASEM, 2015). A brief summary of that report's key findings and conclusions is included in Appendix G.

The following subsections describe how the committee used its statement of task to guide its review and analysis and to determine the inclusion or exclusion of related or noteworthy topics.

Speech and Language Disorders and Corresponding Treatments

Numerous childhood speech and language disorders and other conditions associated with these disorders are worthy of rigorous examination. Similarly, many approaches are used to treat childhood speech and language disorders. As noted above, however, this report does not provide an exhaustive review of all such disorders or of their corresponding treatments.

BOX 1-1
Statement of Task

An ad hoc committee will conduct a study to address the following task order objectives:

- Identify past and current trends in the prevalence and persistence of speech disorders and language disorders for the general U.S. population under age 18 and compare those trends to trends in the Supplemental Security Income (SSI) childhood disability population; and
- Provide an overview of the current status of the diagnosis and treatment of speech disorders and language disorders, and the levels of impairment in the U.S. population under age 18.

To accomplish this goal, the committee will:

- Compare the national trends in the number of children with speech disorders and language disorders under age 18 with the trends in the number of children receiving SSI on the basis of speech disorders and language disorders; and describe the possible factors that may contribute to any differences between the two groups; and
- Identify current professional standards of pediatric and adolescent health care for speech disorders and language disorders and identify the kinds of care documented or reported to be received by children in the SSI childhood disability population.

To perform the above activities, the committee shall do the following with respect to the two child populations:

- Identify national trends in the prevalence of speech disorders and language disorders in children and assess factors that influence these trends.
- Identify the causes of speech disorders and language disorders and determine how often these disorders are the result of known causes.
- Identify the average age of onset and the gender distribution and assess the levels of impairment within age groups.
- Assess how age, development, and gender may play a role in the progression of some speech disorders and language disorders.
- Identify common comorbidities among pediatric speech disorders and language disorders.
- Identify which speech disorders and language disorders are most amenable to treatment and assess typical or average time required for improvement in disorder to manifest following diagnosis and treatment.
- Identify professionally accepted standards of care (such as diagnostic evaluation and assessment, treatment planning and protocols, and educational interventions) for children with speech disorders and with language disorders.

Rather, in accordance with the committee's statement of task, this report describes primary categories of childhood speech and language disorders that occur most commonly in the population of children served by the SSI program and provides an overview of treatments for these disorders. Therefore, the exclusion of any conditions or treatments should not be viewed as an oversight, but as a necessary narrowing of the focus of this study to the issues of greatest relevance to the SSI program.

Data and Data Sources

The committee consulted a variety of data sources to identify trends in the prevalence and persistence of speech and language disorders (prevalence and trends in prevalence are discussed below). These sources included data from clinical samples (i.e., Pennington and Bishop, 2009), population-based studies (i.e., Law et al., 2000; Tomblin et al., 1997), nationally representative surveys (e.g., the National Survey of Children's Health), and administrative or service-based data from federal programs (Medicaid Analytic eXtract [MAX] data, Individuals with Disabilities Education Act [IDEA] child count data, and the SSA's program data). These sources differ substantially with respect to how they define and/or designate speech and language disorders in children, how they collect information (e.g., parental reporting, medical records, test results), which variables are examined (e.g., level of severity or duration of disorders, child and/or family demographic information), and the period(s) of time examined, among other factors. As a result, readers of this report will encounter numbers and estimates that appear quite different from chapter to chapter. Recognizing the challenge this variation presents to readers, the committee carefully describes the different types of data and how estimates were derived throughout the report. (A full discussion of data limitations is included in Chapter 5.)

In addition to the challenges that the committee encountered in using available data, the absence of other relevant data limited the committee's ability to generate more precise population estimates, to compare changes over time, and to conduct further analyses. This absence of data included data sources and data collection efforts that do not currently exist, as well as data that were unavailable to the committee (or to the general public).

For example, the committee's efforts to determine prevalence estimates of children with speech and language disorders could have been improved by access to a national data source derived from health services or health insurance records. Similarly, the committee's efforts to describe trends in childhood speech and language disorders could have been improved through an analysis of longitudinal data from programs (i.e., Medicaid and SSI) or national surveys. At this time, no such national-level data sources or longitudinal data collection efforts exist for these conditions.

Furthermore, the committee's efforts to document the persistence of speech and language disorders among children who receive SSI benefits and the types of treatment received by these children would have been improved by access to certain types of unpublished SSA administrative data, such as age-18 redeterminations and continuing disability reviews. However, these data were not available to the committee for the purpose of this study. Finally, the committee had access to an analysis of MAX data that included limited analyses related to speech and language disorders (see Chapter 5). Because these data are drawn from a study that was commissioned for another report (see NASEM, 2015), this committee was unable to conduct additional analyses, which would have allowed for comparisons between speech and language disorders and other health conditions.

Severity of Speech and Language Disorders

This report frequently refers to "severe" speech and language disorders in children. However, the word "severe" has different meanings depending on the context in which it is used. In clinical research, severity may be measured according to how far below average children score on tests compared with children of the same age (i.e., in standard deviations from a norm-referenced score or quotient) or "percentage of delay" relative to chronological age. In the context of the SSI program, however, the word "severe" has a specific legal meaning that is related to the standard of disability for children in the Social Security Act. Specifically, the regulations explain that "an impairment or combination of impairments must cause 'marked and severe functional limitations' in order to be found disabling."[5] Elsewhere, the regulations explain that "a child's impairment or combination of impairments is 'of listing-level severity' if it causes marked limitation in two areas of functioning or extreme limitation in one such area."[6] These areas of functioning include acquiring and using information, attending to and completing tasks, interacting and relating with others, moving about and manipulating objects, caring for himself or herself, and maintaining health and physical well-being. Chapter 4 includes an in-depth review of how children are evaluated for disability as part of the SSI eligibility determination process. Readers of the report should therefore consider the word "severe" as a clinical expression of impairment level except when it is used in the context of the SSI program.

[5] 20 C.F.R. 416.902.

[6] 20 C.F.R. 416.925(b)(2).

Identifying Severe Speech and Language Disorders

When prevalence estimates (for any condition) are based on a threshold or cutoff score imposed on a continuous normal distribution, the cutoff score will necessarily determine the percentage of individuals falling above and below it. The committee used cutoffs (two and three standard deviations below the mean) that are consistent both with conventional definitions of severe disorders in medicine, psychology, and other fields and with the quantitative standards used by the SSA for defining severe speech and language disorders (see Chapter 4). Many researchers and organizations have noted the need to consider additional sources of evidence, including subjective judgments of functioning, in addition to norm-referenced cutoff scores. For example, the World Health Organization's *International Classification of Functioning, Disability and Health* is one widely accepted approach to describing the severity of medical and developmental conditions (WHO, 2001). This, too, is consistent with the SSA's approach, which requires qualitative evidence that is consistent with quantitative scores when the latter are available. Unfortunately, high-quality data from large, representative populations that have been assessed with both quantitative and qualitative metrics are not available.

Prevalence and Trends in Prevalence

As part of its charge, the committee was asked to "identify past and current trends in the prevalence and persistence of speech disorders and language disorders for the general U.S. population (under age 18) and compare those trends to trends in the SSI childhood disability population." Prevalence is defined as "the number or proportion of cases or events or attributes among a given population" (CDC, 2014). The term "prevalence" is often used to describe "point prevalence," which refers to "the amount of a particular disease present in a population at a single point in time" (CDC, 2014).

Given the lack of longitudinal data on speech and language disorders in SSI administrative data and the paucity of similar data for the general population, the committee determined that the best way to identify trends in prevalence using available data sources would be to examine trends in point prevalence—that is, the number of children with speech and language disorders at a given time and over time both for the general U.S. population (under age 18) and in the SSI childhood disability population. To identify trends in prevalence in these groups, the committee reviewed multiple estimates of point prevalence over time from a variety of sources, including studies using clinical samples, nationally representative surveys, and administrative or service data from federal programs (see Chapter 5).

When these estimates are arranged in chronological order, they produce a trend line—or a trend in prevalence.

However, comparing trends in prevalence between these two populations posed a number of challenges beyond a lack of longitudinal data. These challenges, described in Chapters 4 and 5, include inherent differences in the sample populations (e.g., socioeconomic status, levels of severity) and differences in how children with speech and language disorders are identified and categorized. In addition, many of the estimates of prevalence and trends in prevalence presented in this report lack statements of precision, such as confidence intervals or error bars. Recognizing this limitation, the committee provides detailed information regarding sample sizes and methods used to calculate estimates. These can be found in Chapters 2 and 5 and Appendixes C and D. Despite the numerous challenges and limitations, the committee used the available data to describe changes in both groups[7] over time, in accordance with its charge.

Poverty

Because financial need is a basic condition of eligibility for SSI, the first step in determining eligibility is assessment of family financial status. As a result, the majority of children who receive SSI benefits are from families with a household income less than 200 percent of the federal poverty level (FPL). The number of families with incomes less than 200 percent of the FPL changes over time. That is, as economic conditions deteriorate, more families join the ranks of those with incomes at or below a defined poverty level. This most recently occurred following the 2008-2009 recession in the United States. Table 1-1 presents the absolute number of children under age 18 living in poverty and the percentage of children who were below the FPL annually from 2004 to 2013. The pattern shows that the percentage of children in poverty increased after 2006, peaked in 2010, and declined afterward, although by 2013 it was well above the 2006 level (NASEM, 2015).

This pattern suggests that more children would have met the financial eligibility criteria for SSI benefits during the period that followed the 2008-2009 recession in the United States. Thus, an increase in the number of children with speech and language disorders receiving SSI may not reflect an increase in these disorders, but instead may arise from an increased number of children with these disorders who meet the poverty threshold for SSI eligibility (NASEM, 2015). However, there are no reliable estimates of the

[7] In accordance with the committee's charge, this includes children with speech and language disorders of any level of severity in the general population and children with these disorders in the SSI population, whose impairments are inherently severe.

TABLE 1-1 U.S. Children Living in Poverty (below 100 percent of the federal poverty level), 2004-2013 (numbers in thousands)

		Below the Federal Poverty Level	
Year	Total Number of Children in General U.S. Population	Number of Children	Percent of Total
2004	73,241	13,041	17.8
2005	73,285	12,896	17.6
2006	73,727	12,827	17.4
2007	73,996	13,324	18.0
2008	74,068	14,068	19.0
2009	74,579	15,451	20.7
2010	73,873	16,286	22.0
2011	73,737	16,134	21.9
2012	73,719	16,073	21.8
2013	73,625	14,659	19.9

SOURCE: DeNavas-Walt et al., 2014.

number of children living in poverty who also have speech and language disorders.

Therefore, this report examines the interaction of poverty and disability as well as changes in childhood poverty rates and the changes observed in the SSI program for children with speech and language disorders. Additional data provided in this report allow for comparisons and analyses of SSI determinations, allowances, and total child SSI recipients as a proportion of low-income populations within the United States. This discussion can be found in Chapters 4 and 5.

Limitation of Review of the SSI Program to Children Under Age 18

As noted in the committee's statement of task, this review was limited to children under age 18, the age range served by the SSI childhood program. Therefore, data on redetermination at age 18 are not included in this report, although at age 18, SSI recipients must be reevaluated for eligibility to continue receiving SSI disability benefits as adults. One notable exception is that the committee includes program data on children and youth with disabilities served under IDEA Parts B and C; these data, which could not be disaggregated, include children and youth aged 0-21. Data related to topics beyond the scope of this review, such as continuing disability reviews and age-18 redeterminations, were not made available to the committee by the SSA.

Age of Onset

As part of its task, the committee was asked to identify the average age of onset of speech and language disorders. The onset of a disorder and its chronicity may have important implications related to the burden placed by the disorder on an individual and his or her family, as well as the types and duration of supports an individual will require. Chapter 3 reviews the evidence on persistence of speech and language disorders in children. However, the committee found that in most cases, a simplistic concept of onset does not apply to speech and language or other developmental disorders. The notion of onset of a condition implies that prior to the onset, affected individuals had these functions but then experienced a decline or loss of function. In general, developmental disorders are identified when expected functional skills in children fail to emerge. These expectations usually are based on ages when children typically begin to show these skills. The criteria for determining that a child is presenting severe and long-lasting developmental problems often allow for a period of uncertainty. The underlying factors that contribute to developmental disorders are likely to have been present well before the signs are manifest in the child's development. For example, the babbling of infants who later display severe speech disorders often lacks the consonant-like sounds (closants) seen in typically developing children (Oller et al., 1999). However, there is considerable variability in typical development, so that babbling features alone cannot be used as an accurate diagnostic test for speech disorder.

A major effort in clinical research on developmental disorders has been to identify early risk factors and subclinical signs, so as to support earlier identification and treatment. This research also supports the general assumption that for most developmental disorders, identification is likely to occur during very early stages of development. Therefore, this report reviews what is known about the age of identification of speech and language disorders as it relates to expected developmental milestones. It is generally more accurate to describe the "age of identification" of a speech or language disorder than to focus on the "age of onset." It is worth noting that the age at which a speech or language disorder is identified may be further influenced by a number of factors, including access to care, socioeconomic status, and other demographic factors.

Gender

The committee was charged with identifying the "gender distribution" of speech and language disorders in children and with assessing "how gender may play a role in the progression" of these disorders. This report highlights findings on gender distribution from clinical research and national survey data. However, the evidence base on the effects of gender on the efficacy of treatment and the progression or persistence of speech and language disorders is limited. In its review of the literature, the committee found that few studies examined differential effects of treatment on males and females or included longitudinal data that demonstrated gender differences in the persistence or progression of speech and language disorders.

State-to-State Variation in the SSI Program

Determinations of eligibility for the SSI program are managed at the state level. Through its examination of the evidence, the committee became aware that states vary considerably in the number and rate of applications leading to determinations and in the rate of allowances. This report includes some state-level data to provide an overall perspective, but it does not explore the potential factors contributing to state-to-state variation in the rates of SSI disability, which was beyond the scope of this study. Readers can refer to a recent research brief by the Office of the Assistant Secretary for Planning and Evaluation, *The Child SSI Program and the Changing Safety Net* (Wittenburg et al., 2015), or to *Mental Disorders and Disabilities Among Low-Income Children* (NASEM, 2015) for further information on geographic variation in child SSI program growth and participation.

Exclusion of Recommendations

Finally, the committee was not asked to provide the SSA with recommendations on the SSI program for children. Doing so would be beyond not only the scope of this study as laid out in the statement of task but also the expertise of this committee. Rather, the committee was tasked with gathering information and reporting on the current state of knowledge on the diagnosis, prognosis, and treatment of speech and language disorders in children, as well as trends in the prevalence of these disorders in children. The information presented in this report (and in the recent Academies report on trends in low-income children with mental disorders in the SSI program [NASEM, 2015]) provides a solid evidentiary basis that can inform the SSA's programs and policies, as well as the work of an array of related stakeholders.

STUDY APPROACH

The study committee included 13 members with expertise in speech-language pathology, auditory pathology, pediatrics, developmental-behavioral pediatrics, epidemiology, biostatistics, neurology, neurodevelopmental disabilities, adolescent health, health policy, and special education. (See Appendix H for biographies of the committee members.)

A variety of sources informed the committee's work. The committee met in person five times: two of those meetings included public workshops to provide the committee with input from a broad range of experts and stakeholders, including parents and professional organizations; federal agencies (e.g., the Centers for Disease Control and Prevention, the SSA, and the National Institute of Deafness and Other Communication Disorders); and researchers from a range of relevant disciplines, including speech and language pathology and epidemiology. In addition, the committee conducted a review of the literature to identify the most current research on the etiology, epidemiology, and treatment of pediatric speech and language disorders. The committee made every effort to include the most up-to-date research in peer-reviewed publications. However, strong evidence was sometimes found in older studies that had not been replicated in recent years. In these instances, the older studies are cited. The committee also reviewed findings from a supplemental study using Medicaid data to create an approximate national comparison group for the SSI child population.[8] (See Chapter 5 for additional information about this supplemental study.) Finally, the committee reviewed data collected from SSI case files of children who were eligible for SSI benefits under the category of "speech and language impairment." (See Chapter 4 and Appendix C for more information about this review.)

DEFINITIONS OF KEY TERMS

Language has long been described as a verbal or written code for conveying information to others, and speech refers to oral communication (Bloomfield, 1926). All languages include words (vocabulary), word endings (morphology), and sentence structure (syntax), and speech includes the pronunciation of the sounds (phonemes) of the language. Language development also encompasses acquisition of the social rules for communicating and conversing in society (pragmatics). These rules include participating appropriately in conversations, as well as using and comprehending appropriate gestures and facial expressions during social interaction (Gallagher and Prutting, 1983). The communication and social aspects of speech and language must be coordinated rapidly and fluently when one is speaking.

Given the complex nature of speech and language development, multiple factors can contribute to deficits in their acquisition and use (e.g., motor impairments, processing deficits, cognitive impairments). Disruptions

[8] This supplemental study was commissioned by the Committee on the Evaluation of the Supplemental Security Income Disability Program for Children with Mental Disorders.

in communication development are broadly classified as speech disorders and language disorders.

Speech disorder is defined as disruption in the production of the phonetic aspects of words, phrases, and sentences so that communication is partially or, in severe cases, completely unintelligible to listeners. Stuttering is a form of speech disorder that involves disruptions in the rate and/or fluency of speaking due to hesitations and repetitions of speech sounds, words, and/or phrases.

Language disorder is defined as impairment of expression and comprehension because of a disruption in the acquisition of vocabulary (words), word endings, and sentence structure. In severe cases of language disorder, a child experiences extreme difficulty using correct words and proper grammar and may also have difficulty comprehending what others are saying.

Box 1-2 presents the clinical definitions of speech and language disorders.

BOX 1-2
Clinical Definitions of Speech and Language Disorders

Speech: the production (pronunciation) of meaningful sounds from the complex coordinated movements of the oral mechanism

Speech disorders: deficits that may cause speech to sound abnormal or prevent it altogether

Examples of disordered speech:
Mild to moderate—speaking with a lisp, substituting or deleting sounds in words (e.g., saying "twee" for "three," saying "jo" for "joke")
Severe—making multiple pronunciation errors so that speech is largely or even totally unintelligible

Language: the code or system of symbols for representing ideas in various modalities, including understanding (comprehending) and speaking, reading, and writing

Language disorders: conditions that interfere with the ability to understand the code, to produce the code, or both

Examples of disordered language:
Mild to moderate—omitting word endings, using an incorrect pronoun
Severe—very low vocabulary, inability to comprehend, grossly inaccurate word order

BOX 1-3
Primary Versus Secondary Speech and Language Disorders

Primary speech and language disorders: no other etiology or "cause" is evident

Examples of primary speech and language disorders:
- Speech sound disorders
- Voice disorders
- Stuttering
- Expressive language disorder
- Receptive language disorder
- Combined receptive and expressive language disorder
- Social communication disorder

Secondary speech and language disorders: can be attributed to another condition

Examples of contributors to secondary speech and language disorders:
- Hard of hearing or deaf
- Intellectual disability
- Autism spectrum disorder
- Cleft palate
- Cerebral palsy

Furthermore, speech and language disorders can be categorized as primary, meaning the disorder does not arise from an underlying medical condition (e.g., cerebral palsy, Down syndrome, hearing impairment), or secondary, meaning the disorder can be attributed to another condition (see Box 1-3). This report discusses both primary and secondary speech and language disorders, but it focuses mainly on speech and language disorders that are identified as the primary condition. This corresponds with the categories of speech and language disorders in the SSI program that the report examines.

SIGNIFICANCE AND IMPACT OF SEVERE SPEECH AND LANGUAGE DISORDERS

Speech and language disorders can have a significant adverse impact on a child's ability to have meaningful conversations and engage in age-appropriate social interaction. These disorders are serious disabilities with long-term ramifications for cognitive and social-emotional development and for literacy and academic achievement and have lifelong economic and social impacts, and these disruptions are evidenced in increased risk for learning disabilities, behavior disorders, and related psychiatric conditions. The following sections describe the variety of ways in which speech and language disorders can impact children and their families.

Impact on Social-Emotional and Cognitive Development

Child development is best viewed in the context of a dynamic interaction between social-emotional and cognitive development (Karmiloff-Smith et al., 2014). A seminal paper by Sameroff (1975) brought attention to the critical role of parent–child interactions and social-communicative exchanges in children's social and emotional development. In this communicative-interactive model, social development is the direct product of parent–child (or caregiver–child) interaction (Sameroff, 2009). Specifically, parent–child communication interactions, including speech and language skills, are foundational to emotional attachment, social learning, and cognitive development in addition to communication development. Communication interactions—social "back and forth" exchanges—are a natural part of parent-child communication, with more than 1 million of these parent–child exchanges occurring in the first 5 years of a child's life (Hart and Risley, 1995). Figure 1-1 illustrates how social interaction between parent and child leads to the development of speech.

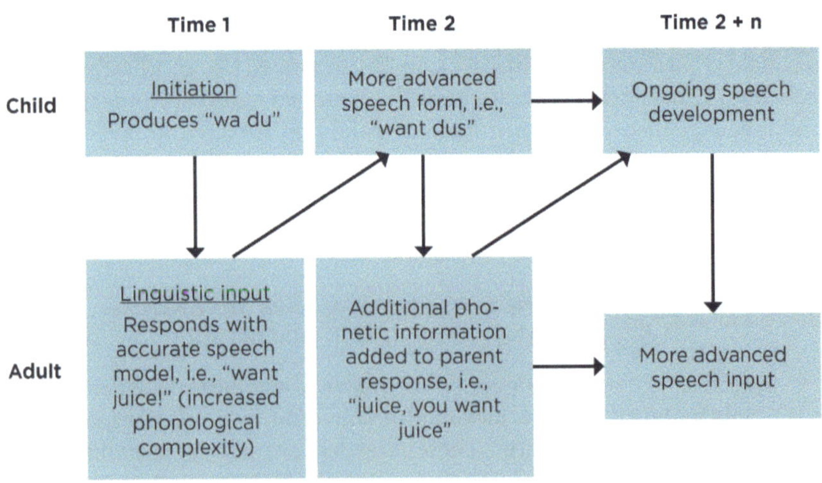

FIGURE 1-1 Example of communication-interaction for speech development.

In the decades since Sameroff's (1975) original article, the communication-interaction model has been applied to multiple aspects of development, including speech (Camarata, 1993), language (Nelson, 1989), the development of self (Damon and Hart, 1982), and cognitive development (Karmiloff-Smith et al., 2012). Karmiloff-Smith (2011) adapted the communication-interaction perspective as a means of mapping developmental processes across multiple domains of genetics and neuroimaging, as well as cognitive and linguistic abilities. In essence, she argues that dynamic communication interactions between parent and child serve not only as learning opportunities but also as the core of the genetically mediated neural phenomena occurring for childhood brain development, often referred to as neural plasticity and remodeling. Viewed in this way, communicative interchanges are fundamental to the developmental experiences that shape a child's neural architecture and, more important, brain function. Severe speech and language disorders can derail this typical cascade of development and have profound and wide-ranging adverse impacts (Clegg et al., 2005).

Impacts on Literacy and Academic Achievement

Figure 1-2 illustrates the importance of language development for the development of literacy skills and the relationship of both to academic achievement across a range of subject areas. Considerable data suggest that severe speech and language disorders are associated with reading disabilities and general disruptions in literacy (Fletcher-Campbell et al., 2009). In

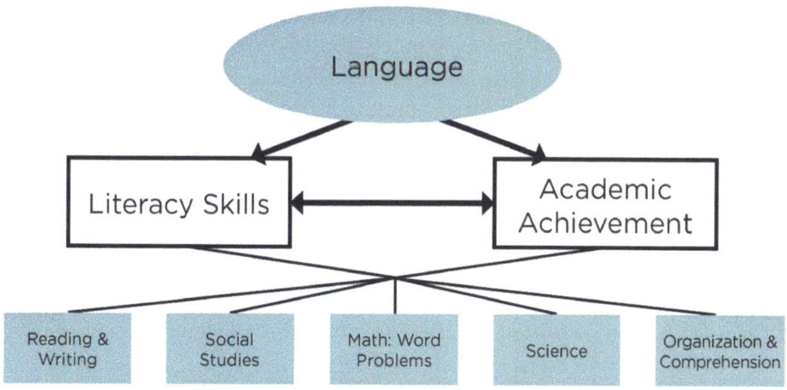

FIGURE 1-2 The relationship among language development, literacy skills, and academic achievement.

essence, reading involves mapping visual symbols (letters) onto linguistic forms (words). When the acquisition and mastery of oral vocabulary are impaired, it is not surprising that the mapping of symbols such as letters onto words is also disrupted. In addition, broader language and speech disorders can make processing the visual symbols much less efficient and disrupt their mapping onto meaning. Even after vocabulary has been acquired, cognitive problems with translating text to language can continue (Briscoe et al., 2001). In languages such as English that use phonetic text, severe speech disorders also can disrupt the phonological processing associated with reading (Pennington and Bishop, 2009). In sum, severe speech and language disorders often have direct or indirect adverse impacts on the development of literacy and fluid reading.

In addition to their direct impact on literacy, severe speech and language disorders can have a deleterious cascading effect on other aspects of academic achievement. To illustrate, in a 15-year follow-up study of children with speech and language disorders, a high percentage (52 percent) of the children initially identified with such disorders had residual learning disabilities and poor academic achievement later in life (King, 1982). Similarly, Hall and Tomblin (1978) report poor overall long-term achievement in language-impaired children. More recently, a study of preterm infants with language disorders indicated multiple disruptions in subsequent achievement (Wolke et al., 2008). And Stoeckel and colleagues (2013) found a strong correlation between early language problems and later diagnosis of written-language disorders. Because so much of academic achievement is predicated on acquiring information through reading and listening comprehension, early severe speech and language disorders often are associated with poor achievement beyond reading problems.

As illustrated in Figure 1-3, the most recent data from the Institute of Education Sciences of the U.S. Department of Education indicate that 21 percent of all special education eligibility in the United States is for speech and language impairments—three times greater than eligibility for autism or intellectual disability. Speech and language disorders are among the highest-incidence conditions among children in special education. Moreover, these data may underestimate the prevalence of speech and language disorders because the highest-incidence condition—specific learning disability—includes many students who were previously categorized as having a speech or language impairment (Aram and Nation, 1980; Catts et al., 2002). Although mild speech and language impairments in preschool will sometimes be transient, severe forms of the disorders have a high probability of being long-term disabilities (Beitchman et al., 1994; Bishop and Edmundson, 1987), with that probability rising with the disorder's severity.

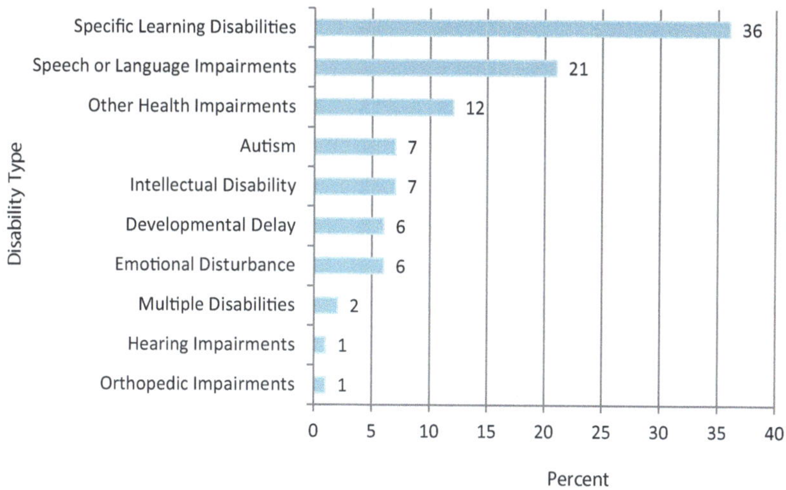

FIGURE 1-3 Percentage distribution of children aged 3-21 served under the Individuals with Disabilities Education Act (IDEA) Part B, by disability type: school year 2011-2012.
SOURCE: Kena et al., 2014.

Economic and Family Impacts

In a review of the economic impact of communication disorders on society, Ruben (2000, p. 241) estimates that "communication disorders may cost the United States from $154 billion to $186 billion per year." Severe speech and language disorders elevate risk for a wide variety of adverse economic and social outcomes, such as lifelong social isolation and psychiatric disorders, learning disabilities, behavior disorders, academic failure, and chronic underemployment (Aram and Nation, 1980; Baker and Cantwell, 1987; Beitchman et al., 1996; Johnson et al., 1999; Stothard et al., 1998; Sundheim and Voeller, 2004). Following a cohort of individuals with severe language disorders in childhood longitudinally through school age and adolescence and into early adulthood, Clegg and colleagues (2005, p. 128) found that "in their mid-30s, those who had language disorders as children had significantly worse social adaptation with prolonged unemployment and a paucity of close friendships and love relationships."

Research shows that children living in poverty are at greater risk for a disability relative to their wealthier counterparts, and that childhood disability increases the risk of a family living in poverty (Emerson and Hatton, 2005; Farran, 2000; Fujiura and Yamaki, 2000; Lustig and Strauser, 2007; Msall et al., 2006; NASEM, 2015; Parish and Cloud, 2006). For example, data from the U.S. Census 2010 showed that families raising children with a disability experienced poverty at higher rates than families raising children without a disability (21.8 and 12.6 percent, respectively) (Wang, 2005). At the same time, childhood poverty and the accompanying deprivations have significant adverse implications for children with disabilities and their families. Families with children with disabilities are also more likely to incur increased out-of-pocket expenses; for example, for child care or for transportation to locations with specialized medical care (Kuhlthau et al., 2005; Newacheck and Kim, 2005). Data from the National Survey of Children with Special Health Care Needs help illustrate the impact on families of caring for children with communication disorders. For example, the survey asked whether family members cut back on or stopped working because of their child's health needs. Fifty-two percent of the survey respondents whose children had "a lot of difficulty speaking, communicating, or being understood" responded affirmatively to this question (Wells, 2015).

In sum, given the complex multidimensional nature of language acquisition and the integral role of speech and language across multiple domains of early child development, speech and language disorders occur at relatively high rates (Kena et al., 2014). In 2011-2012, 21 percent of children served under IDEA Part B had speech or language impairments (Kena et al., 2014). These disorders also are associated with a wide range of other conditions (Beitchman et al., 1996), such as intellectual disabilities (Georgieva, 1996), autism spectrum disorder (Geurts and Embrechts, 2008; Sturm et al., 2004), hearing loss (Yoshinaga-Itano et al., 1998), learning disabilities (Pennington and Bishop, 2009; Schuele, 2004), ADHD (Cohen et al., 2000), and severe motor conditions such as cerebral palsy (Pirila et al., 2007).

NOTABLE PAST WORK

As noted earlier, in the period between 2000 and 2011, speech and language impairments were among the three most prevalent impairments in children in the SSI disability program (preceded by ADHD and followed by autism spectrum disorder) (GAO, 2012). In an effort to understand these trends in comparison with trends in the general population, the SSA requested that the IOM conduct two studies: the previously mentioned study on childhood mental disorders (including ADHD and autism spectrum disorder)[9] and this study on childhood speech and language disorders. While these impairments frequently co-occur and may have similar

[9] Information on the Committee on the Evaluation of the Supplemental Security Income Disability Program for Children with Mental Disorders can be found online at http://iom.nationalacademies.org/activities/mentalhealth/ssidisabilityprograms.aspx.

diagnostic characteristics, the separate studies allowed two independent committees to examine distinct literatures and data sources and to review different standards of care and treatment protocols. The study on children with mental health disorders was conducted from January 2014 through August 2015; the final report of that study was released in September 2015 (NASEM, 2015).

While this report is the first examination of the SSI disability program for children with speech and language disorders conducted by the Academies, the IOM, and the National Research Council (NRC) have a long history of studying issues related to disability in children and adults and the SSA's disability determination process. In addition to the recently released *Mental Disorders and Disabilities Among Low-Income Children* (NASEM, 2015), earlier reports by the IOM and the NRC that informed this committee's work include *The Dynamics of Disability: Measuring and Monitoring Disability for Social Security Programs* (IOM and NRC, 2002), *The Future of Disability in America* (IOM, 2007b), *Improving the Social Security Disability Decision Process* (IOM, 2007a), *HIV and Disability: Updating the Social Security Listings* (IOM, 2010b), *Cardiovascular Disability: Updating the Social Security Listings* (IOM, 2010a), and *Psychological Testing in the Service of Disability Determination* (IOM, 2015). Along with this earlier work of the Academies, the committee drew important lessons from the body of data and research aimed at identifying trends in the prevalence and persistence of speech and language disorders, as well as addressing diagnosis and treatment of and levels of impairment associated with these disorders.

FINDINGS AND CONCLUSIONS

Findings

1-1. Developmental disorders are identified when expected functional skills in children fail to emerge.

1-2. Underlying factors that contribute to developmental disorders are likely to have been present well before the signs are manifest in the child's development.

1-3. In a 15-year follow-up study of children with speech and language disorders, 52 percent of the children initially identified with such disorders had residual learning disabilities and poor academic achievement later in life.

1-4. Twenty-one percent of all special education eligibility in the United States is for speech and language impairments—three times greater than eligibility for autism or intellectual disability.

Conclusions

1-1. It is generally more accurate to describe the "age of identification" of a speech or language disorder than to focus on the "age of onset."

1-2. Mild speech and language impairments in preschool will sometimes be transient; severe forms of these disorders have a high probability of being long-term disabilities.

ORGANIZATION OF THE REPORT

This report consists of six chapters. It is organized to provide readers with important background information on speech and language disorders in children in the general population before describing the subset of children with severe speech and language disorders who receive SSI benefits. To take readers through this progression, the report describes the SSI program in some detail. This description is intended to orient readers to the determination process that shapes the population served by the program: children with severe speech and language disorders who are also from low-income, resource-limited families. The report then compares changes over time in the prevalence of speech and language disorders in the general and SSI child populations, based on the best evidence available. The report culminates with a summary of the committee's overall findings and conclusions. The contents of each chapter are as follows:

- Chapter 2 provides an overview of childhood speech and language disorders in the general U.S. population. The chapter begins with an overview of speech and language development in children. It then examines the diagnosis of speech and language disorders in children, causes and risk factors, and prevalence. The chapter also includes evidence related to common comorbidities of childhood speech and language disorders.
- Chapter 3 reviews what is known about the treatment and persistence of speech and language disorders in children. This review includes current standards of care for these disorders, an overview of treatment approaches for different speech and language disorders, and expected responses to treatment.
- Chapter 4 provides an overview of the SSI program for children, how it has changed over time, and how those changes have shaped the population of children receiving SSI benefits. It describes the eligibility determination process and the speech and language-related criteria that are used to evaluate children. Finally, the chapter includes case examples and a review of a random sample of case files

of children who receive SSI benefits based on speech and language disorders. This information offers insight into the characteristics of children with speech and language disorders who apply for SSI and helps demonstrate the evidence considered by the SSA when making a disability determination for a case.

- Chapter 5 compares trends in speech and language disorders among children (under age 18) in the general population with trends in these disorders among participants in the SSI childhood disability program. The chapter reviews the data sources used by the committee to describe the epidemiology of speech and language disorders in children in both populations. It also identifies gaps in the evidence that impede more precise estimates of trends in prevalence for speech and language disorders and comorbid conditions.
- Finally, Chapter 6 provides a summary of the committee's overall findings and conclusions and their implications in the following three areas: speech and language disorders in children in the general population, speech and language disorders among children who receive SSI benefits, and comparisons between these two groups.

The report includes several appendixes. Appendix A provides a glossary of terms used throughout the report, while Appendix B includes summaries of data sources that informed the committee's work. Appendix C includes administrative/service data that the committee used to examine changes in program participation over time and national survey data that the committee used to estimate changes in prevalence over time. Appendix D provides the methods that the committee used to calculate trends in the national survey data. Appendix E includes a description of the methods used to review case files, and Appendix F lists the agendas and speakers for the committee's public workshops. A brief summary of *Mental Disorders and Disabilities Among Low-Income Children*, the report of the Committee on the Evaluation of the Supplemental Security Income Disability Programs for Children with Mental Disorders, is included in Appendix G. Finally, Appendix H contains biographical sketches of the committee members.

REFERENCES

Aram, D. M., and J. E. Nation. 1980. Preschool language disorders and subsequent language and academic difficulties. *Journal of Communication Disorders* 13(2):159-170.

Baker, L., and D. P. Cantwell. 1987. A prospective psychiatric follow-up of children with speech/language disorders. *Journal of the American Academy of Child & Adolescent Psychiatry* 26(4):546-553.

Beitchman, J. H., E. Brownlie, A. Inglis, J. Wild, R. Mathews, D. Schachter, R. Kroll, S. Martin, B. Ferguson, and W. Lancee. 1994. Seven-year follow-up of speech/language-impaired and control children: Speech/language stability and outcome. *Journal of the American Academy of Child & Adolescent Psychiatry* 33(9):1322-1330.

Beitchman, J. H., B. Wilson, E. Brownlie, H. Walters, and W. Lancee. 1996. Long-term consistency in speech/language profiles: I. Developmental and academic outcomes. *Journal of the American Academy of Child & Adolescent Psychiatry* 35(6):804-814.

Bishop, D. V. M., and A. Edmundson. 1987. Language-impaired 4-year-olds: Distinguishing transient from persistent impairment. *Journal of Speech and Hearing Disorders* 52(2): 156-173.

Bloomfield, L. 1926. *A set of postulates for the science of language*. Indianapolis, IN: Bobbs-Merrill.

Briscoe, J., D. V. M. Bishop, and C. F. Norbury. 2001. Phonological processing, language, and literacy: A comparison of children with mild-to-moderate sensorineural hearing loss and those with specific language impairment. *Journal of Child Psychology and Psychiatry* 42(3):329-340.

Camarata, S. 1993. The application of naturalistic conversation training to speech production in children with speech disabilities. *Journal of Applied Behavior Analysis* 26(2):173-182.

Catts, H. W., M. E. Fey, J. B. Tomblin, and X. Zhang. 2002. A longitudinal investigation of reading outcomes in children with language impairments. *Journal of Speech Language and Hearing Research* 45(6):1142-1157.

CDC (Centers for Disease Control and Prevention). 2014. *Principles of epidemiology glossary*. http://www.cdc.gov/ophss/csels/dsepd/SS1978/Glossary.html (accessed August 11, 2015).

Clegg, J., C. Hollis, L. Mawhood, and M. Rutter. 2005. Developmental language disorders—a follow-up in later adult life. Cognitive, language and psychosocial outcomes. *Journal of Child Psychology and Psychiatry* 46(2):128-149.

Cohen, N. J., D. D. Vallance, M. Barwick, N. Im, R. Menna, N. B. Horodezky, and L. Isaacson. 2000. The interface between ADHD and language impairment: An examination of language, achievement, and cognitive processing. *Journal of Child Psychology and Psychiatry* 41(3):353-362.

Damon, W., and D. Hart. 1982. The development of self-understanding from infancy through adolescence. *Child Development* 53(4):841-864.

DeNavas-Walt, C., B. D. Proctor, and J. C. Smith. 2014. *Income and poverty in the United States: 2013*. Washington, DC: U.S. Census Bureau.

Emerson, E., and C. Hatton. 2005. The socio-economic circumstances of families with disabled children. *Disability and Society* 22(6):563-580.

Farran, D. 2000. Another decade of intervention for children who are low-income or disabled: What do we know now? In *Handbook of early childhood intervention* (2nd ed.), edited by J. P. Shonkoff and S. J. Meisels. Cambridge, England: Cambridge University Press. Pp. 510-548.

Fletcher-Campbell, F., J. Soler, and G. Reid. 2009. *Approaching difficulties in literacy development assessments, pedagogy and programmes*. Thousand Oaks, CA: Sage Publications.

Fujiura, G. T., and K. Yamaki. 2000. Trends in demography of childhood poverty and disability. *Exceptional Children* 66(2):187-199.

Gallagher, T. M., and C. A. Prutting. 1983. *Pragmatic assessment and intervention issues in language*. San Diego, CA: College-Hill Press.

GAO (U.S. Government Accountability Office). 2012. *Supplemental security income: Better management oversight needed for children's benefits: Report to congressional requesters*. http://purl.fdlp.gov/GPO/gpo25551 (accessed June 12, 2015).

Georgieva, D. 1996. *Speech and language disorders in children with intellectual disability [microform]*, edited by M. Cholakova. Washington, DC: ERIC Clearinghouse.

Geurts, H. M., and M. Embrechts. 2008. Language profiles in ASD, SLI, and ADHD. *Journal of Autism and Developmental Disorders* 38(10):1931-1943.

Hall, P. K., and J. B. Tomblin. 1978. A follow-up study of children with articulation and language disorders. *Journal of Speech and Hearing Disorders* 43(2):227-241.

Hart, B., and T. R. Risley. 1995. *Meaningful differences in the everyday experience of young American children*. Baltimore, MD: Paul H. Brookes Publishing Co.

IOM (Institute of Medicine). 2007a. *Improving the social security disability decision process*, edited by J. D. Stobo, M. McGeary, and D. K. Barnes. Washington, DC: The National Academies Press.

IOM. 2007b. *The future of disability in America*, edited by M. J. Field and A. M. Jette. Washington, DC: The National Academies Press.

IOM. 2010a. *Cardiovascular disability: Updating the social security listings*. Washington, DC: The National Academies Press.

IOM. 2010b. *HIV and disability: Updating the social security listings*. Washington, DC: The National Academies Press.

IOM. 2015. *Psychological testing in the service of disability determination*. Washington, DC: The National Academies Press.

IOM and NRC (National Research Council). 2002. *The dynamics of disability: Measuring and monitoring disability for social security programs*, edited by G. S. Wunderlich, D. P. Rice, and N. L. Amado. Washington, DC: National Academy Press.

Johnson, C. J., J. H. Beitchman, A. Young, M. Escobar, L. Atkinson, B. Wilson, E. B. Brownlie, L. Douglas, N. Taback, I. Lam, and M. Wang. 1999. Fourteen-year follow-up of children with and without speech/language impairments. *Journal of Speech Language and Hearing Research* 42(3):744.

Karmiloff-Smith, A. 2011. Static snapshots versus dynamic approaches to genes, brain, cognition, and behavior in neurodevelopmental disabilities. In *Early development in neurogenetic disorders*, Vol. 40, edited by D. J. Fidler. London, UK: Elsevier. Pp. 1-15.

Karmiloff-Smith, A., D. D'Souza, T. M. Dekker, J. Van Herwegen, F. Xu, M. Rodic, and D. Ansari. 2012. Genetic and environmental vulnerabilities in children with neurodevelopmental disorders. *Proceedings of the National Academy of Sciences of the United States of America* 109:17261-17265.

Karmiloff-Smith, A., B. J. Casey, E. Massand, P. Tomalski, and M. S. C. Thomas. 2014. Environmental and genetic influences on neurocognitive development: The importance of multiple methodologies and time-dependent intervention. *Clinical Psychological Science* 2(5):628-637.

Kena, G., S. Aud, F. Johnson, X. Wang, J. Zhang, A. Rathbun, S. Wilkinson-Flicker, and P. Kristapovich. 2014. *The condition of education 2014*. NCES 2014-083. Washington, DC: U.S. Department of Education, National Center for Education Statistics.

King, R. R. 1982. In retrospect: A fifteen-year follow-up report of speech-language-disordered children. *Language, Speech, and Hearing Services in Schools* 13(1):24-32.

Kuhlthau, K., K. Hill, R. Yucel, and J. Perrin. 2005. Financial burden for families of children with special health care needs. *Maternal and Child Health Journal* 9(2):207-218.

Law, J., J. Boyle, F. Harris, A. Harkness, and C. Nye. 2000. Prevalence and natural history of primary speech and language delay: Findings from a systematic review of the literature. *International Journal of Language & Communication Disorders/Royal College of Speech & Language Therapists* 35(2):165-188.

Lustig, D. C., and D. R. Strauser. 2007. Causal relationships between poverty and disability. *Rehabilitation Counseling Bulletin* 50(4):194-202.

Msall, M. E., F. Bobis, and S. Field. 2006. Children with disabilities and supplemental security income: Guidelines for appropriate access in early childhood. *Infants & Young Children* 19(1):2-15.

NASEM (National Academies of Sciences, Engineering, and Medicine). 2015. *Mental disorders and disabilities among low-income children.* Washington, DC: The National Academies Press.

Nelson, K. E. 1989. Strategies for first language teaching. In *The teachability of language*, edited by M. Rice and R. L. Schiefelbusch. Baltimore, MD: Paul H. Brookes Publishing Co. Pp. 263-310.

Newacheck, P. W., and S. E. Kim. 2005. A national profile of health care utilization and expenditures for children with special health care needs. *Archives of Pediatric and Adolescent Medicine* 159(1):10-17.

Oller, D. K., R. E. Eilers, A. R. Neal, and H. K. Schwartz. 1999. Precursors to speech in infancy: The prediction of speech and language disorders. *Journal of Communication Disorders* 32(4):223-245.

Oller, J. W., S. D. Oller, and L. C. Badon. 2006. *Milestones: Normal speech and language development across the life span.* San Diego, CA: Plural Publishing.

Parish, S. L., and J. M. Cloud. 2006. Financial well-being of young children with disabilities and their families. *Social Work* 51(3):223-232.

Pennington, B. F., and D. V. Bishop. 2009. Relations among speech, language, and reading disorders. *Annual Review of Psychology* 60:283-306.

Pirila, S., J. van der Meere, T. Pentikainen, P. Ruusu-Niemi, R. Korpela, J. Kilpinen, and P. Nieminen. 2007. Language and motor speech skills in children with cerebral palsy. *Journal of Communication Disorders* 40(2):116-128.

Ruben, R. J. 2000. Redefining the survival of the fittest: Communication disorders in the 21st century. *The Laryngoscope* 110(2):241-245.

Sameroff, A. 1975. Transactional models in early social relations. *Human Development* 18(1-2):65-79.

Sameroff, A. 2009. *The transactional model.* Washington, DC: American Psychological Association.

Schuele, C. M. 2004. The impact of developmental speech and language impairments on the acquisition of literacy skills. *Mental Retardation and Developmental Disabilities Research Reviews* 10(3):176-183.

SSA (Social Security Administration). 2015. *SSI monthly statistics, December 2014.* http://www.ssa.gov/policy/docs/statcomps/ssi_monthly/2014/index.html (accessed February 18, 2015).

Stoeckel, R. E., R. C. Colligan, W. J. Barbaresi, A. L. Weaver, J. M. Killian, and S. K. Katusic. 2013. Early speech-language impairment and risk for written language disorder: A population-based study. *Journal of Developmental and Behavioral Pediatrics* 34(1):38.

Stothard, S. E., M. J. Snowling, D. Bishop, B. B. Chipchase, and C. A. Kaplan. 1998. Language-impaired preschoolers: A follow-up into adolescence. *Journal of Speech, Language, and Hearing Research* 41(2):407-418.

Sturm, H., E. Fernell, and C. Gillberg. 2004. Autism spectrum disorders in children with normal intellectual levels: Associated impairments and subgroups. *Developmental Medicine & Child Neurology* 46(7):444-447.

Sundheim, S. T., and K. K. Voeller. 2004. Psychiatric implications of language disorders and learning disabilities: Risks and management. *Journal of Child Neurology* 19(10):814-826.

Tomblin, J. B., N. L. Records, P. Buckwalter, X. Xhang, E. Smith, and M. O'Brien. 1997. Prevalence of specific language impairment in kindergarten children. *Journal of Speech, Language, and Hearing Research* 40:1245-1260.

Wang, Q. 2005. Disability and American families: 2000. *Bulletin* 62(4):21-30.

Wells, N. 2015. Families of Children/Youth with Special Health Care Needs. Workshop presentation to the Committee on the Evaluation of the Supplemental Security Income (SSI) Disability Program for Children with Speech Disorders and Language Disorders on March 9, Washington, DC.

WHO (World Health Organization). 2001. *International classification of functioning, disability and health*. Geneva, Switzerland: WHO.

Williams, F. 2013. *Language and poverty: Perspectives on a theme*. Philadelphia, PA: Elsevier.

Wittenburg, D., J. Tambornino, E. Brown, G. Rowe, M. DeCamillis, and G. Crouse. 2015. *The Child SSI Program and the changing safety net*. Washington, DC: Mathematica Policy Research.

Wolke, D., M. Samara, M. Bracewell, N. Marlow, and E. S. Group. 2008. Specific language difficulties and school achievement in children born at 25 weeks of gestation or less. *The Journal of Pediatrics* 152(2):256-262.

Yoshinaga-Itano, C., A. L. Sedey, D. K. Coulter, and A. L. Mehl. 1998. Language of early- and later-identified children with hearing loss. *Pediatrics* 102(5):1161-1171.

2

Childhood Speech and Language Disorders in the General U.S. Population

Speech and language disorders in children include a variety of conditions that disrupt children's ability to communicate. Severe speech and language disorders are particularly serious, preventing or impeding children's participation in family and community, school achievement, and eventual employment. This chapter begins by providing an overview of speech and language development and disorders. It then addresses the following topics within the committee's charge: (1) current standards of care for assessing and diagnosing speech and language disorders; (2) causes of and risk factors for these disorders; (3) their prevalence and its relationship to age, development, and gender; and (4) common comorbidities (i.e., other co-occurring conditions).

OVERVIEW OF CHILDHOOD SPEECH AND LANGUAGE DISORDERS

Differentiating Language from Speech

The words "language" and "speech" are often used interchangeably in casual conversation, but in the context of communication disorders, it is important to understand the differences between them. *Language* refers to the code, or symbol system, for transforming unobservable mental events, such as thoughts and memories, into events that can be perceived by other people. Being a competent language user requires two essential capabilities. One, known as *expressive language* or *language production*, is the ability to encode one's ideas into language forms and symbols. The other, known as *receptive language* or *language comprehension*, is the ability to understand the meanings that others have expressed using language. People commonly express themselves by speaking and understand others' meanings by listening. However, language also can be expressed and understood in other ways—for example, by reading, writing, and signing (Crystal, 2009).

Speech has a narrower meaning than *language* because it refers specifically to sounds produced by the oral mechanism, including the lips, tongue, vocal cords, and related structures (Caruso and Strand, 1999). Speech is the most common way to transmit language and, unlike language, can be observed directly. Speech disorders are sometimes mistakenly equated with language disorders, and conversely, normal speech is sometimes assumed to reflect normal language. In fact, speech disorders and language disorders can occur separately or together. For example, a child might have a speech disorder, such as extremely poor articulation, yet have intact language skills. Another child might have a language disorder, such as extremely poor comprehension, yet be able to produce speech sounds normally. Finally, some children have both language disorders and speech disorders. In young children who are producing little if any speech, it can be difficult to determine whether a speech disorder, a language disorder, or both are present. As noted in Chapter 3 on treatment, early intervention for such children generally is designed to facilitate both language and speech skills. When children reach an age that allows each area to be assessed separately, it becomes possible to narrow the focus of treatment according to whether deficits are found only in speech, only in language, or in both.

In this report, the terms "speech disorders," "language disorders," and "speech and language disorders" are used (see Box 1-2). The terms "speech disorders" and "language disorders" are used only to refer to these disorders as defined in this chapter, while the term "speech and language disorders" denotes all of the disorders encompassed by these two categories.

Overview of Speech and Language Development and Disorders

The foundations for the development of speech and language begin in utero, with the growth of the anatomical structures and physiological processes that will eventually support sensory, motor, attention, memory, and learning skills. As discussed in the later section of this chapter on causes and risk factors, virtually every factor that threatens prenatal development of the fetus—from genetic abnormalities, to nutritional deficiencies, to exposure to environmental toxins—is associated with an increased risk of developing speech and/or language disorders. Before the end of the prenatal period, fetuses are able to hear, albeit imperfectly, speech and other environmental sounds, and within a few minutes after birth they show special attention to human faces and voices. This early interest in other people appears to set the stage for forming relationships with caregivers, who scaffold the child's growing ability to anticipate, initiate, and participate in social routines (e.g., Locke, 2011). The social experiences and skills that occur during the infant's first months of life are important precursors to pragmatic language skills: the infant first learns to engage in reciprocal interactions and to convey communicative intentions through nonlinguistic means such as gestures, and begins to accomplish these same goals through language forms such as early words. In the first few months of life, infants show improvement in their ability to recognize increasingly detailed patterns of speech, a precursor to linking spoken words with their meanings. Also in the first months of life, infants begin to use their oral mechanisms to produce nonspeech sounds, such as cooing and squealing, as they develop control of their muscles and movements. Thus, they are able to produce increasingly consistent combinations of speech-like sounds and syllables (babbling), a precursor to articulating recognizable words (e.g., Kent, 1999).

Evidence from neurophysiological habituation, neuroimaging, and preferential looking studies shows that children begin to recognize speech patterns that recur in their environments early in the first year of life (Friedrich et al, 2015; Pelucchi et al., 2009; Werker et al., 2012). When tested using behavioral measures, most 12- to 18-month-old children show that they can understand at least a few words in the absence of gestural or other cues to their meaning (e.g., Miller and Paul, 1995). They also can produce at least a few intelligible words during this period (e.g., Squires et al., 2009), showing that they are acquiring both expressive language and speech skills. Their speech skills progress in a systematic fashion over the next few years, as they learn first to say relatively simpler consonants (e.g., "m," "d," "n") and later to say more challenging consonants (e.g., "s," "th," "sh") and consonant clusters (e.g., "bl," "tr," "st") (Shriberg, 1993). Receptive language, expressive language, and speech all develop at a rapid pace through the preschool period as children learn to understand and say thousands of individual words, as well as learn the grammatical (or morpho-syntactic) rules that enable them to understand and produce increasingly lengthy, sophisticated, intelligible, and socially acceptable combinations of words in phrases and sentences (e.g., Fenson et al., 2007). These speech and language skills enable children to achieve communication goals as diverse as understanding a simple story, taking a turn in a game, expressing an emotion, sharing a personal experience, and asking for help (e.g., Boudreau, 2008). By the end of the preschool period, children's ability to understand the language spoken by others and to speak well enough for others to understand them provides the scaffolding for their growing independence.

The end of the preschool period is also when most children show signs that they can think consciously about sounds and words, an ability known as *metalinguistic awareness* (Kim et al., 2013). Awareness of the phonological (sound) characteristics of words, for example, enables children to identify words that rhyme or words that begin or end with the same speech sound. Such phonological awareness skills have been linked to children's ability to learn that speech sounds can be represented by printed letters—one of the skills necessary for learning to read words (Troia, 2013). Reading requires more than recognizing individual words, however. Competent readers also must understand how words combine to express meanings in connected text, such as phrases, sentences, and paragraphs. Strong evidence shows that children's receptive language skills—such as their knowledge of vocabulary and grammar—are important contributors as well to this aspect of reading comprehension (Catts and Kamhi, 2012; Duke et al., 2013).

In short, by the time children enter elementary school, the speech and language skills they have acquired through listening and speaking provide the foundation for reading and writing. These new literacy skills are critical for learning and social development through the school years and beyond. At the same time, ongoing growth in spoken language skills contributes to building personal and professional relationships and participating independently in society.

It is worth noting that children's speech and language experiences may vary substantially depending on the values and expectations of their culture, community, and family. This point is most obvious for children being raised in multilingual environments, who acquire more than one language. Although the majority of people in the world speak two languages, bilingualism currently is not the norm in the United States, and bilingualism has sometimes been assumed to increase the risk of speech and language disorders. However, there is no evidence that speech or language disorders are more prevalent in bilingual than in monolingual children with similar biological and sociodemographic profiles (Gillam et al., 2013; Goldstein and Gildersleeve-Neumann, 2012; Kohnert and Derr, 2012).

Similarly, some investigators have reported differences in the amounts and kinds of language experienced by children according to their socioeconomic circumstances, and some of these differences have been associated with scores on later tests that emphasize language skills, including tests of vocabulary and verbal intelligence (Hart and Risley, 1995; Hurtado et al., 2014). The language spoken to children certainly influences their language skills, and some aspects of language have been linked to parents' socioeconomic and educational backgrounds (e.g., Hoff, 2013). However, the range of language variations observed to date has not been found to increase the risk of speech or language disorders independent of other factors associated with low socioeconomic status, including inadequate or poor-quality health care, hunger, reduced educational and social resources, and increased exposure to environmental hazards (Harrison and McLeod, 2010; Parish et al., 2010; Pentimonti et al., 2014).

Speech Disorders

As described above, *speech* refers to the production of meaningful sounds (words and phrases) from the complex coordinated movements of the oral mechanism. Speech requires coordinating breathing (respiration) with movements that produce voice (phonation) and sounds (articulation). Respiration yields a stream of breath, which is set into vibration by laryngeal mechanisms (voice box, vocal cords) to yield audible phonation or voicing. Exquisitely timed and coordinated movements by the articulatory mechanisms, including the jaw, lips, tongue, soft palate, teeth, and upper airway (pharynx), then modify this voiced stream to yield the speech sounds, or phonemes, of the speaker's native language (Caruso and Strand, 1999). *Speech disorders* are deficits that may prevent speech from being produced at all, or result in speech that cannot be understood or is abnormal in some other way. This broad category includes three main subtypes: speech sound disorders, voice disorders, and stuttering. Speech sound disorders can be further classified into articulation disorders, dysarthria, and childhood apraxia of speech. The speech variations produced by speakers of different dialects and non-native speakers of English are not defined as speech disorders unless they significantly impede communication or educational achievement.

Speech sound disorders, often termed articulation or phonological disorders, are deficits in the production of individual speech sounds, or sequences of speech sounds, caused by inadequate planning, control, or coordination of the structures of the oral mechanism. *Dysarthria* is a speech sound disorder caused by medical conditions that impair the muscles or nerves that activate the oral mechanism (Caruso and Strand, 1999). Dysarthric speech may be difficult to understand as a result of speech movements that are weak, imprecise, or produced at abnormally slow or rapid rates (Morgan and Vogel, 2008; Pennington et al., 2009). Neuromuscular conditions, including stroke, infections (e.g., polio, meningitis), cerebral palsy, and trauma, can cause dysarthria. Another rare speech sound disorder, *childhood apraxia of speech*, is caused by difficulty with planning and programming speech movements (ASHA, 2007). Children with this disorder may be delayed in learning the speech sounds expected for their age, or they may be physically capable of producing speech sounds but fail to produce the same sounds correctly when attempting to use them in words, phrases, or sentences.

Voice disorders (also known as *dysphonias*) occur when the laryngeal structures, including the vocal cords, do not function correctly (Carding et al., 2006). For example, a voice that sounds hoarse or breathy may be due to growths on the vocal cords, allergies, paralysis, infection, or excessive vocal abuse when speaking. A complete inability to produce any sound, called *aphonia*, may be caused by inflammation, infection, or injury to the vocal cords.

Stuttering (also known as *fluency disorder* or *dysfluency*) is a speech disorder that disrupts the ability to speak as smoothly as desired. Dysfluent speech contains an excessive amount of repetitions of sounds, words, and phrases, and involuntary breaks, or "blocks." Severe stuttering can effectively prevent a speaker from speaking at all; it may also lead to other abnormal physical and emotional behaviors as the speaker struggles to end a particular block or avoid blocks in the future (Conture, 2001).

Language Disorders

As described above, *language* refers to the code, or system of symbols, for representing ideas in various modalities, including hearing and speaking, reading, and writing. Language may also refer to the ability to interpret and produce manual communication, such as American Sign Language. *Language disorders* interfere with a child's ability to understand the code, to produce the code, or both (American Psychiatric Association, 2013; WHO, 1992). Children with *expressive language disorders* have difficulty in formulating their ideas and messages using language. Children with *receptive language disorders* have difficulty understanding messages encoded in language. Children with *expressive-receptive language disorders* have difficulty both understanding and producing messages coded in language.

Language disorders may also be classified according to whether they affect *pragmatics, semantics,* or *grammar.* Pragmatic language disorders may be seen in children who generally lack social reciprocity, a contributor to the dynamic turn-taking exchanges that typify the earliest communicative interactions (e.g., Sameroff, 2009). A child with a receptive pragmatic language disorder may have difficulty understanding messages that involve abstract ideas, such as idioms, metaphors, and irony. A child with an expressive pragmatic disorder may have difficulty producing messages that are socially appropriate for a given listener or context. A child with a receptive semantic disorder may not understand as many vocabulary words as expected for his or her age, while a child with an expressive semantic disorder may find it difficult to produce the right word to convey the intended meaning accurately. A child with a receptive grammatical deficit may not understand the differences between word endings that indicate concepts such as past (*walked*) or present (*walking*), or may not understand complex sentences (e.g., *The man that the boy saw was running away*). Similarly, a child with an expressive grammatical disorder may produce short, incomplete sentences that lack the grammatical endings or structures necessary to express ideas clearly or completely.

Language disorders can interfere with any of these subsystems, singly or in combination. For example, children with severe pragmatic deficits may appear uninterested in communicating with others. Other children may try to communicate, but suffer from semantic disorders that prevent them from acquiring the words they need to express their messages. Still other children have normal pragmatic skills and vocabularies, but produce grammatical errors when they attempt to combine words into phrases and sentences. Finally, children with phonological disorders may be delayed in learning which sounds belong in words.

As mentioned earlier, language disorders first identified in the preschool period have been linked to learning disabilities when children enter school (Sun and Wallach, 2014). In fact, the Individuals with Disabilities Education Act (IDEA) (Section 300.8) defines a specific learning disability as "a disorder in one or more of the basic psychological processes involved in understanding or in using language, spoken or written, that may manifest itself in the imperfect ability to listen, think, speak, read, write, spell, or to do mathematical calculations." Strong evidence suggests that early language disorders increase the risk of poor literacy, mental health, and employment outcomes well into adulthood (e.g., Atkinson et al., 2015; Clegg et al., 2015; Law et al., 2009). For this reason, children with a history of language disorders as preschoolers are monitored closely when they enter elementary school, so that services can be provided to those whose language disorders adversely affect literacy, learning, and academic achievement.

Box 2-1 summarizes the major types of speech and language disorders in children.

Co-occurring Speech and Language Disorders

Speech and language disorders may co-occur in children, and in children with severe disorders it is plausible that less obvious deficits in other aspects of development, such as cognitive and sensorimotor processing, may also be implicated. In the first few years of life it may be particularly difficult to determine whether a child's failure to speak is the result of a speech disorder, of a language disorder, or of both. For one thing, many speech and language abilities emerge during the early years of development, and disorders cannot be identified until children have reached the ages at which various speech and language abilities are expected. This difficulty is compounded by the fact that children under the age of approximately 30 months are often difficult to evaluate because they may be reluctant or unable to engage in formal standardized tests of their speech and language skills.

BOX 2-1
Types of Speech and Language Disorders in Children

Speech Disorders

Speech Sound Disorders

Articulation/Phonological Disorder

- Impaired production of individual speech sounds or sequences
- Cause may be known structural abnormality (e.g., cleft palate), inadequate knowledge of speech sound patterns, or unknown

Dysarthria

- Speech may be abnormally slow, fast, weak, slurred, or imprecise
- Caused by medical conditions that interfere with muscles and nerves that control speech

Childhood Apraxia of Speech

- Deficits in planning and coordination of speech sound sequences rather than inability to articulate individual speech sounds
- Cause is usually unknown

Voice Disorders (Dysphonia)

- Impaired functioning of laryngeal structures leads to abnormal voice quality or complete inability of the vocal cords to vibrate to produce sound
- Cause may be known medical condition (e.g., trauma, abnormal growth) or unknown

Stuttering (Fluency Disorder, Dysfluency)

- Excessive disruptions (repetitions, breakdowns) of the forward flow of speech
- Cause usually unknown; in some cases, onset coincides with neurological condition

Language Disorders

Expressive Language Disorder

- Impaired ability to formulate ideas and messages using words and sentences
- Cause may be known neurological condition or unknown

Receptive Language Disorder

- Impaired ability to understand messages encoded in words and sentences
- Cause may be known neurological condition or unknown

Expressive-Receptive Language Disorder

- Combination of deficits in understanding and producing messages
- Cause may be known neurological condition or unknown

Fortunately, effective treatments for very young nonspeaking children exist that do not depend on differentiating speech from language disorders, and a child's rate of progress in treatment may provide important evidence on the nature and severity of the disorders.

DIAGNOSING SPEECH AND LANGUAGE DISORDERS

Speech and language disorders can accompany or result from any of the conditions that interfere with the development of perceptual, motor, cognitive, or socioemotional function. Accordingly, conditions as varied as Down syndrome, fragile X syndrome, autism spectrum disorder, traumatic brain injury, and being deaf or hard of hearing are known to increase the potential for childhood speech and/or language disorders, and many children with such conditions will also have speech and language disorders. In addition, studies of children with primary speech and language disorders often reveal that they have abnormalities in other areas of development. For example, studies by Brumbach and Goffman (2014) suggest that children with primary language impairment show general deficits in gross and fine motor performance, and such children also show deficits in working memory and procedural learning (Lum et al., 2014). Conversely, some children who have primary speech sound disorders as preschoolers have deficits in reading and spelling during their elementary school years (Lewis et al., 2011). In short, considerable evidence suggests that spoken language skills, including speech sound production, constitute an integrated system and that clear deficits in one area may coexist with deficits in other areas that can compromise future development in language-related domains such as literacy. Intensive monitoring of speech and language development in such children is important for early detection and intervention to lessen the effects of speech and language disorders.

In many children, however, speech and language disorders occur for unknown reasons. In such children, diagnosing speech and language disorders is a complex process that requires assessing not only speech and language skills but also cognitive, perceptual, motor, and socioemotional development; biological, medical, and socioeconomic circumstances; and cultural and linguistic environments. Best-practice guidelines recommend evaluating across multiple domains and obtaining information from multiple sources, including a combination of formal, standardized, or norm-referenced tests; criterion-referenced observations by speech-language pathologists and other professionals; and judgments of familiar caregivers about the child's speech and language competence relative to community expectations for children of the same age (ASHA, 2004; Nelson et al., 2006, 2008; Royal College of Speech & Language Therapists, 2005; Shevell et al., 2003; Wilkinson et al., 2013).

On norm-referenced tests, children's scores are compared with average scores from large, representative samples of children of the same age. Children scoring below a cutoff value are defined as having a deficit, and severity is defined according to how far below average their scores fall. Deficits can range from mild to severe. In clinical practice, scores that fall more than two but less than three standard deviations below the mean are described as severely or extremely low; only 2.14 percent of children would be expected to score this poorly. Scores that fall three or more standard deviations below the mean are extraordinarily low; only 0.13 percent of children would be expected to score this poorly (Urbina, 2014). Figure 2-1 represents these numbers in graphic terms. It shows that only 1 child in 1,000 would be expected to score three or more standard deviations below the mean, and only about 22 children in 1,000 would score more than two but less than three standard deviations below the mean.

In practice, few norm-referenced speech and language tests include a separate severity category for scores that are three or more standard deviations below the mean; all scores two or more standard deviations below the mean are classified together as "severe" or "very low" (Spaulding et al., 2012). As noted in Chapter 1, these clinical criteria for defining severity are not identical to the legal standards for severity specified in the regulations for the Supplemental Security Income (SSI) program, which also considers functional limitations (that are the result of the interactive and cumulative effects of all impairments) to determine the severity. Chapter 4 includes an in-depth review of how children are evaluated for disability in the SSI eligibility determination process.

Norm-referenced testing is not always possible because children may be too young or too disabled to participate in formal standardized testing procedures. In children younger than 3 years and others incapable of formal testing, behaviors and skills are compared with those of typically developing children using criterion-referenced measures or observational checklists (Salvia et al., 2012). Some criterion-referenced measures involve detailed observations of specific skills, such as parent checklists of the number of words that children say. For example, 3-year-old children are expected to say 50 or more different words; those who fail to reach this criterion may be identified as having a significant vocabulary delay. Similarly, by 9-10 months of age, children are expected to communicate with their caregivers using nonlinguistic signals such as pointing and clapping; a 12-month-old who appears uninterested in others and fails to produce such basic communicative precursors to language may be identified as having a significant delay in the pragmatic domain of language. Still other criterion-referenced measures involve more global judgments of whether the child's language abilities are generally commensurate with those of peers, such as asking parents whether they are concerned about their child's ability to talk

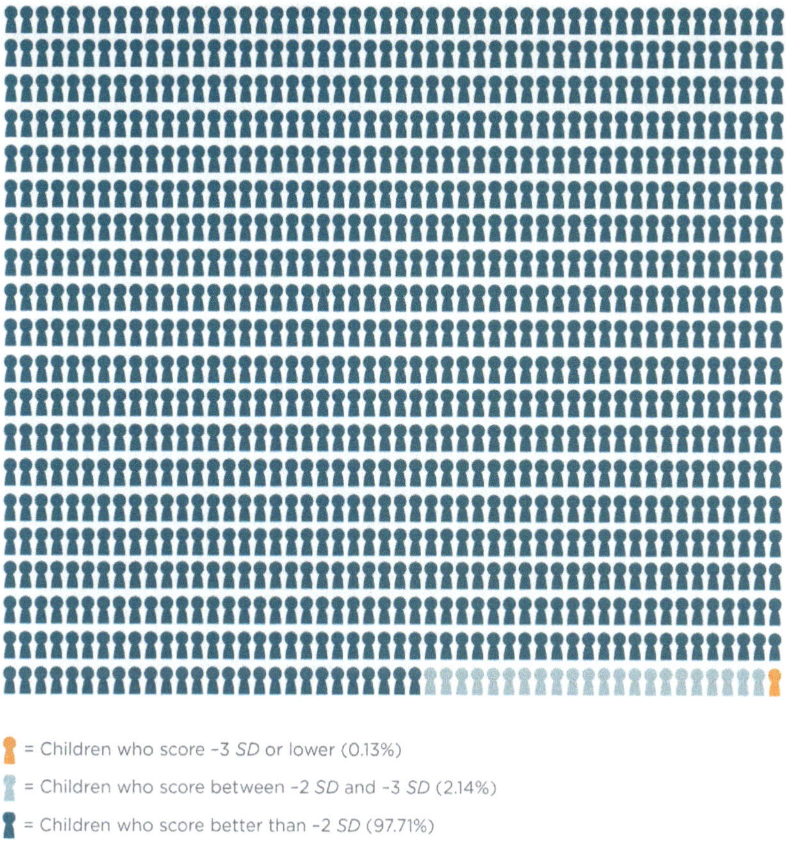

FIGURE 2-1 In a normative sample of 1,000 children, only 1 child (shown in orange) is expected to score three or more standard deviations below the mean. Another 22 children (shown in light green) are expected to score more than two but less than three standard deviations below the mean. The remaining 977 children (shown in dark green) are not expected to have scores as low as two standard deviations below the mean.
SOURCE: Based on data in Urbina, 2014.

or understand as well as other children of the same age. In many cases, children are diagnosed as having language delays when their level of performance on some criterion-referenced skill is inconsistent with age to a significant degree, usually defined as a "percentage of delay" relative to chronological age. For example, a 24-month-old with the skills of children half her age (i.e., 12-month-old children) can be described as having a

50 percent delay; if her skills are comparable to those of 18-month-olds, she is described as having a 25 percent delay. In many states, delays of more than 20-25 percent are used to identify children under age 3 years for early intervention under Part C of the 2004 IDEA (Ringwalt, 2015).

Validated norm-referenced tests may not be available for children who are members of cultural and linguistic communities that are not represented adequately in normative samples (e.g., AERA et al., 2014; Roseberry-McKibbin, 2014). In addition, norm-referenced test scores may be influenced by such extraneous factors as additional or confounding deficits (e.g., poor vision, inability to respond actively to test items), fatigue, and emotional state on a given day (Urbina, 2014). Finally, norm-referenced testing may not adequately reflect the functional limitations that speech and language deficits impose on the child's ability to participate in some demanding, real-world contexts. For example, a child with a speech sound disorder may be able to articulate a single word reasonably clearly on a norm-referenced speech test, but be incapable of coordinating the many events necessary to produce an intelligible sentence in fast-paced, dynamic conversation. Similarly, a child with an expressive language disorder may be able to produce single words and short phrases successfully elicited by a norm-referenced test, but be incapable of producing grammatical sentences, much less stories that include them. And a child with a receptive language disorder may understand words presented individually and point to a picture on a norm-referenced test, but be unable to comprehend sentences, especially if the sentences are lengthy, complex, spoken at the normal rate of two to four words per second, or spoken in noisy or distracting environments. For all of these reasons, best diagnostic practices require that evidence from norm- and criterion-referenced testing by professionals be considered in conjunction with judgments made by people who are familiar with the child's usual functioning in his or her daily environment (e.g., Paul and Norbury, 2012).

CAUSES AND RISK FACTORS

This chapter now turns to an overview of known underlying causes of speech and language disorders, followed by a summary of factors that have been associated with an increased risk of speech and language disorders having no known cause. Although prevalence estimates are available for some of the causes described below, and speech and language disorders are frequently mentioned among their sequelae, evidence on the percentage of speech and language disorders attributable solely to the underlying condition is not available. For example, Down syndrome, a chromosomal disorder with a prevalence of 1:700 live births, causes deficits spanning multiple areas of development, including not only speech and language but also cognition and sensorimotor skills, making it difficult to quantify the syndrome's causal role specifically in speech and language disorders.

Speech and Language Disorders with Known Causes

Determining the underlying etiology of a speech or language disorder is essential to providing the child with an appropriate set of interventions and the parents with an understanding of the cause and natural history of their child's disability. A variety of congenital and acquired conditions may result in abnormal speech and/or language development. These conditions include primary disorders of hearing, as well as specific genetic diseases, brain malformation syndromes, inborn errors of metabolism, toxic exposures, nutritional deficiencies, injuries, and epilepsy.

Children who are deaf or hard of hearing provide an especially clear example of the interrelationships among the many causes and consequences of speech and language disorders in childhood (Fitzpatrick, 2015). Because adequate hearing is critically important for developing and using receptive language, expressive language, and speech, being deaf or hard of hearing can lead to speech and language disorders, which in turn contribute to socioemotional and academic disabilities. This is particularly the case when the onset of hearing problems is either congenital or acquired during the first several years of life. Therefore, it is essential that hearing be assessed in children being evaluated for speech and language disorders.

Childhood hearing loss may result from or be associated with a wide variety of causes, which are categorized in Box 2-2. Hearing may be affected by disorders of either the sensory component of the auditory system (i.e., peripheral) or the processing of auditory information within the brain (i.e., central). Peripheral causes may be either unilateral or bilateral and are subdivided into conductive types, which are due to developmental or acquired abnormalities of the structures of the outer or middle ear, and sensorineural types, which are due to a variety of disorders affecting the sound-sensing organ—the cochlea—and its nerve that goes to the brain—the cochlear nerve.

Conductive-related causes of reduced hearing levels include congenital structural malformations of the outer and inner ear, consequences of acute or recurrent middle-ear infections, eustachian tube dysfunction, tumors, and trauma. Sensorineural types are even more diverse. A variety of genetic disorders have been identified that affect the function of the cochlea or cochlear nerve, and the disorder may be sporadic or inherited in an autosomal dominant, autosomal recessive, or X-linked manner, depending on the specific gene. Sensorineural types may be secondary to medical illness or even treatments for babies who must be placed in neonatal intensive care units because of either prematurity or a variety of perinatal disorders, such as

BOX 2-2
Examples of Conditions Affecting Hearing Early in Life That May Affect the Development of Speech and Language

Impact on Peripheral Hearing

Conductive (abnormal function or structure of outer or middle ear)

Abnormal development of the outer- or middle-ear structures

Pierre Robin sequence (e.g., Glynn et al., 2011)
Microtia (e.g., Luquetti et al., 2012)
Exposure to teratogens (e.g., thalidomide) (e.g., Shiga et al., 2015)
Other malformation syndromes

Acquired middle-ear dysfunction

Chronic otitis media (e.g., Patterson and Paparella, 1999) and eustachian tube dysfunction (e.g., Swarts and Bluestone, 2003)
Skull fracture (e.g., Dunklebarger et al., 2014)

Sensorineural (abnormal structure or function of cochlea or cochlear nerve)

Genetic* (e.g., Parker and Bitner-Glindzicz, 2015)

Alport (e.g., *COL4A*)
Pendred (e.g., *SLC26A4*)
Stickler (e.g., *COL2A1*, *COL11A1*, *COL9A1*)
Usher type 1-3 (e.g., *USH1C*, *USH2A*, *CLRN1*)
Waardenburg types 1-4 (e.g., *PAX3*)
Perrault (e.g., *HSD17B4*)
Connexin 26

Acquired etiologies

Hypoxia-ischemia (e.g., Robertson and Finer, 1985)
Congenital (maternal) infection with toxoplasmosis, cytomegalovirus, or rubella (e.g., Cohen et al., 2014; Goderis et al., 2014)
Hyperbilirubinemia (kernicterus) (e.g., Corujo-Santana et al., 2015)
Neonatal meningitis or sepsis-direct infection and ototoxic drug exposure (e.g., aminoglycosides) (e.g., Caye-Thomasen et al., 2012; Jing et al., 2015)
Skull fracture (e.g., Dunklebarger et al., 2014)
Pediatric tumors (e.g., medulloblastoma and vestibular schwannomas) (e.g., Schreiber et al., 2014)

Impact on Central Hearing

Landau-Kleffner Syndrome (acquired epileptic aphasia) (e.g., Plyler and Harkrider, 2013)
Hyperbilirubinemia (kernicterus)

---

* Genetic conditions can affect hearing at multiple locations.

hypoxia (oxygen deficiency), disturbances of blood flow, infections, or hyperbilirubinemia (excessive bilirubin levels that lead to jaundice and brain dysfunction known as kernicterus). Prenatal infections due to maternal cytomegalovirus, toxoplasmosis, or rubella (TORCH infections) can have a significant congenital impact on the sensorineural hearing mechanism, as can postnatal infectious illnesses such as meningitis (inflammation of membranes around the brain and spinal cord). Ironically, the treatment of meningitis or other bacterial infections with certain antibiotics can result in decreased hearing levels, as some of these life-saving drugs are ototoxic (i.e., harmful to structures of the ear). The impact of antibiotics on central hearing function is much less common in childhood and generally does not lead to total deafness.

The best-recognized cause affecting central hearing is Landau-Kleffner syndrome, or acquired epileptic aphasia, a rare condition that typically presents in early childhood with either minimal speech and language development or loss of previously acquired speech and language due to cortical deafness secondary to persistent epileptiform activity in the electroencephalogram, even in the absence of clinical seizures. Lastly, neonatal hyperbilirubinemia (kernicterus) can impact both sensorineural and central hearing, the latter as a result of dysfunction at the level of the brainstem. Importantly, in addition to the causes described above, many factors that impact hearing are themselves caused by, or co-occur with, underlying conditions that affect other aspects of children's development.

Apart from being deaf or hard of hearing, there are a diverse set of conditions that should be considered as other potential causes of speech and language disorders, as summarized in Box 2-2. As is the case with hearing, abnormal development of anatomic structures critical to the proper generation of speech may lead to speech sound disorders or voice disorders. For example, articulation and phonological disorders may result from cleft palate. A wide variety of genetic syndromes are known to be associated with disordered speech and language development. These include well-characterized conditions that are due to an abnormal number of a specific chromosome, such as Down syndrome (associated with three rather than two copies of chromosome 21) (Tedeschi et al., 2015) or Klinefelter syndrome (which occurs in boys who have a normal Y chromosome together with two or more X chromosomes, rather than one X chromosome).

Well-recognized genetic syndromes due to a mutation in a single gene (such as fragile X syndrome, neurofibromatosis type I, Williams syndrome, and tuberous sclerosis) are associated with speech or language disorders, and current research has demonstrated that alterations in small groups of genes (copy number variations such as 16p11.2 deletion) may increase the risk of a speech or language disability. In general, when indicated by history and clinical examination, these genetic conditions can be detected with clinically available blood-based laboratory tests. Primary malformations of the central nervous system—such as hydrocephalus (an expansion of the fluid-filled cavities within the brain), agenesis of the corpus callosum (the absence of the main structure that connects the right and left hemispheres of the brain), and both gross and microscopic abnormalities of cortical development (cortical dysplasia, an abnormal layering or location of neurons)—also may be associated with speech and language disorders. In general, these primary disruptions in brain anatomy may be diagnosed by magnetic resonance imaging (MRI) and in some cases discovered via an in utero maternal-fetal ultrasound examination.

A variety of prenatal and postnatal toxic exposures may result in abnormal brain development with resultant neurodevelopmental consequences. Maternal alcohol and other substance use are well recognized in this regard, as is postnatal exposure to lead. Similarly, abnormal prenatal growth, postnatal nutritional deprivation, and hypothyroidism (underactive thyroid) have developmental consequences. Injuries to the developing brain, such as perinatal stroke from brain hemorrhages or ischemia (inadequate blood supply), accidental trauma, and nonaccidental trauma (child abuse), must also be considered, as must such neoplastic conditions as primary brain tumors, metastatic disease, and the consequences of oncological therapies (e.g., chemotherapy and radiation). Some children with cerebral palsy (a condition that results in abnormal motor development and that has numerous causes) may also have an associated speech or language disorder. In addition, speech and language disorders may be secondary to poorly controlled epilepsy associated with a variety of causes, including structural abnormalities in cortical development, genetic disorders (e.g., mutations in ion channel genes), and complex epileptic encephalopathies (e.g., West, Lennox-Gastault, or Landau-Kleffner syndromes) (Campbell et al., 2003; Feldman and Messick, 2009).

Box 2-3 presents a listing of examples of speech and language disorders with known causes.

Risk Factors Associated with Speech and Language Disorders with No Known Cause

In addition to the etiologies described above, a number of variables have been associated with an increased risk of childhood speech and/or language disorders with no known cause. Findings in this literature are somewhat inconsistent (Harrison and McLeod, 2010; Nelson et al., 2006), varying with characteristics of the children examined (e.g., age, phenotype, severity, comorbidity) and with research design features (e.g., sample size, control for confounding, statistical analyses).

Studies of speech and language disorders in children, such as speech sound disorders (Lewis et al., 2006, 2007) and specific language impairment (Barry et al., 2007; Bishop, 2006; Bishop and Hayiou-Thomas, 2008; Rice, 2012; Tomblin and Buckwalter, 1998), show that these conditions are familial (i.e., risk for these disorders is elevated for family members of affected individuals) and that this familiality is partially heritable (i.e., genetic factors shared among biological family members contribute to family aggregation). However, heritability estimates (i.e., the proportion of phenotypic variance that can be attributed to genetic variance) for some speech and language disorders, such as specific language impairment, have been inconsistent (Bishop and Hayiou-Thomas, 2008). For example, twin studies on heritability of language disorders have shown a range of estimates of heritability, from 45 percent for deficient language achievement (Tomblin and Buckwalter, 1998) to 25 percent for specific language impairment (DeThorne et al., 2005). One study of 579 4-year-old twins with low language performance and their co-twins found heritability was greater for more severe language impairment, suggesting a stronger influence of genes at the lower end of language ability (Viding et al., 2004). Finally, a review of twin data found that the environment shared by the twins was "relatively unimportant" in causing specific language impairment compared with genetic factors (Bishop, 2006). Overall, the evidence suggests that susceptibility to speech and language disorders results from interactions between genetic and environmental factors (Newbury and Monaco, 2010).

To date, the evidence best supports a cumulative risk model in which increases in risk are larger for combinations of risk factors than for individual factors (Harrison and McLeod, 2010; Lewis et al., 2015; Pennington and Bishop, 2009; Reilly et al., 2010; Whitehouse et al., 2014). In a study of speech sound disorders, for example, Campbell and colleagues (2003) found that three variables—male sex, low maternal education, and positive family history of developmental communication disorders—were individually associated with increased odds of speech sound disorder, but the odds of such a disorder were nearly eight times larger in a child with all three risk factors than in a child with none of them. Based on a national database in the United Kingdom, Dockrell and colleagues (2014) report higher odds (2.5) of speech, language, and communication needs in boys than in girls, and they document a strong social gradient for childhood speech, language, and communication disorders in which the odds were 2.3 times greater for children entitled to free school lunches and living in more deprived neighborhoods than for children without these factors. It is important to note that risk indices such as odds ratios cannot provide evidence on the proportion of cases of the disorder that are caused by the factor in question, both because they could reflect the influence of some other, unknown causal factor and because they are influenced by the composition of the samples (e.g., base rate, severity) in which they are calculated.

BOX 2-3
Examples of Speech and Language Disorders with Known Causes

Abnormal Development of Facial and Pharyngeal Structures
Cleft palate (e.g., Mildinhall, 2012)
Velocardiofacial syndrome (e.g., Ford et al., 2000)

Genetic Disorders Associated with Neurodevelopmental Impairment
Chromosomal disorders
Klinefelter syndrome (XXY) (e.g., Simpson et al., 2014)
Turner syndrome (monosomy X) (e.g., Simpson et al., 2014)
Down syndrome (trisomy 21) (e.g., Næss et al., 2015)
Copy number variants (e.g., Hanson et al., 2015)
16p11.2
15p11
1q21.1 (expressive language affected more than receptive language)
Single gene disorders resulting in brain malformation, abnormalities of synaptic transmission, abnormalities of DNA synthesis, or inborn errors of intermediary metabolism
X-linked
ARGHEF 9 (disorder of GABA)
Neuroligin (*NLGN3* and *NLGN4*) (e.g., Yan et al., 2005)
Autosomal
Neurexin (*NRXN1*) (e.g., Béna et al., 2013)
Forkhead Box P1 (*FOXP1*) (Lozano et al., 2015)
Forkhead Box P2 (*FOXP2*) (Takahashi et al., 2010)
Phenylketonuria (e.g., Gejão et al., 2009; Soleymani et al., 2015)
Epigenetic mechanisms

Brain Malformations and Cortical Dysplasia (neuropathologically defined, some with genetic causes identified)
Polymicrogyria (e.g., Chang et al., 2007; Saporta et al., 2011)
Hydrocephalus (e.g., Vinchon et al., 2012)
Agenesis of the corpus callosum (e.g., Paul, 2011)
Neurofibromatosis type I (e.g., Klein-Tasman et al., 2014)
Tuberous sclerosis (e.g., Gallagher et al., 2013)

Research has shown a strong association between poverty and developmental delays, such as language delays. For example, in a study of 513 3-year-olds who had been exposed to risk factors that included inadequate income, lack of social supports, poor maternal prenatal care, and high family stress, King and colleagues (2005) found that 10 percent of children—four times the expected 2.5 percent—had severe delays, scoring two or more standard deviations below the mean on a norm-referenced

Neoplastic Disorders (e.g., Dennis, 2010; Hudson and Murdoch, 1990)

Congenital brain tumors

Brain tumors (primary or metastatic) that present during the period of speech and language development

Consequences of oncological therapies (chemotherapy and radiation) (e.g., Moleski, 2000)

Injuries and Exposures (e.g., Dennis, 2010)

Prenatal

Toxins (e.g., tobacco, alcohol, stimulants) (e.g., McGee et al., 2009)

Abnormal fetal growth (small for gestational age, prematurity)

Poverty (e.g., lack of or poor prenatal care) (e.g., King et al., 2005; Walker et al., 2011)

Perinatal

Neonatal encephalopathy/hypoxic ischemic encephalopathy (e.g., Robertson and Finer, 1985)

Postnatal

Complications of prematurity (e.g., Adams-Chapman et al., 2015)

Focal brain lesions due to stroke (e.g., Ilves et al., 2014)

Toxins (lead, pesticides) (e.g., Jurewicz et al., 2013)

Trauma

Abuse and/or severe deprivation (e.g., Perry et al., 2008)

Poverty (e.g., Hart and Risley, 1995)

Hypothyroidism (e.g., Gejão et al., 2009)

Nutritional deficiencies

Consequences of epilepsy and epileptic encephalopathy (e.g., Jambaque et al., 2012)

language test. Walker and colleagues (2011) showed that experiences in early life affect the structure and functioning of the brain. For example, a malnourished expectant mother who faces barriers in accessing prenatal care is at risk of having a child who is premature, is small for his or her gestational age, or experiences perinatal complications (Adams et al., 1994; Walker et al., 2011). Children exposed to such factors in the womb are at increased risk for developing a disability such as specific language impairment (Spitz et al., 1997; Stanton-Chapman et al., 2004). Lastly, a variety of other psychosocial factors—including deprivation of appropriate stimuli from parents and caretakers (Akca et al., 2012; Fernald et al., 2013; Hart and Risley, 1995), excess media (television and screen time) exposure (Christakis et al., 2009; Zimmerman et al., 2007), and poor sleep hygiene (Earle and Myers, 2014)—need to be considered as potential risk factors for speech and language disorders.

PREVALENCE

Law and colleagues (2000) found that there existed no systematic synthesis of the evidence concerning the prevalence of pediatric speech and language disorders with primary causes; their observation remains true in 2015 (Wallace et al., 2015). Estimating the prevalence of these disorders with confidence is difficult for several reasons. First, because the characteristics of these disorders differ with age, the diagnostic tools by which they are identified necessarily vary in format, ranging from simple parental reports at the earliest ages to formal standardized testing at later ages. Second, because these disorders can vary in scope—from problems with relatively discrete skills (e.g., producing individual speech sounds) to problems with broader and less observable sets of abilities (e.g., drawing inferences from or comprehending language that is ambiguous, indirect, or nonliteral)—there exists no single diagnostic tool capable of addressing the full range of pediatric speech and language skills. Third, as with many pediatric psychological and behavioral disorders, diagnostic criteria involve integrating observations from multiple sources and time points.

As a result, there currently is no single reference standard for identifying pediatric speech and language disorders of primary origin in children of all ages. Instead, prevalence estimates come from studies that focused on different ages and used different diagnostic tools and criteria. Law and colleagues (2000) found a median prevalence of 5.95 percent in the four studies they reviewed; they observe that this value is consistent with several other estimates, but emphasize the need for caution pending additional evidence from well-designed population studies.

The following subsections describe prevalence estimates from studies that have attempted to distinguish speech disorders from language disorders. However, these estimates also must be viewed with caution, given differences among studies in sample composition and diagnostic criteria.

Speech Disorders

Consistent with the varying expectations for speech skills in children of different ages, estimates of the incidence (i.e., the risk of acquiring a disorder for an individual in a specified population) and prevalence (i.e., the percentage of individuals affected by a disorder in a specified population at a specific point in time) of speech disorders vary according to age, the presence of other neurodevelopmental disorders, and the diagnostic criteria employed.

Most of the literature on the prevalence of speech disorders has focused on children with articulation or phonological disorders due to unknown causes. Shriberg and colleagues (1999, cited in Pennington and Bishop, 2009) report a mean prevalence of 8.2 percent for such disorders; Bishop (2010) estimates prevalence at 10 percent. The prevalence of these disorders varies with age, however, decreasing from 15-16 percent at age 3 (Campbell et al., 2003) to approximately 4 percent at age 6 (Shriberg et al., 1999). Evidence suggests that speech sound disorders affect more boys than girls (Eadie et al., 2015), particularly in early life. In preschoolers, the ratio of affected boys to girls is 2 or 3:1, declining by age 6 to 1.2:1 (Pennington and Bishop, 2009; Shriberg et al., 1999). Although many children with speech sound disorders as preschoolers will progress into the normal range by the time of school entry, the close ties between spoken and written language have motivated many studies of the extent to which speech sound disorders are associated with an increased risk of reading, writing, or spelling disorders. To date, evidence from several studies (e.g., Lewis et al., 2015; Pennington and Bishop, 2009; Skebo et al., 2013) suggests that in comparison with their unaffected peers, children with speech sound disorders but normal-range language skills may have somewhat lower reading scores than their peers, but they rarely meet eligibility criteria for a reading disability (Skebo et al., 2013). However, severity has not been considered to date in studies of the relationship between speech sound disorders and reading skills (Skebo et al., 2013).

Little evidence is available concerning the epidemiology of voice disorders in children (dysphonias) not attributable to other developmental disorders. In a prospective population-based cohort of 7,389 8-year-old British children, 6-11 percent were identified as dysphonic; male sex, number of siblings, asthma, and frequent upper respiratory infections were among the factors associated with an increased risk of voice disorders (Carding et al., 2006).

Stuttering is estimated to have a lifetime incidence of 5 percent but a population prevalence of just under 1 percent (Bloodstein and Ratner, 2008). The prevalence of stuttering before the age of 6 years is much higher than that at later ages; evidence from several sources suggests that rates of natural recovery from stuttering in children before age 6 may be as high as 85 percent (Yairi and Ambrose, 2013). Evidence indicates that stuttering affects only slightly more boys than girls during the preschool period, although higher ratios of affected males to females have been observed at later ages. Finally, approximately 60 percent of cases of developmental stuttering co-occur with other speech and language disorders (Kent and Vorperian, 2013).

Language Disorders

As with speech disorders, estimates of the prevalence of language disorders vary across studies by age, the presence of other neurodevelopmental disorders, and the diagnostic criteria employed. Language disorders with no known cause, sometimes referred to as "specific" (or "primary") language impairments (e.g., Reilly et al., 2014), are highly prevalent, affecting 6-15 percent of children when identified through formal norm-referenced testing in population-based samples (Law et al., 2000). This is consistent with the cutoff values of 1.0-1.5 standard deviations below the mean employed in several investigations (e.g., Tomblin et al., 1997b). By contrast, prevalence estimates are generally higher when based on parent or teacher reports. For example, in a survey of parents and teachers conducted in a nationally representative sample of 4,983 4- to 5-year-old children in Australia, McLeod and Harrison (2009) found that prevalence estimates based on parent and teacher reports were somewhat higher than those based on norm-referenced testing, with 22-25 percent of children perceived as having deficits in talking (expressive language) and 10-17 percent as having deficits in understanding (receptive language). As noted by Law and colleagues (2000), the discrepancy between prevalence rates defined according to norm- and criterion-referenced methods could be due to a number of factors, including the inability of norm-referenced tests to capture or reflect the child's language functioning in relatively more challenging situations, such as classrooms and conversations.

Language disorders that have no known cause have been reported to affect more boys than girls, but it appears that the gender imbalance is greater in clinical than in population-based samples (e.g., Pennington and Bishop, 2009). For example, the ratio of affected males to females has ranged from 2:1 to 6:1 across several clinical samples, but boys were only slightly more likely to be affected than girls (1.3:1) in a large population-based sample of U.S. kindergarten children (Tomblin et al., 1997b).

As noted earlier, many aspects of literacy depend heavily on the language knowledge and skills that children acquire before they enter school (Catts and Kamhi, 2012), and children with severe language disorders have a substantially increased risk of deficits in reading and academic achievement. Estimates vary, but children diagnosed with language disorders with no known cause as preschoolers are at least four times more likely to have reading disabilities than their unaffected peers (Pennington and Bishop, 2009). Similarly, evidence from a large-scale, prospective methodologically sound cohort study of kindergarteners followed longitudinally showed that the majority of those with language disorders with no known cause continued to exhibit language and/or academic difficulties through adolescence (Tomblin and Nippold, 2014).

One study that helped frame the committee's understanding of prevalence estimates of speech and language disorders was a study of specific language impairment conducted by Tomblin and colleagues (1997b). This study selected a geographic region in the upper Midwest of the United States and sampled rural, suburban, and urban schools within that region. All eligible 5- to 6-year-old children were systematically screened and followed up with diagnostic testing for specific language impairment. Children were not included if they spoke a language other than English, failed a hearing test, or demonstrated low functioning in nonverbal intelligence (suggesting overall lower intellectual functioning). When a cutoff 1.25 standard deviations below the mean (i.e., approximately the 10th percentile, or the lowest 10 percent of the normative sample) on at least two language scores was used, the prevalence rate of specific language impairment was estimated at 7.4 percent of kindergarten children. The prevalence of specific language impairment for boys was 8 percent and for girls was 6 percent.

When the cutoff was set at two standard deviations below the mean (i.e., approximately the 2nd percentile), the prevalence estimate dropped to 1.12 percent. Using 1.25 standard deviations below the mean as the criterion, there were slightly higher rates of specific language impairment among African American and Native American children relative to white and Hispanic children. Only 29 percent of the parents of the kindergarteners diagnosed with specific language impairment reported having been informed that their children had speech or language problems. It is important to note that large-scale epidemiological studies on autism spectrum disorder, learning disorders, and attention deficit hyperactivity disorder have clearly demonstrated that active case-finding strategies lead to higher and more accurate rates of identification of children with neurodevelopmental disorders (Barbaresi et al., 2002, 2005, 2009; CDC, 2014; Katusic et al., 2001) relative to studies depending only on parent reports. Studies that followed this sample of children with specific language impairment into their school years demonstrated that as a group, they also experienced lower academic achievement.

The Tomblin et al. (1997a) study underscores several methodological issues relevant for the current report: differences in severity level for case identification, comorbidity with other disorders considered primary disabilities, and differences in prevalence related to gender and racial or ethnic identity. Subsequent studies with the children included in this study identified low maternal and paternal education and paternal history of speech,

TABLE 2-1 Estimates of the Prevalence of Speech and Language Disorders from Studies of U.S. Children

Study Source	Condition	How the Child's Condition Is Identified	Ages	Sample Size	Prevalence (% positive)
Tomblin et al., 1997b	Specific language impairment	−1.25 standard deviations (SD) on >2 language composites or −2 SD on one Test of Language Development (TOLD) subtest	5-6 yrs.	7,218 screened; 2,084 tested	7.4% (confidence interval [CI] 6.3, 8.5)
King et al., 2005	Language delay	Preschool Language Scale-3 total score; severe delay: ≥2 SD	36-40 mos.	513 at risk	10%
Campbell et al., 2003	Speech delay	Continuous speech sample analyzed with Speech Disorders Classification System (SDCS)	36-38 mos.	639	15.6%
Shriberg et al., 1999	Speech delay	Validated algorithm applying SDCS to TOLD Word Articulation subtest	5-6 yrs.	1,328 (subsample of 2,084 tested in Tomblin et al. [1997] study)	3.8% (CI 2.9, 5.0)
Pinborough-Zimmerman et al., 2007	Communication disorder	Medical/educational records reviewed for *International Classification of Diseases, Ninth Edition, Clinical Modification* (ICD-9-CM) codes (315.3, 315.31, 315.32) and/or school designation of special education exceptionality of communication disorder	8 yrs.	26,518	6.3% (CI 6.0, 6.6)

NOTES: The Test of Language Development (TOLD) assesses spoken language in young children. It has nine subtests that measure aspects of oral language: picture vocabulary, relational vocabulary, oral vocabulary, syntactic understanding, sentence imitation, morphological completion, word discrimination, word analysis, and word articulation. The Speech Disorders Classification System (SDCS) is the primary qualitative system for classifying speech disorders from 2 years of age through adulthood (Shriberg, 1993).

SOURCES: Campbell et al., 2003; King et al., 2005; Pinborough-Zimmerman et al., 2007; Shriberg, 1993; Shriberg et al., 1999; Tomblin et al., 1997b.

learning, or intellectual difficulties as risk factors for specific language impairment (Tomblin et al., 1997a).

Table 2-1 provides a summary of prevalence estimates from the studies of U.S. children that the committee also reviewed. This list is not the result of a meta-analysis, nor is it exhaustive; rather, the table includes a number of well-designed studies that employed clear and consistent definitions. The committee reviewed numerous well-designed studies and meta-analyses from other countries (e.g., Beitchman et al., 1996a,b,c [Canada]; Law et al., 2000 [United Kingdom, others]; McLeod and Harrison, 2009 [Australia]). For the purposes of this study, however, the committee limited the summary of prevalence estimates to U.S. children. Table 2-1 includes the populations and conditions studied, the diagnostic criteria used to identify the conditions, and the prevalence of the conditions (or percent positive). Confidence intervals are included when available. As noted earlier, and as is evident from the table, the studies reviewed vary greatly in terms of ages, diagnostic tools or criteria, and methods used. The estimates presented in the table (in addition to estimates based on national survey data presented in Chapter 5) indicate that speech and language disorders affect between 3 and 16 percent of U.S. children.

COMMON COMORBIDITIES

An examination of comorbidities (i.e., other co-occurring conditions) of speech and language disorders is complicated by the central role of language and communication in the development and behavior of children and adolescents. Speech and language disorders are a definitional component of certain conditions, most prominently autism spectrum disorder (American Psychiatric Association, 2013). Other neurodevelopmental disorders, including cognitive impairment, are universally associated with varying degrees of delays and deficits in language and communication skills (American Psychiatric Association, 2013). In addition to their co-occurrence with a wide range of neurodevelopmental disorders, speech and language delays in toddlers and preschool-age children are associated with a significantly increased risk for long-term developmental challenges, such as language-based learning disorders (Beitchman et al., 1996a,b,c, 1999, 2001, 2014; Brownlie et al., 2004; Stoeckel et al., 2013; Voci et al., 2006; Young et al., 2002). While specific language impairments (i.e., those not associated with other diagnosable neurodevelopmental disorders) are relatively common, it is likely that substantially greater numbers of children and adolescents experience significant speech and/or language impairment associated with other diagnosable disorders. Finally, speech and language delays and deficits may lead to impairments in other aspects of a child's functional skills (e.g., social interaction, behavior, academic achievement) even when not associated with other diagnosable disorders (Beitchman et al., 1996c, 2001, 2014; Brownlie et al., 2004; Voci et al., 2006; Young et al., 2002). This section, therefore, examines the association of speech and language disorders from the following perspectives: (1) speech and language disorders that are comorbid with other diagnosable disorders, and (2) speech and language disorders in early childhood that confer a quantifiable risk for the later development of comorbid conditions. Together, these two perspectives create a comprehensive picture of the association of speech and language disorders with other neurodevelopmental disorders.

Autism spectrum disorder is a highly prevalent neurodevelopmental disorder, affecting an estimated 1 in 68 8-year-old children in the United States (CDC, 2014). By definition, all children with autism spectrum disorder have deficits in communication, ranging from a complete absence of verbal and nonverbal communication skills, to atypical language (e.g., echolalia or "scripted" language), to more subtle deficits in pragmatic (i.e., social) communication (American Psychiatric Association, 2013). The formal diagnostic criteria for autism spectrum disorder require documentation of deficits in the social-communication domain (American Psychiatric Association, 2013). In clinical practice, when children present with significant delays in the development of communication skills, autism spectrum disorder is one of the primary diagnostic considerations (Myers and Johnson, 2007).

All children and adolescents with intellectual disability have varying degrees of impairment in communication skills (American Psychiatric Association, 2013). Among those with mild intellectual disability, deficits in communication may be relatively subtle, including inability to understand or employ highly abstract language or impairment in social communication. In contrast, children and adolescents with severe or profound levels of intellectual disability may be able only to communicate basic requests, understand concrete instructions, and communicate with simple phrases or single words; others may be unable to employ or understand spoken language. A number of specific genetic disorders are directly associated with varying degrees of intellectual disability together with abnormalities of speech and language (see Box 2-3). Some of these genetic conditions often are also associated with specific profiles of speech and language impairment (Feldman and Messick, 2009). Examples include dysfluent speech in children with Down syndrome, echolalia in boys with fragile X syndrome, and fluent but superficial social language in children with Williams syndrome (Feldman and Messick, 2009).

Language-based learning disorders, including reading and written language disorders, are often associated with speech and language disorders. The association between language impairment and reading disorders has been demonstrated in studies examining the likelihood that family members of subjects with language impairment are at increased risk for reading disorder (Flax et al., 2003). Both epidemiologic and clinic-based studies have demonstrated that children with speech sound disorders and language disorders are at increased risk for reading disorder (Pennington and Bishop, 2009). Similarly, multiple studies have demonstrated a strong association between attention deficit hyperactivity disorder and speech and language disorders (Pennington and Bishop, 2009; Tomblin, 2014).

The comorbidity of speech and language disorders and other neurodevelopmental disorders may not be apparent in pre-school-age children, since these very young children may not yet manifest the developmental lags or symptoms required to make comorbid diagnoses of such conditions as learning disorders and attention deficit hyperactivity disorder. In their prospective community-based study, for example, Beitchman and colleagues (1989) found significant differences in measures of "reading readiness" among 5-year-old children with poor language comprehension compared with children with either high overall speech and language ability or isolated articulation difficulties (Beitchman et al., 1989). Similarly, there was a tendency for 5-year-olds with a combination of low articulation and poor language comprehension to have higher teacher ratings of hyperactivity and inattention and lower maternal ratings of social competence (Beitchman et al., 1989). By age 12, the children who earlier had shown combined deficits in speech and language had significantly lower levels of reading achievement and higher rates of diagnosed psychiatric disorders (57.1 percent versus 23.7 percent for children with normal speech and language at age 5) (Beitchman et al., 1994). By age 19, children with documented language impairment at age 5 had significantly higher rates of reading disorder (36.8 percent versus 6.4 percent), math disorder (53.9 percent versus 12.2 percent), and psychiatric disorders (40 percent versus 21 percent) compared with their peers with normal language ability at age 5 (Young et al., 2002).

In summary, speech and language disorders are frequently identified in association with (i.e., comorbid with) a wide range of other neurodevelopmental disorders. Children with comorbid conditions can be expected to be more severely impaired and to experience greater functional limitations (due to the interactive and cumulative effects of multiple conditions) than children who do not have comorbid conditions. Furthermore, young children with language impairments are at high risk for later manifestation of learning and psychiatric disorders. It is therefore important both to carefully examine the speech and language skills of children with other developmental disorders and to identify other neurodevelopmental disorders among children presenting with speech and language impairment. Among populations of children with conditions as diverse as autism spectrum disorder, attention deficit hyperactivity disorder, traumatic brain injury, and genetic disorders, speech and language disorders may be the most easily identified impairments because of the central role of language and communication in the functional capacity of children and adolescents.

FINDINGS AND CONCLUSIONS

Findings

2-1. Speech and language disorders are prevalent, affecting between 3 and 16 percent of U.S. children. Prevalence estimates vary according to age and the diagnostic criteria employed, but best evidence suggests that approximately 2 percent of children have speech and/or language disorders that are severe according to clinical standards.

2-2. Some speech and language disorders result from known biological causes.

2-3. In many cases, these disorders have no identifiable cause, but factors including male sex and reduced socioeconomic and educational resources have been associated with an increased risk of the disorders.

2-4. Diagnosing speech and language disorders in children is a complex process that requires integrating information on speech and language with information on biological and medical factors, environmental circumstances, and other areas of development.

2-5. Speech and language disorders frequently co-occur with other neurodevelopmental disorders and may be among the earliest symptoms of serious neurodevelopmental conditions.

2-6. Children with severe speech and language disorders have an increased risk of a variety of adverse outcomes, including mental health and behavior disorders, learning disabilities, poor academic achievement, and limited employment and social participation.

Conclusions

2-1. Severe speech and language disorders represent serious threats to children's social, emotional, educational, and employment outcomes.

2-2. Severe speech and language disorders are debilitating at any age, but their impacts on children are particularly serious because of their widespread adverse effects on development and the fact that these negative consequences cascade and build on one another over time.

2-3. Severe speech and language disorders may be one of the earliest detectable symptoms of other serious neurodevelopmental conditions; for this reason, they represent an important point of entry to early intervention and other services.

2-4. It is critically important to identify such disorders for two reasons: first, because they may be an early symptom of other serious neurodevelopmental disorders, and second, so that interventions aimed at forestalling or minimizing their adverse consequences can be undertaken.

REFERENCES

Adams, C. D., N. Hillman, and G. R. Gaydos. 1994. Behavioral difficulties in toddlers: Impact of socio-cultural and biological risk factors. *Journal of Clinical Child Psychology* 23(4):373-381.

Adams-Chapman, I., C. Bann, S. L. Carter, and B. J. Stoll. 2015. Language outcomes among ELBW infants in early childhood. *Early Human Development* 91(6):373-379.

AERA (American Educational Research Association), APA (American Psychological Association), and NCME (National Council on Measurement in Education). 2014. *Standards for educational and psychological testing*. Washington, DC: AERA.

Akca, O. F., C. Ugur, M. Colak, O. O. Kartal, A. S. Akozel, G. Erdogan, and R. I. Uslu. 2012. Underinvolved relationship disorder and related factors in a sample of young children. *Early Human Development* 88(6):327-332.

American Psychiatric Association. 2013. *Diagnostic and statistical manual of mental disorders: DSM-5* (5th ed.). Washington, DC: American Psychiatric Association.

ASHA (American Speech-Language-Hearing Association). 2004. *Preferred practice patterns for the profession of speech-language pathology*. http://www.asha.org/policy/PP2004-00191.htm (accessed September 29, 2015).

ASHA. 2007. *Childhood apraxia of speech*. http://www.asha.org/policy/TR2007-00278.htm (accessed September 29, 2015).

Atkinson, L., J. Beitchman, A. Gonzalez, A. Young, B. Wilson, M. Escobar, V. Chisholm, E. Brownlie, J. E. Khoury, J. Ludmer, and V. Villani. 2015. Cumulative risk, cumulative outcome: A 20-year longitudinal study. *PLoS ONE* 10(6):e0127650.

Barbaresi, W. J., S. K. Katusic, R. C. Colligan, V. Shane Pankratz, A. L. Weaver, K. J. Weber, D. A. Mrazek, and S. J. Jacobsen. 2002. How common is attention-deficit/hyperactivity disorder? Incidence in a population-based birth cohort in Rochester, Minn. *Archives of Pediatrics and Adolescent Medicine* 156(3):217-224.

Barbaresi, W. J., S. K. Katusic, R. C. Colligan, A. L. Weaver, and S. J. Jacobsen. 2005. Math learning disorder: Incidence in a population-based birth cohort 1976-82, Rochester, Minn. *Ambulatory Pediatrics* 5(5):281-289.

Barbaresi, W. J., R. C. Colligan, A. L. Weaver, and S. K. Katusic. 2009. The incidence of clinically diagnosed versus research-identified autism in Olmsted County, Minnesota, 1976-1997: Results from a retrospective, population-based study. *Journal of Autism and Developmental Disorders* 39(3):464-470.

Barry, J. G., I. Yasin, and D. V. Bishop. 2007. Heritable risk factors associated with language impairments. *Genes, Brain, and Behavior* 6(1):66-76.

Beitchman, J. H., J. Hood, J. Rochon, M. Peterson, T. Mantini, and S. Majumdar. 1989. Empirical classification of speech/language impairment in children: I. Identification of speech/language disorders. *Journal of the American Academy of Child & Adolescent Psychiatry* 28(1):112-117.

Beitchman, J. H., E. B. Brownlie, A. Inglis, J. Wild, R. Mathews, D. Schachter, R. Kroll, S. Martin, B. Ferguson, and W. Lancee. 1994. Seven-year follow-up of speech/language-impaired and control children: Speech/language stability and outcome. *Journal of the American Academy of Child & Adolescent Psychiatry* 33(9):1322-1330.

Beitchman, J. H., B. Wilson, E. B. Brownlie, H. Walters, and W. Lancee. 1996a. Long-term consistency in speech/language profiles: I. Developmental and academic outcomes. *Journal of the American Academy of Child & Adolescent Psychiatry* 35(6):804-814.

Beitchman, J. H., B. Wilson, E. B. Brownlie, H. Walters, A. Inglis, and W. Lancee. 1996b. Long-term consistency in speech/language profiles: II. Behavioral, emotional and social outcomes. *Journal of the American Academy of Child & Adolescent Psychiatry* 35(6):815-825.

Beitchman, J. H., E. B. Brownlie, A. Inglis, J. Wild, R. Mathews, D. Schachter, R. Kroll, S. Martin, B. Ferguson, and W. Lancee. 1996c. Seven-year follow-up of speech/language impaired and control children: Psychiatric outcomes. *Journal of the American Academy of Child & Adolescent Psychiatry* 37(8):961-970.

Beitchman, J. H., L. Douglas, B. Wilson, C. Johnson, A. Young, L. Atkinson, M. Escobar, and N. Taback. 1999. Adolescent substance use disorders: Findings from a 14-year follow-up of speech/language-impaired and control children. *Journal of Clinical Child & Adolescent Psychology* 28(3):312-321.

Beitchman, J. H., B. Wilson, C. J. Johnson, L. Atkinson, A. Young, E. Adlaf, M. Escobar, and L. Douglas. 2001. Fourteen-year follow-up of speech/language-impaired and control children: Psychiatric outcome. *Journal of the American Academy of Child & Adolescent Psychiatry* 40(1):75-82.

Beitchman, J. H., E. B. Brownlie, and L. Bao. 2014. Age 31 mental health outcomes of childhood language and speech disorders. *Journal of the American Academy of Child & Adolescent Psychiatry* 53(10):1102-1110.

Béna, F., D. L. Bruno, M. Eriksson, C. van Ravenswaaij-Arts, Z. Stark, T. Dijkhuizen, E. Gerkes, S. Gimelli, D. Ganesamoorthy, A. C. Thuresson, A. Labalme, M. Till, F. Bilan, L. Pasquier, A. Kitzis, C. Dubourgm, M. Rossi, A. Bottani, M. Gagnebin, D. Sanlaville, B. Gilbert-Dussardier, M. Guipponi, A. van Haeringen, M. Kriek, C. Ruivenkamp, S. E. Antonarakis, B. M. Anderlid, H. R. Slater, and J. Schoumans. 2013. Molecular and clinical characterization of 25 individuals with exonic deletions of NRXN1 and comprehensive review of the literature. *American Journal of Medical Genetics Part B: Neuropsychiatric Genetics* 162(4):388-403.

Bishop, D. V. M. 2006. What causes specific language impairment in children? *Current Directions in Psychological Science* 15(5):217-221.

Bishop, D. V. M. 2010. Which neurodevelopmental disorders get researched and why? *PLoS ONE* 5(11):e15112.

Bishop, D. V. M., and M. E. Hayiou-Thomas. 2008. Heritability of specific language impairment depends on diagnostic criteria. *Genes, Brain, and Behavior* 7(3):365-372.

Bloodstein, O., and N. B. Ratner. 2008. *A handbook on stuttering* (6th ed.). New York: Thomson Delmar.

Boudreau, D. 2008. Narrative abilities: Advances in research and implications for clinical practice. *Topics in Language Disorders* 28(2):99-114.

Brownlie, E. B., J. H. Beitchman, M. Escobar, A. Young, L. Atkinson, C. Johnson, B. Wilson, and L. Douglas. 2004. Early language impairment and young adult delinquent and aggressive behavior. *Journal of Abnormal Child Psychology* 32(4):453-467.

Brumbach, A. C. D., and L. Goffman. 2014. Interaction of language processing and motor skill in children with specific language impairment. *Journal of Speech, Language, and Hearing Research* 57(1):158-171.

Campbell, T. F., C. A. Dollaghan, H. E. Rockette, J. L. Paradise, H. M. Feldman, L. D. Shriberg, D. Sabo, and M. Kurs-Lasky. 2003. Risk factors for speech delay in three-year-old children. *Child Development* 74:346-357.

Carding, P. N., S. Roulstone, K. Northstone, and the ALSPAC Study Team. 2006. The prevalence of childhood dysphonia: A cross-sectional study. *Journal of Voice* 20(4):623-630.

Caruso, A. J., and E. A. Strand. 1999. Motor speech disorders in children: Definitions, background, and a theoretical framework. In *Clinical management of motor speech disorders in children*, edited by A. Caruso and E. Strand. New York: Thieme. Pp. 1-27.

Catts, H. W., and A. G. Kamhi. 2012. *Language and reading disabilities*. Boston, MA: Pearson.

Caye-Thomasen, P., M. S. Dam, S. H. Omland, and M. Mantoni. 2012. Cochlear ossification in patients with profound hearing loss following bacterial meningitis. *Acta Oto-Laryngologica* 132(7):720-725.

CDC (Centers for Disease Control and Prevention). 2014. Developmental disabilities monitoring network surveillance year 2010 principal investigators. Prevalence of autism spectrum disorder among children aged 8 years—Autism and Developmental Disabilities Monitoring Network, 11 sites, United States, 2010. *Morbidity and Mortality Weekly Report Surveillance Summaries* 63(2):1-21.

Chang, B., C. A. Walsh, K. Apse, and A. Bodell. 2007. *Polymicrogyria overview*. Seattle, WA: GeneReviews.

Christakis, D. A., J. Gilkerson, J. A. Richards, F. J. Zimmerman, M. M. Garrison, D. Xu, S. Gray, and U. Yapanel. 2009. Audible television and decreased adult words, infant vocalizations, and conversational turns: A population-based study. *Archives of Pediatrics and Adolescent Medicine* 163(6):554-558.

Clegg, J., J. Law, R. Rush, T. J. Peters, and S. Roulstone. 2015. The contribution of early language development to children's emotional and behavioral functioning: An analysis of data from the Children in Focus sample from the ALSPAC birth cohort. *Journal of Child Psychology and Psychiatry* 56(1):67-75.

Cohen, B. E., A. Durstenfeld, and P. C. Roehm. 2014. Viral causes of hearing loss: A review for hearing health professionals. *Trends in Hearing* 18.

Conture, E. G. 2001. *Stuttering: Its nature, assessment, and treatment*. Needham Heights, MA: Allyn & Bacon.

Corujo-Santana, C., J. Falcón-González, S. Borkoski-Barreiro, D. Pérez-Plasencia, and Á. Ramos-Macías. 2015. The relationship between neonatal hyperbilirubinemia and sensorineural hearing loss. *Acta Otorrinolaringologica Espanola* 66(6):326-331.

Crystal, D. 2009. *Dictionary of linguistics and phonetics*. Hoboken, NJ: Wiley-Blackwell.

Dennis, M. 2010. Language disorders in children with central nervous system injury. *Journal of Clinical and Experimental Neuropsychology* 32(4):417-432.

DeThorne, L. S., S. A. Petrill, M. E. Hayiou-Thomas, and R. Plomin. 2005. Low expressive vocabulary: High heritability as a function of more severe cases. *Journal of Speech, Language, and Hearing Research* 48(4):792-804.

Dockrell, J., G. Lindsay, S. Roulstone, and J. Law. 2014. Supporting children with speech, language and communication needs: An overview of the results of the Better Communication Research Programme. *International Journal of Language & Communication Disorders* 49(5):543-557.

Duke, N. K., K. B. Cartwright, and K. R. Hilden. 2013. Difficulties with reading comprehension. In *Handbook of language and literacy: Development and disorders* (2nd ed.), edited by C. A. Stone, E. R. Silliman, B. J. Ehren, and G. P. Wallach. New York: Guilford Press. Pp. 451-468.

Dunklebarger, J., B. Branstetter, A. Lincoln, M. Sippey, M. Cohen, B. Gaines, and D. Chi. 2014. Pediatric temporal bone fractures: Current trends and comparison of classification schemes. *The Laryngoscope* 124(3):781-784.

Eadie, P., A. Morgan, O. C. Okoumunne, K. T. Eecen, M. Wake, and S. Reilly. 2015. Speech sound disorder at 4 years: Prevalence, comorbidities, and predictors in a community cohort of children. *Developmental Medicine and Child Neurology* 57(6):578-584.

Earle, F. S., and E. B. Myers. 2014. Building phonetic categories: An argument for the role of sleep. *Frontiers in Psychology* 5:1192.

Feldman, H. M., and C. Messick. 2009. Language and speech disorders. In *Developmental-behavioral pediatrics* (4th ed.), edited by W. B. Carey, A. C. Crocker, W. L. Coleman, E. R. Elias, and H. M. Feldman. Philadelphia, PA: Saunders. Pp. 717-729.

Fenson, L., V. A. Marchman, D. J. Thal, P. S. Dale, J. S. Reznick, and E. Bates. 2007. *MacArthur-Bates communicative development inventories* (2nd ed.). Baltimore, MD: Paul H. Brookes Publishing Co.

Fernald, A., V. A. Marchman, and A. Weisleder. 2013. SES differences in language processing skill and vocabulary are evident at 18 months. *Developmental Science* 16(2):234-248.

Fitzpatrick, E. 2015. Neurocognitive development in congenitally deaf children. In *Handbook of clinical neurology*, Ch. 19, Vol. 129, edited by M. J. Aminoff, F. Boller, and D. F. Swaab. Philadelphia, PA: Elsevier. Pp. 335-356.

Flax, J. F., T. Realpe-Bonilla, L. S. Hirsch, L. M. Brzustowicz, C. W. Bartlett, and P. Tallal. 2003. Specific language impairment in families: Evidence for co-occurrence with reading impairments. *Journal of Speech, Language, and Hearing Research* 46(3):530-543.

Ford, L. C., S. L. Sulprizio, and B. M. Rasgon. 2000. Otolaryngological manifestations of velocardiofacial syndrome: A retrospective review of 35 patients. *The Laryngoscope* 110(3):362-367.

Friedrich, M., I. Wilhelm, J. Born, and A. D. Friederici. 2015. Generalization of word meanings during infant sleep. *Nature Communications* 6.

Gallagher, A., N. Tanaka, N. Suzuki, H. Liu, E. A. Thiele, and S. M. Stufflebeam. 2013. Diffuse cerebral language representation in tuberous sclerosis complex. *Epilepsy Research* 104(1):125-133.

Gejão, M. G., A. T. Ferreira, G. K. Silva, F. D. L. Anastácio-Pessan, and D. A. C. Lamônica. 2009. Communicative and psycholinguistic abilities in children with phenylketonuria and congenital hypothyroidism. *Journal of Applied Oral Science* 17(Suppl.):69-75.

Gillam, R. B., E. D. Peña, L. M. Bedore, T. M. Bohman, and A. Mendez-Perez. 2013. Identification of specific language impairment in bilingual children. Part 1: Assessment in English. *Journal of Speech, Language, and Hearing Research* 56:1813-1823.

Glynn, F., D. Fitzgerald, M. J. Earley, and H. Rowley. 2011. Pierre Robin sequence: An institutional experience in the multidisciplinary management of airway, feeding and serous otitis media challenges. *International Journal of Pediatric Otorhinolaryngology* 75(9):1152-1155.

Goderis, J., E. De Leenheer, K. Smets, H. Van Hoecke, A. Keymeulen, and I. Dhooge. 2014. Hearing loss and congenital CMV infection: A systematic review. *Pediatrics* 134(5):972-982.

Goldstein, B. A., and C. Gildersleeve-Neumann. 2012. Phonological development and disorders. In *Bilingual language development and disorders in Spanish-English speakers*, edited by B. A. Goldstein. Baltimore, MD: Paul H. Brookes Publishing Co. Pp. 285-309.

Hanson, E., R. Bernier, K. Porche, F. I. Jackson, R. P. Goin-Kochel, L. G. Snyder, A. V. Snow, A. S. Wallace, K. L. Campe, Y. Zhang, Q. Chen, D. D'Angelo, A. Moreno-De-Luca, P. T. Orr, K. B. Boomer, D. W. Evans, S. Kanne, L. Berry, F. K. Miller, J. Olson, E. Sherr, C. L. Martin, D. H. Ledbetter, J. E. Spiro, W. K. Chung, and C. Simons. 2015. The cognitive and behavioral phenotype of the 16p11.2 deletion in a clinically ascertained population. *Biological Psychiatry* 77(9):785-793.

Harrison, L. J., and S. McLeod. 2010. Risk and protective factors associated with speech and language impairment in a nationally representative sample of 4- to 5-year-old children. *Journal of Speech, Language, and Hearing Research* 53(2):508-529.

Hart, B., and T. Risley. 1995. *Meaningful differences in the everyday experiences of young American children.* Baltimore, MD: Paul H. Brookes Publishing Co.

Hoff, E. 2013. Interpreting the early language trajectories of children from low-SES and language minority homes: Implications for closing achievement gaps. *Developmental Psychology* 49(1):4-14.

Hudson, L. J., and B. Murdoch. 1990. Speech and language disorders in childhood brain tumours. *Acquired Neurological Speech/Language Disorders in Childhood* 245-268.

Hurtado, N., T. Grüter, V. A. Marchman, and A. Fernald. 2014. Relative language exposure, processing efficiency and vocabulary in Spanish-English bilingual toddlers. *Bilingualism: Language and Cognition* 17(1):189-202.

Ilves, P., T. Tomberg, J. Kepler, R. Laugesaar, M.-L. Kaldoja, K. Kepler, and A. Kolk. 2014. Different plasticity patterns of language function in children with perinatal and childhood stroke. *Journal of Child Neurology* 29(6):756-764.

Jambaque, I., C. Pinabiaux, and M. Lassonde. 2012. Cognitive disorders in pediatric epilepsy. *Handbook of Clinical Neurology* 111:691-695.

Jing, W., H. Zongjie, F. Denggang, H. Na, Z. Bin, Z. Aifen, H. Xijiang, Y. Cong, D. Yunping, and H. Z. Ring. 2015. Mitochondrial mutations associated with aminoglycoside ototoxicity and hearing loss susceptibility identified by meta-analysis. *Journal of Medical Genetics* 52(2):95-103.

Jurewicz, J., K. Polanska, and W. Hanke. 2013. Chemical exposure early in life and the neurodevelopment of children—an overview of current epidemiological evidence. *Annals of Agricultural and Environmental Medicine* 20(3):465-486.

Katusic, S. K., R. C. Colligan, W. J. Barbaresi, D. J. Schaid, and S. J. Jacobsen. 2001. Incidence of reading disability in a population-based birth cohort, 1976-1982, Rochester, Minn. *Mayo Clinic Proceedings* 76(11):1081-1092.

Kent, R. D. 1999. Motor control: Neurophysiology and functional development. In *Clinical management of motor speech disorders in children*, edited by A. J. Caruso and E. A. Strand. New York: Thieme. Pp. 29-71.

Kent, R. D., and H. K. Vorperian. 2013. Speech impairment in Down syndrome: A review. *Journal of Speech, Language, and Hearing Research* 56(1):178-210.

Kim, Y-S., K. Apel, and S. Al Otaiba. 2013. The relation of linguistic awareness and vocabulary to word reading and spelling for first-grade students participating in response to intervention. *Language, Speech, and Hearing Services in Schools* 44(4):337-347.

King, T. M., L. A. Rosenbert, L. Fuddy, E. McFarlane, C. Sia, and A. K. Duggan. 2005. Prevalence and early identification of language delays among at-risk three year olds. *Journal of Developmental and Behavioral Pediatrics* 26(4):293-303.

Klein-Tasman, B. P., K. M. Janke, W. Luo, C. L. Casnar, S. J. Hunter, J. Tonsgard, P. Trapane, F. van der Fluit, and L. A. Kais. 2014. Cognitive and psychosocial phenotype of young children with neurofibromatosis-1. *Journal of the International Neuropsychological Society* 20(1):88-98.

Kohnert, K., and A. Derr. 2012. Language intervention with bilingual children. In *Bilingual language development and disorders in Spanish-English speakers*, edited by B. A. Goldstein. Baltimore, MD: Paul H. Brookes Publishing Co. Pp. 337-356.

Law, J., J. Boyle, F. Harris, A. Harkness, and C. Nye. 2000. Prevalence and natural history of primary speech and language delay: Findings from a systematic review of the literature. *International Journal of Language & Communication Disorders* 35(2):165-188.

Law, J., R. Rush, I. Schoon, and S. Parsons. 2009. Modeling developmental language difficulties from school entry into adulthood: Literacy, mental health, and employment outcomes. *Journal of Speech, Language, and Hearing Research* 52(6):1401-1416.

Lewis, B. A., L. D. Shriberg, L. A. Freebairn, A. J. Hansen, C. M. Stein, H. G. Taylor, and S. K. Iyengar. 2006. The genetic bases of speech sound disorders: Evidence from spoken and written language. *Journal of Speech, Language, and Hearing Research* 49(6):1294-1312.

Lewis, B. A., L. A. Freebairn, A. J. Hansen, L. Miscimarra, S. K. Iyengar, and H. G. Taylor. 2007. Speech and language skills of parents of children with speech sound disorders. *American Journal of Speech-Language Pathology* 16(2):108-118.

Lewis, B. A., A. A. Avrich, L. A. Freebairn, A. J. Hansen, L. E. Sucheston, I. Kuo, H. G. Taylor, S. K. Iyengar, and C. M. Stein. 2011. Literacy outcomes of children with early childhood speech sound disorders: Impact of endophenotypes. *Journal of Speech, Language, and Hearing Research* 54(6):1628-1643.

Lewis, B. A., L. Freebairn, J. Tag, A. A. Ciesla, S. K. Iyengar, C. M. Stein, and H. G. Taylor. 2015. Adolescent outcomes of children with early speech sound disorders with and without language impairment. *American Journal of Speech-Language Pathology/American Speech-Language-Hearing Association* 24(2):150-163.

Locke, J. 2011. The development of linguistic systems: Insights from evolution. In *Handbook of psycholinguistic and cognitive processes: Perspectives in communication disorders*, edited by J. Guendouzi, F. Loncke, and M. J. Williams. New York: Psychology Press. Pp. 3-29.

Lozano, R., A. Vino, C. Lozano, S. E. Fisher, and P. Deriziotis. 2015. A de novo FOXP1 variant in a patient with autism, intellectual disability and severe speech and language impairment. *European Journal of Human Genetics* 23(12):1702-1707.

Lum, J. A., G. Conti-Ramsden, A. T. Morgan, and M. T. Ullman. 2014. Procedural learning deficits in specific language impairment (SLI): A meta-analysis of serial reaction time task performance. *Cortex* 51:1-10.

Luquetti, D. V., C. L. Heike, A. V. Hing, M. L. Cunningham, and T. C. Cox. 2012. Microtia: Epidemiology and genetics. *American Journal of Medical Genetics Part A* 158A(1):124-139.

McGee, C. L., O. A. Bjorkquist, E. P. Riley, and S. N. Mattson. 2009. Impaired language performance in young children with heavy prenatal alcohol exposure. *Neurotoxicology and Teratology* 31(2):71-75.

McLeod, S., and L. J. Harrison. 2009. Epidemiology of speech and language impairment in a nationally representative sample of 4- to 5-year-old children. *Journal of Speech, Language, and Hearing Research* 52(5):1213-1229.

Mildinhall, S. 2012. Speech and language in the patient with cleft palate. *Frontiers of Oral Biology* 16:137-146.

Miller, J. F., and R. Paul. 1995. *The clinical assessment of language comprehension*. Baltimore, MD: Paul H. Brookes Publishing Co.

Moleski, M. 2000. Neuropsychological, neuroanatomical, and neurophysiological consequences of CNS chemotherapy for acute lymphoblastic leukemia. *Archives of Clinical Neuropsychology* 15(7):603-630.

Morgan, A. T., and A. P. Vogel. 2008. Intervention for dysarthria associated with acquired brain injury in children and adolescents. *Cochrane Database of Systematic Reviews* (3):CD006279.

Myers, S. M., and C. P. Johnson. 2007. Management of children with autism spectrum disorders. *Pediatrics* 120(5):1162-1182.

Næss, K. A. B., A. Lervåg, S. A. H. Lyster, and C. Hulme. 2015. Longitudinal relationships between language and verbal short-term memory skills in children with Down syndrome. *Journal of Experimental Child Psychology* 135:43-55.

Nelson, H. D., P. Nygren, M. Walker, and R. Panoscha. 2006. Screening for speech and language delay in preschool children: Systematic evidence review of the US Preventive Services Task Force. *Pediatrics* 117(2):e298-e319.

Nelson, H. D., C. Bougatsos, and P. Nygren. 2008. Universal newborn hearing screening: systematic review to update the 2001 US Preventive Services Task Force Recommendation. *Pediatrics* 122(1):e266-e276.

Newbury, D. F., and A. P. Monaco. 2010. Genetic advances in the study of speech and language disorders. *Neuron* 68(2):309-320.

Parish, S. L., M. Grinstein-Weiss, Y. H. Yeo, R. A. Rose, and A. Rimmerman. 2010. Assets and income: Disability-based disparities in the United States. *Social Work Research* 34(2):71-82.

Parker, M., and M. Bitner-Glindzicz. 2015. Genetic investigations in childhood deafness. *Archives of Disease in Childhood* 100(3):271-278.

Patterson, M., and M. M. Paparella. 1999. Otitis media with effusion and early sequelae: Flexible approach. *Otolaryngologic Clinics of North America* 32(3):391-400.

Paul, L. K. 2011. Developmental malformation of the corpus callosum: A review of typical callosal development and examples of developmental disorders with callosal involvement. *Journal of Neurodevelopmental Disorders* 3(1):3-27.

Paul, R., and C. F. Norbury. 2012. *Language disorders from infancy through adolescence: Listening, speaking, reading, writing, and communicating* (4th ed.). St. Louis, MO: Elsevier.

Pelucchi, B., J. F. Hay, and J. R. Saffran. 2009. Statistical learning in a natural language by 8-month-old infants. *Child Development* 80(3):674-685.

Pennington, B. F., and D. V. M. Bishop. 2009. Relations among speech, language, and reading disorders. *Annual Review of Psychology* 60:283-306.

Pennington, L., N. Miller, and S. Robson. 2009. Speech therapy for children with dysarthria acquired before three years of age. *Cochrane Database of Systematic Reviews* (4):CD006937.

Pentimonti, J. M., L. J. Justice, and J. N. Kaderavek. 2014. School-readiness profiles of children with language impairment: Linkages to home and classroom experiences. *International Journal of Language & Communication Disorders* 49(5):567-583.

Perry, B. D., T. Beauchaine, S. P. Hinshaw. 2008. Child maltreatment: A neurodevelopmental perspective on the role of trauma and neglect in pyschopathology. *Child and Adolescent Psychopathology* 93-129.

Pinborough-Zimmerman J., R. Satterfield, J. Miller, D. Bilder, S. Hossain, W. McMahon. 2007. Communication disorders: Prevalence and comorbid intellectual disability, autism, and emotional/behavioral disorders. *American Journal of Speech-Language Pathology* 16(4):359-367.

Plyler, E., and A. W. Harkrider. 2013. Serial auditory-evoked potentials in the diagnosis and monitoring of a child with Landau-Kleffner syndrome. *Journal of the American Academy of Audiology* 24(7):564-571.

Reilly, S., M. Wake, O. C. Ukoumunne, E. Bavin, M. Prior, E. Cini, L. Conway, P. Eadie, and L. Bretherton. 2010. Predicting language outcomes at 4 years of age: Findings from Early Language in Victoria Study. *Pediatrics* 126(6):e1530-e1537.

Reilly, S., B. Tomblin, J. Law, C. McKean, F. Mensah, A. Morgan, S. Goldfield, J. Nicholson, and M. Wake. 2014. Specific language impairment: A convenient label for whom? *International Journal of Language & Communication Disorders* 49(4):415-433.

Rice, M. L. 2012. Toward epigenetic and gene regulation models of specific language impairment: Looking for links among growth, genes, and impairments. *Journal of Neurodevelopmental Disorders* 4(1):1.

Ringwalt, S. 2015. *Summary table of states' and territories' definitions of/criteria for IDEA Part C eligibility*. Chapel Hill, NC: Early Childhood Technical Assistance Center.

Robertson, C., and N. Finer. 1985. Term infants with hypoxic-ischemic encephalopathy: Outcome at 3.5 years. *Developmental Medicine & Child Neurology* 27(4):473-484.

Roseberry-McKibbin, C. 2014. *Multicultural students with special language needs* (4th ed.). Oceanside, CA: Academic Communication Associates.

Royal College of Speech & Language Therapists. 2005. Preschool children with communication, language & speech needs. In *Clinical guidelines* (Ch. 5.2), edited by S. Taylor-Groh. Bicester, UK: Speechmark Publishing Ltd. Pp. 19-24.

Salvia, J., J. Ysseldyke, and S. Bolt. 2012. *Assessment: In special and inclusive education*. Boston, MA: Cengage Learning.

Sameroff, A. 2009. *The transactional model*. Washington, DC: American Psychological Association.

Saporta, A. S., A. Kumar, R. M. Govindan, S. K. Sundaram, and H. T. Chugani. 2011. Arcuate fasciculus and speech in congenital bilateral perisylvian syndrome. *Pediatric Neurology* 44(4):270-274.

Schreiber, J. E., J. G. Gurney, S. L. Palmer, J. K. Bass, M. Wang, S. Chen, H. Zhang, M. Swain, M. L. Chapieski, M. J. Bonner, D. J. Mabbott, S. J. Knight, C. L. Armstrong, R. Boyle, and A. Gajjar. 2014. Examination of risk factors for intellectual and academic outcomes following treatment for pediatric medulloblastoma. *Neuro-Oncology* 16(8):1129-1136.

Shevell, M., S. Ashwal, D. Donley, J. Flint, M. Gingold, D. Hirtz, A. Majnemer, M. Noetzel, and R. D. Sheth. 2003. Practice parameter: Evaluation of the child with global developmental delay. Report of the Quality Standards Subcommittee of the American Academy of Neurology and The Practice Committee of the Child Neurology Society. *Neurology* 60(3):367-380.

Shiga, T., T. Shimbo, and A. Yoshizawa. 2015. Multicenter investigation of lifestyle-related diseases and visceral disorders in thalidomide embryopathy at around 50 years of age. *Birth Defects Research. Part A, Clinical and Molecular Teratology* 103(9):787-793.

Shriberg, L. D. 1993. Four new speech and prosody-voice measures for genetics research and other studies in developmental phonological disorders. *Journal of Speech and Hearing Research* 36:105-140.

Shriberg, L. D., J. B. Tomblin, and J. L. McSweeny. 1999. Prevalence of speech delay in 6-year-old children and comorbidity with language impairment. *Journal of Speech, Language, and Hearing Research* 42(6):1461-1481.

Simpson, N. H., L. Addis, W. M. Brandler, V. Slonims, A. Clark, J. Watson, T. S. Scerri, E. R. Hennessy, P. F. Bolton, G. Conti-Ramsden, B. P. Fairfax, J. C. Knight, J. Stein, J. B. Talcott, A. O'Hare, G. Baird, S. Paracchini, S. E. Fisher, and D. F. Newbury. 2014. Increased prevalence of sex chromosome aneuploidies in specific language impairment and dyslexia. *Developmental Medicine & Child Neurology* 56(4):346-353.

Skebo, C. M., B. A. Lewis, L. A. Freebairn, J. Tag, A. A. Ciesla, and C. M. Stein. 2013. Reading skills of students with speech sound disorders at three stages of literacy development. *Language, Speech, and Hearing Services in Schools* 44(4):360-373.

Soleymani, Z., N. Keramati, F. Rohani, and S. Jalaei. 2015. Factors influencing verbal intelligence and spoken language in children with phenylketonuria. *Indian Pediatrics* 52(5):397-401.

Spaulding T. J., M. S. Szulga, and C. Figueroa. 2012. Using norm-referenced tests to determine severity of language impairment in children: Disconnect between U.S. policy makers and test developers. *Language, Speech, and Hearing Services in Schools* 43(2):176-190.

Spitz, R. V., P. Tallal, J. Flax, and A. A. Benasich. 1997. Look Who's Talking: A Prospective Study of Familial Transmission of Language Impairments. *Journal of Speech, Language, and Hearing Research* (40)5:990-1001.

Squires, J., E. Twombly, D. Bricker, and L. Potter. 2009. *ASQ-3: Ages & Stages Questionnaires* (3rd ed.). Baltimore, MD: Paul H. Brookes Publishing Co.

Stanton-Chapman, T. L., D. A. Chapman, A. P. Kaiser, and T. B. Hancock. 2004. Cumulative risk and low-income children's language development. *Topics in Early Childhood Special Education* 24(4):227-237.

Stoeckel, R. E., R. C. Colligan, W. J. Barbaresi, A. L. Weaver, J. M. Killian, and S. K. Katusic. 2013. Early speech-language impairment and risk for written language disorder: A population-based study. *Journal of Developmental & Behavioral Pediatrics* 34(1):38-44.

Sun, L., and G. P. Wallach. 2014. Language disorders are learning disabilities: Challenges on the divergent and diverse paths to language learning disability. *Topics in Language Disorders* 34(1):25-38.

Swarts, J. D., and C. D. Bluestone. 2003. Eustachian tube function in older children and adults with persistent otitis media. *International Journal of Pediatric Otorhinolaryngology* 67(8):853-859.

Takahashi, H., K. Takahashi, and F.-C. Liu. 2010. FOXP genes, neural development, speech and language disorders. In *Forkhead Transcription Factors: Vital Elements in Biology and Medicine*, edited by K. Maiese. New York: Springer. Pp. 117-129.

Tedeschi, A. S., N. J. Roizen, H. G. Taylor, G. Murray, C. A. Curtis, and A. S. Parikh. 2015. The prevalence of congenital hearing loss in neonates with Down syndrome. *The Journal of Pediatrics* 166(1):168-171.

Tomblin, J. B. 2014. Educational and psychosocial outcomes of language impairment in kindergarten. In *Understanding individual differences in language development across the school years*, edited by J. B. Tomblin and M. A. Nippold. New York: Psychology Press. Pp. 166-203.

Tomblin, J. B., and P. R. Buckwalter. 1998. Heritability of poor language achievement among twins. *Journal of Speech, Language, and Hearing Research* 41(1):188-199.

Tomblin, J. B., and M. A. Nippold (eds.). 2014. *Understanding individual differences in language development across the school years.* New York: Psychology Press.

Tomblin, J. B., E. Smith, and X. Zhang. 1997a. Epidemiology of specific language impairment: Prenatal and perinatal risk factors. *Journal of Communication Disorders* 30(4):325-344.

Tomblin, J. B., N. L. Records, P. Buckwalter, X. Xhang, E. Smith, and M. O'Brien. 1997b. Prevalence of specific language impairment in kindergarten children. *Journal of Speech, Language, and Hearing Research* 40(6):1245-1260.

Troia, G. A. 2013. Phonological processing deficits and literacy learning. In *Handbook of language and literacy: Development and disorders* (2nd ed.), edited by C. A. Stone, E. R. Silliman, B. J. Ehren, and G. P. Wallach. New York: Guilford Press. Pp. 227-245.

Urbina, S. 2014. *Essentials of behavioral science: Essentials of psychological testing* (2nd ed.). Somerset, NJ: Wiley.

Viding, E., F. M. Spinath, T. S. Price, D. V. Bishop, P. S. Dale, and R. Plomin. 2004. Genetic and environmental influence on language impairment in 4-year-old same-sex and opposite-sex twins. *Journal of Child Psychology and Psychiatry* 45(2):315-325.

Vinchon, M., H. Rekate, and A. V. Kulkarni. 2012. Pediatric hydrocephalus outcomes: A review. *Fluids and Barriers of the CNS* 9(1):18.

Voci, S. C., J. H. Beitchman, E. B. Brownlie, and B. Wilson. 2006. Social anxiety in late adolescence: The importance of early childhood language impairment. *Journal of Anxiety Disorders* 20(7):915-930.

Walker, S. P., T. D. Wachs, S. Grantham-McGregor, M. M. Black, C. A. Nelson, S. L. Huffman, and H. Baker-Henningham. 2011. Inequality in early childhood: risk and protective factors for early child development. *Lancet* 9799 (378):1325-1338.

Wallace, I. F., N. D. Berkman, L. R. Watson, T. Coyne-Beasley, C. T. Wood, K. Cullen, and K. N. Lohr, 2015. Screening for speech and language delay in children 5 years old and younger: A systematic review. *Pediatrics* 136(2):e448-e462.

Werker, J. F., H. H. Yeung, and K. A. Yoshida. 2012. How do infants become experts at native-speech perception? *Current Directions in Psychological Science* 21(4):221-226.

Whitehouse A. J. O., W. M. R. Shelton, C. Ing, and J. P. Newnham. 2014. Prenatal, perinatal, and neonatal risk factors for specific language impairment: A prospective pregnancy cohort study. *Journal of Speech, Language, and Hearing Research* 57(4):1418-1427.

Wilkinson, J., C. Bass, S. Diem, A. Gravley, L. Harvey, M. Maciosek, K. McKeon, L. Milteer, J. Owens, P. Rothe, L. Snellman, L. Solberg, and P. Vincent. 2013. *Institute for Clinical Systems Improvement health care guideline: Preventive services for children and adolescents.* https://www.icsi.org/_asset/x1mnv1/PrevServKids-Interactive0912.pdf (accessed September 29, 2015).

WHO (World Health Organization). 1992. *The ICD-10 classification of mental and behavioral disorders: Clinical descriptions and diagnostic guidelines.* Geneva, Switzerland: WHO.

Yairi, E., and N. Ambrose. 2013. Epidemiology of stuttering: 21st century advances. *Journal of Fluency Disorders* 38(2):66-87.

Yan, J., G. Oliveira, A. Coutinho, C. Yang, J. Feng, C. Katz, J. Sram, A. Bockholt, I. R. Jones, N. Craddock, E. H. Cook, Jr., A. Vicente, and S. S. Sommer. 2005. Analysis of the neuroligin 3 and 4 genes in autism and other neuropsychiatric patients. *Molecular Psychiatry* 10(4):329-332.

Young, A. R., J. H. Beitchman, C. Johnson, L. Douglas, L. Atkinson, M. Escobar, and B. Wilson. 2002. Young adult academic outcomes in a longitudinal sample of early identified language impaired and control children. *Journal of Child Psychology and Psychiatry* 43(5):635-645.

Zimmerman, F. J., D. A. Christakis, and A. N. Meltzoff. 2007. Associations between media viewing and language development in children under age 2 years. *The Journal of Pediatrics* 151(4):364-368.

3

Treatment and Persistence of Speech and Language Disorders in Children

This chapter addresses three topics within the committee's charge: current standards of care for speech and language disorders in children; which of the disorders are amenable to treatment and the typical time course required for this treatment; and the persistence of these disorders in children. The discussion is limited to those childhood speech and language disorders that are most common in the Supplemental Security Income (SSI) population; it is not intended to be a comprehensive review of interventions for or the persistence of speech and language disorders. The chapter begins with an overview of the factors that influence treatment of speech and language disorders in children. This is followed by a summary of policies and guidelines that influence the provision of treatment services. Next is an age-based description of treatment approaches. The chapter ends with discussion of the persistence of childhood speech and language disorders and the committee's findings and conclusions.

Before beginning it is important to emphasize that treatment is considered to be essential for all children with speech and language disorders, but with few exceptions, it is most effective for less severe disorders. Nevertheless, even children with the most severe disorders can develop enhanced, functionally important communication skills that have a meaningful impact on their lives even though their speech and language disorders have not been completely resolved.

FACTORS THAT INFLUENCE TREATMENT FOR SPEECH AND LANGUAGE DISORDERS

Speech and language treatment programs employ a variety of approaches that are dependent on the particular needs and circumstances of the child. Several important factors shape the appropriate intervention program for any given child. These include treatment objectives based on the severity of the disorder, the developmental level of the child, the individuals involved in the intervention (or "agents of change"), the setting in which treatment is provided, and certain key properties of speech and language. Each of these factors is described in turn below.

Objectives of Treatment Based on the Severity of the Disorder

For children with severe speech and language disorders, it often is not possible to alter underlying limitations in developmental processes and systems, partly because of the current state of knowledge in developmental and learning sciences. For some children, conventional means of communication are impossible given the child's level of development and severity of communication difficulties. In these cases, compensatory means of communication, such as picture cards or computer-based communication systems, are employed. Furthermore, parents of children with severe speech and language disorders often are in need of support as well (Zebrowski and Schum, 1993).

Developmental Level of the Child

Treatment programs must be adapted to the child's current developmental status with respect to both speech and language skills and general social, emotional, and physical development. Treatment programs are, therefore, designed to build on the child's developmental level, regardless of the child's age (Brown and Ferrara, 1999). Thus, for example, a 5-year-old child who is functioning at a 3-year-old level in language is unlikely to be able to acquire the language skills of a typical 5-year-old without having accumulated the intermediary skills normally acquired between ages 3 and 5.

Agent(s) of Change

Treatment programs for speech and language disorders nearly always require that someone, usually an adult, provide an environmental milieu that promotes speech and language growth (Paul and Norbury, 2012). Some computer-based programs that require a minimum of adult interaction have been developed (Tallal et al., 1996), but there is no consensus on their effectiveness (Cohen et al., 2005; Gillam et al., 2008; Strong et al., 2011). Thus, speech and language therapy usually requires that the child be engaged with a partner (clinician, parent, peer) who is a competent speaker/listener of the language. This engagement becomes the means of producing learning and behavior change. Various types of individuals can be considered agents of change for and integral to speech and language treatment for children, including professionally trained and certified speech-language pathologists, parents, early childhood educators or teachers, and peers. In some cases, the role of the speech-language clinician may be as a consultant and educator for others who are the primary agents of change.

Treatment Setting

Treatment may occur in a number of settings or environments because speech and language skills develop within the context of a child's daily communication activities—for example, at home, in the neighborhood, and in school. Each setting provides opportunities for communication and interaction. In the past, speech and language therapy was provided almost exclusively in therapy rooms and classrooms where the speech-language clinician engineered the environment to promote learning (McWilliam, 1995). In the past two decades, however, speech and language intervention has moved out of these special-purpose environments (Peña and Quinn, 2003). This practice is predicated in part on the belief that treating in these natural settings will promote generalization of learning to these settings. For children younger than 3 years of age, services may be provided in the home (Mahoney et al., 1999). Preschoolers may be served in an early childhood or daycare setting, while treatment programs for school-age children usually are integrated into the classroom.

Key Properties of Speech and Language

Chapter 2 describes language as involving several interrelated systems used together to accomplish communication. Box 3-1 briefly defines these systems, explaining how they make it possible to *understand* the meaning and intent of utterances spoken by others and to use words and sentences to *express* meaning and intent to others. What is heard and what is said can be thought of as the superficial manifestations of communication. Underlying these manifestations are complex knowledge systems stored in memory systems in the brain. This complex combination of knowledge and skills that must be acquired by a child is the common target of speech and language therapy.

BOX 3-1
Basic Systems and Subsystems That Enable Human Communication

Phonology: the sounds of a language that distinguish one word from another (e.g., *cat* versus *sat*), as well as the allowable sequences of these sounds

Vocabulary: sound combinations in a language that are associated with meaning

Grammar: the principles in a language governing arrangements of words that convey propositional meaning (e.g., who does what to whom, when, why, and/or how)

Pragmatics: principles that govern how the above systems are employed effectively and appropriately to accomplish the social functions of communication

Speech and Language Knowledge Is Implicit

The typical child develops speech and language knowledge quickly and with little conscious effort and, importantly, with little intentional instruction by his or her parents (Pinker, 1984). As an example, consider the following sentence: "The basketball player dribble ball." Most native English-speaking adults would revise the sentence and automatically change "dribble ball" to "dribbles the ball." Although these kinds of judgments of mature English speakers are common, many adults cannot explain why they make these judgments. This kind of knowledge is often called *implicit knowledge*—knowledge that is acquired through experience or exposure, rather than from explicit instruction—and much of a young child's speech and language learning develops through this implicit process (Bock and Griffin, 2000; Conway et al., 2010). In this way, much of speech and language learning is akin to learning to tie a shoe or ride a bike—skills that can be acquired only by doing and, in fact, are difficult to explain without demonstrating. This type of learning requires repeated exposure or practice, and the resulting knowledge builds gradually.

Speech and Language Knowledge Is Abstract

The implicit knowledge that accumulates during speech and language development is abstract. Knowledge of grammar appears to require processing such notions as the subject of a sentence, which involves the role of a phrase in a sentence that governs certain grammatical features of the sentence. Words usually refer to classes of referents and phonemes (speech sounds) that comprise categories of specific speech sounds (phones). These abstract relations, roles, and categories allow language to express meanings in consistent but flexible ways. How these abstractions are acquired is a topic of considerable debate (Bates and MacWhinney, 1987; Chomsky, 1986; St Clair et al., 2010). Although sentences involving such abstractions can be provided to a young child, the actual abstraction cannot; instead, the child must create it. Thus, the child can be given the raw material from which language is learned, but the abstract learning product must be generated through mental processes within the child. Unlike a physical therapist, who can physically change the state of a targeted tissue through manipulation, a speech-language clinician cannot make direct contact with these mental processes because they are dynamic learning processes within the brain.

Knowledge Allows for Creativity

Another important characteristic of speech and language knowledge is that it allows for considerable creativity and adaptability. A key feature of language is that what one says is often novel; that is, one can say things one has not heard before. This creative aspect of language can be used to adapt and adjust what one says to a particular situation. This adaptability also is seen in speech production and the ability to produce intelligible speech in a variety of ways. Thus, knowing a language is not simply imitating or storing away a collection of words or sentences to be called up when needed, but using rules or principles and abstract knowledge in flexible and creative ways. As a result, although treatment may target and change relatively specific aspects of speech and language, the child's ability to understand and produce novel utterances that are necessary for communication will be quite limited unless the treatment results in broader changes in underlying skills and knowledge.

POLICIES AND GUIDELINES THAT INFLUENCE THE PROVISION OF SPEECH AND LANGUAGE SERVICES TO CHILDREN

Numerous factors influence the range of treatments and services received by children with speech and language disorders. Within the universe of children with such disorders who receive SSI benefits, several sets of policies might be expected to play an especially prominent role: the Individuals with Disabilities Education Act (IDEA); Medicaid and its special early and periodic screening, diagnosis, and treatment (EPSDT) benefit for children and adolescents up to age 21, to which all children receiving SSI are entitled; and policies established by the leading professional society in the area of speech and language treatment, which guide the provision of treatment under public programs.

Individuals with Disabilities Education Act

IDEA[1] requires that all children with disabilities—including speech and language disorders—be provided a free, appropriate public education in the least restrictive environment possible. Part B of this law applies this mandate to children aged 3-22, whereas Part C extends this mandate to children from birth to 3 years of age.

Within the United States, speech and language services for children usually are provided by school systems as part of special education services (U.S. Bureau of Labor Statistics, 2014). However, speech and language services are not provided exclusively by public school systems; they also can be found in some community-based programs, such as Head Start. Payment for services both within and outside of the school system are covered by Medicaid. Children with speech and language disorders may also receive treatment and services through privately funded programs, such as those supported by Easter Seals or the Scottish Rite Language Clinics.

Medicaid Early and Periodic Screening, Diagnosis, and Treatment Program

Under the Medicaid EPSDT program, children under 21 who are enrolled in Medicaid must be provided appropriate preventive and specialty services for audiology and speech and language disorders (CMS, n.d.). This includes "diagnostic, screening, preventive, or corrective services provided by or under the direction of a speech and language pathologist or audiologist."[2] Specifically, the EPSDT benefit provides coverage for

- the identification of children with speech or language impairments;
- diagnosis and appraisal of specific speech or language impairments;
- referral for medical or other professional attention necessary for rehabilitation of speech or language impairment;
- provision of speech and language services; and
- counseling and guidance of parents, children, and teachers (ASHA, n.d.).

[1] Individuals with Disabilities Education Act of 2004, Public Law 108-446, 108th Cong. (December 3, 2004).

[2] 42 C.F.R. § 440.110(c).

American Speech-Language-Hearing Association

Services for children with speech and language disorders are also influenced by the American Speech-Language-Hearing Association (ASHA), which has issued practice guidelines for speech and language therapy:

> Children receive intervention and/or consultation services when their ability to communicate effectively is impaired because of a communication disorder and when there is a reasonable expectation of benefit in body structure/function and/or activity/participation. Interventions that enhance activity and participation through modification of contextual factors may be warranted even if the prognosis for improved body structure/function is limited. (ASHA, 2004)

With regard to the duration of treatment, ASHA states,

> Intervention extends long enough to accomplish stated objectives/predicted outcomes and ends when there is no expectation for further benefit during the current developmental stage. (ASHA, 2004)

In many cases, the duration of treatment can be protracted, given that throughout childhood, the functional requirements for language and communication continually increase and often outpace the child's growth (see Figure 3-1). Thus, a child with a speech and/or language disorder, although making progress, falls further behind his or her typically developing peers in the ability to meet functional communication expectations. As a result, and in keeping with the ASHA guidelines, treatment often is protracted, particularly for children with severe speech and language disorders.

TREATMENT FOR SPEECH AND LANGUAGE DISORDERS

The primary objective of treatment for speech and language disorders is to ameliorate a child's communication difficulties and thereby reduce or minimize the negative sequelae associated with these disorders. Optimal treatments would be those that resolved or cured the problem and thus resolved the disability. Indeed, some treatments for speech and language disorders may approach this level of efficacy for some children. Two examples are given here.

First, children born with clefts of the lip and palate are at considerable risk for poor speech intelligibility. Advances in early surgical management of clefts of the lip and/or palate have resulted in substantial improvements in the speech outcomes of affected children, often permitting normal levels of speech development (Bzoch, 1997). Although surgery serves as an important treatment, surgery alone is not sufficient in the majority of instances to

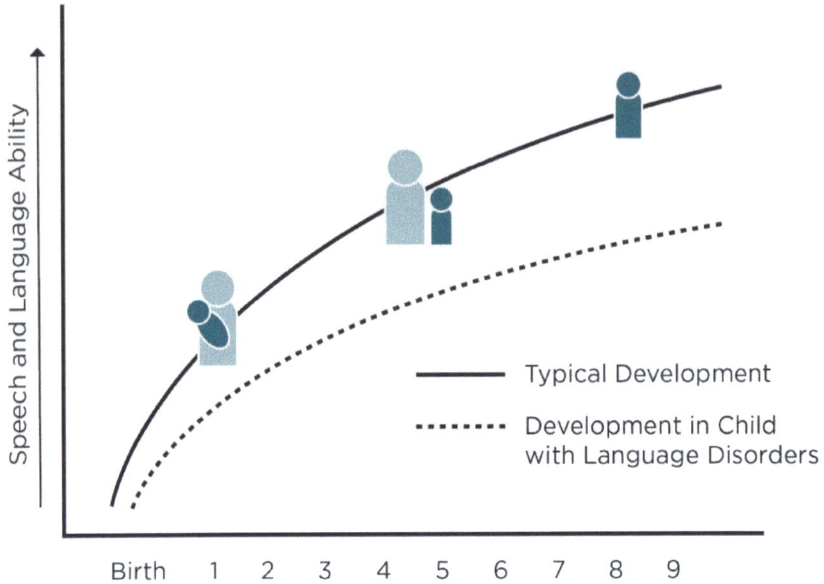

FIGURE 3-1 Persistence of the disparity between growth in functional communication skills for typically developing children and for those with language disorders.

fully resolve the risk for speech impairment, and behavioral treatment (i.e., speech therapy) often is needed as well (Hardin-Jones and Jones, 2005).

Similarly, children who are born deaf or hard of hearing have very high rates of speech and language impairment. During the past several decades, auditory prostheses such as hearing aids and cochlear implants, when paired with appropriate and intensive interventions, have been shown to lead to considerable improvements in the speech and language outcomes of these children (Niparko et al., 2010; Tomblin et al., 2014b). Yet despite the effectiveness of these prostheses, the risk of poor speech and language outcomes remains for some children.

Both surgery for cleft lip and palate and the provision of auditory prostheses are interventions directed at the fundamental cause of the speech/language disorder. Each reflects etiologies impacting peripheral systems for communication (anatomical structures for speech or sensory input) that are relatively amenable to direct intervention. For the vast majority of speech and language disorders, however, the cause is unknown or when known, involves developmental impairments of the brain (see Chapter 2). For these disorders, there currently are no interventions, such as a pharmacological or surgical treatment, that can resolve the cause of the problem and thus result in substantial resolution of the child's disability. Instead, the treatment of these pediatric speech and language disorders consists of behavioral approaches that improve function, and among more severely impaired children, treatment rarely results in resolution of the overall disability.

Early Intervention (Birth to Age 3) for Language and Speech Sound Disorders

Early Intervention Approaches

The need for language intervention may be identified quite early in an infant's life, particularly when the child has comorbid disabilities that are known to be consequential for speech and language development (e.g., Down syndrome, cerebral palsy, fragile X syndrome, autism spectrum disorder, traumatic brain injury, being deaf or hard of hearing). In other cases, infants or young children fail to meet early language or speech milestones (e.g., development of meaningful speech, ability to produce or combine words by 24 months of age), which prompts enrollment in intervention. When children are quite young, language intervention typically is implemented through a family-centered approach. The intervention is carried out by the parents or caregivers, while the speech clinician takes on a support role, providing guidance that helps parents/caregivers develop the knowledge and skills needed to promote the child's development throughout everyday routines and interactions.

These approaches entail providing a context of emotional support for family members, who may be adjusting to the child's developmental challenges and the resulting impact on family life. In addition, family-centered practices recognize the influential role of caregivers and the home context in children's development. For example, a skilled clinician may provide early intervention for 1-2 hours per week, which represents only a fraction of a young child's nearly 100 hours weekly of awake and potential learning time (Warren et al., 2006). The intent of family-centered, parent-implemented approaches is to support the ability of caregivers to promote the child's communicative development throughout everyday routines (Rush and Shelden, 2008).

Very early research on talk to children (Brown and Bellugi, 1964) revealed that parents sometimes rephrase things children say. For example, when a child says, "See doggy," the parent may follow by saying, "Yes, see the doggy." This form of parent behavior was termed "expansion" in that the parent provided a model of a grammatically well-formed sentence by expanding the child's utterance. A variant on expansion called "recasts" entails reformulation of a child's prior well-formed utterance to include additional and more advanced grammatical properties (Nelson et al., 1973). Thus, the child might say, "The doggy is barking," and the adult might follow by saying, "Yes, the doggy is barking very loudly, isn't he?" In one early study, children exposed to increased rates of expansion and recasts showed improved grammatical development (Nelson et al., 1973). Subsequent research showed that children exposed to elevated rates of expansion have better language growth (Cleave et al., 2015; Leonard et al., 2004; Nelson et al., 1996). Other examples of caregiver use of talk that encourages language development include "parallel talk" (e.g., describing in the moment what the child is doing or experiencing, such as "You are swinging so high.") and open-ended questions whose answers are unknown to the caregiver (e.g., "What else do you want?") (Fey et al., 1999; Proctor-Williams et al., 2001; Szagun and Stumper, 2012).

In addition to supporting parents in using responsive language, it is important to reduce the use of caregiver styles that are overly directive and/or controlling of the child, such as leading the child's attention away from current interests, correcting grammar ("Say it this way, not that way."), or withholding an object until the child speaks. Maternal directiveness has been negatively associated with subsequent child language outcomes (Landry et al., 1997, 2000; Rowe, 2008), which has led interventionists to provide caregivers with feedback and support that promote responsive rather than directive interactions.

Enhanced parental confidence is emphasized in interventions focused on caregiver promotion of language abilities throughout daily routines. Early interventionists seek to promote caregivers' *self-efficacy* in their roles in promoting the child's development, defined as the "expectations caregivers hold about their ability to parent successfully" (Jones and Prinz, 2005, p. 342). Caregivers with low levels of self-efficacy may find it difficult to persist when presented with challenges in parenting their child. In contrast, high levels of maternal self-efficacy have been linked to responsiveness to the child and the provision of stimulating interactions (Coleman and Karraker, 2003).

Indeed, promoting caregiver responsiveness to the child and to the child's efforts to communicate is another primary goal of early intervention. This approach builds on decades of research showing that children exposed to conversational talk that is responsive have better rates of language development than those who are not (Cross, 1978; Goldfield, 1987; Landry et al., 2006; Tamis-LeMonda et al., 1996). One form of this responsive communication occurs when the parent or clinician says something that builds on the meaning of the child's prior utterances—referred to as "semantic extensions" (Cleave et al., 2015). The effectiveness of semantic extensions in promoting language growth was first shown by Cazden (1965).

Interventions Focused on Promoting Language Growth in Young Children

The section above focuses on early intervention aimed at supporting caregivers in being responsive and employing qualitative features in their use of language that are known to promote children's linguistic development. Within the early intervention context, numerous intervention approaches have been developed to promote the child's growth along a developmental continuum. It is beyond the scope of this report to provide comprehensive coverage of the multiple goals, approaches, and techniques involved in child-focused interventions. However, commonly selected child targets in early language intervention and treatment goals for meeting those targets are summarized in Box 3-2.

BOX 3-2
Selected Examples of Targets and Treatment Goals in Early Language Intervention (birth to age 3)

Treatment Goals	
Prelinguistic communication	• Increase prelinguistic behaviors that are foundational to language development in preverbal children (Warren et al., 2008; Yoder and Warren, 1998, 2002). – Increase child's use of gestures – Increase use of eye gaze to signal desires, wants – Promote shared attention and joint engagement – Increase child's use of vocalizations – Increase intentional communication attempts – Promote combining communication modes (gesture + vocalization + eye gaze)
Vocabulary development	• Promote child's understanding and use of diverse word types and concepts (e.g., object and person names, verbs, descriptive terms) to strengthen language comprehension and promote word learning and use of word combinations (Girolametto et al., 1998; Lonigan and Whitehurst, 1998; Marulis and Neuman, 2010)
Early word combinations and grammar	• Target grammatical forms that are emerging and represent next developmental steps for the child (Fey et al., 2003); promote word combinations with increasing length and complexity (i.e., including word endings) once the child shows sufficient readiness (Hadley, 2014)

continued

BOX 3-2 Continued

Pragmatics	• Emphasize child's ability to express a range of communicative functions (e.g., request, protest, comment, question [Bates, 1976]) • Adults contingently responsive to child's communicative attempts (in a variety of forms) to promote child's participation in conversational turn-taking interactions (Fey et al., 2006; Landry et al., 2001)
Selected Intervention Strategies	
Enabling environments	• Environment is modified in ways that result in frequent exposure of child to developmentally appropriate language models and opportunities to use emerging language abilities (Finestack and Fey, 2013; Hemmeter and Kaiser, 1994; Warren et al., 2006)
Joint engagement routines with adult responsivity	• Caregivers learn to encourage child's participation in social routines by being responsive and focusing on child's interests (Girolametto et al., 1994; Kasari et al., 2010; Yoder and Warren, 2001)
Focused stimulation	• Clinician identifies specific language targets (e.g., vocabulary, grammar, language functions), and adults provide multiple exposures to child's targets and encourage child to produce the targets (Leonard, 1981) • May include elicitation strategies such as imitation prompts (Camarata et al., 1994; Ingersoll and Lalonde, 2010; Kouri, 2005); emphasis may be placed on targeted forms (Robertson and Weismer, 1999) • Explicit and implicit vocabulary instruction provided through multiple exposures to words in natural contexts (Leonard et al., 1982; Marulis and Neuman, 2010)
Script-based interventions	• Socio-dramatic play routines that engage child in representing familiar event sequences or scripts (Schank and Abelson, 1977) used to foster social and

Interventions for Nonspeaking Children with Profound Hearing Loss

Some children are nonspeaking because of severe-to-profound deafness (Brookhouser and Moeller, 1986). For these children, evidence points to two established options for improving communication skills: sign language and/or cochlear implants. Nonspeaking deaf children have been shown to

	linguistic development; concept is that child's familiarity with event structure frees up cognitive resources to focus on learning new linguistic targets (Nelson and Gruendel, 1986)
Shared/interactive book reading	• Adult–child social interactions during storybook reading tailored to promote a variety of linguistic goals for child (Bradshaw et al., 1998; Whitehurst et al., 1994)
Recast	• Caregiver/therapist repeats what child says in developmentally more advanced form to promote grammatical development (Cleave et al., 2015; Proctor-Williams et al., 2001)
Learning Context	
Clinician support for caregiver	• Emphasis on naturalistic and developmentally appropriate language stimulation throughout daily routines, with a goal of frequent language exposure and frequent opportunities for child to understand and use language
Child-centered	• Emphasis on maintaining communication interactions and embedding teaching in natural, playful communication exchanges
Hybrid	• Combines home-based and clinician-delivered interventions
Parameters of Service Delivery	
Dose of treatment	• Focuses on parent/caregiver implementation in natural daily routines to promote high dosage and generalization
Agent of change	• Parent/caregiver supported in home setting by clinician; clinician may provide child-focused intervention with parent training component
Treatment setting	• Typically focuses on natural environments (home, daycare), but may include clinic or early intervention setting

be quite adept at acquiring sign language, which provides a rich means of communicating with members of the deaf community and others fluent in that form of communication (Newport and Meier, 1985). In recent years, many of these children have been provided with cochlear implants, which have been shown for some to provide very good speech and language outcomes (Niparko et al., 2010; Tomblin et al., 1999).

Efficacy of Early Interventions

Several meta-analyses in the early childhood special education literature demonstrate the impact of family-centered practices on caregiver abilities. One meta-analysis integrated 52 studies to estimate effect sizes in relation to specific family-centered practices (Dunst et al., 2008). It examined the relationships between family-centered help giving and six categories of child and family outcomes (participant satisfaction, self-efficacy, program helpfulness, child functioning, parent–family functioning, and parenting behaviors). The relationships were significant in all six analyses, with average effect sizes ranging from 0.65 to 0.15 across the six outcomes. Overall, results suggest that family-centered practices have either direct effects on family and child functioning, indirect effects mediated through self-efficacy, or both. A more recent meta-analysis suggests that family-centered practices directly influence parental self-efficacy, and that indirect effects of these practices on parent–child interaction and child development are mediated by caregiver self-efficacy (Trivette et al., 2010). The authors reviewed eight studies including 910 infants, toddlers, and preschoolers with and without developmental delays. Results, which were statistically significant, showed that family-centered help-giving practices and family-systems interventions directly influenced parental self-efficacy and well-being and that there were indirect effects on parent–child interaction and child development, mediated by caregiver self-efficacy and parental well-being.

Another meta-analysis focuses on 18 studies evaluating the effects of parent-implemented interventions for toddlers and preschoolers with language impairments (Roberts and Kaiser, 2011). This analysis shows that parent-implemented language interventions have a positive impact on children's receptive and expressive language outcomes relative to a control group. Increasing parent–child turn taking in interactions and improving responsiveness to child communication also are associated with positive outcomes in child language. The effect sizes are statistically significant for receptive language and for expressive grammar. The authors note that the effect sizes for six of the seven language constructs measured are positive and significant. Increasing parent–child turn taking in interactions and improving responsiveness to child communication also are associated with positive outcomes in child language. Law and colleagues (2004) found a significant effect of expressive language intervention compared with no therapy. They also found that speech-language interventions administered to children by speech-language pathologists and interventions administered by parents trained by speech-language pathologists were comparable in effectiveness, suggesting that caregivers can become effective agents of change.

Because most of these studies involved parents of relatively high socioeconomic status, more research is needed to understand how these approaches are working or may need to be adapted with caregivers in circumstances of low income.

Preschool Intervention

The preschool period marks a time of transition for children. During this period, children begin to spend more time outside the home and in play-based settings with peers. By 3 years of age, many preschoolers can sit and attend for at least short intervals, and by the end of the preschool period, the typically developing child is expected to be capable of participating in group activities and attending to and following the instructions of an adult (Paul and Norbury, 2012). For the preschooler with developmental disorders, the preschool years also mark a time when clinical services are likely to move out of the home and into centers and clinics. However, parent-based programs are common during these years. The following subsections summarize the treatment modalities that make up the typical standards of care for the preschool child with speech and/or language disorders and the evidence for their efficacy.

Treatment for Preschool-Age Children with Severe Language Disorders

Children with severe language disorders are likely to engage with others to accomplish a variety of communication acts, such as talking about things around them, asking questions, and expressing preferences (e.g., by saying "no"). Their language is likely to be characteristic of a younger child, with limited vocabulary and simple or immature sentences. Importantly, children with severe language disorders also are likely to understand things said to them at this lower level. If this gap in achievement persists into the early school years, these children are likely to enter school with language skills similar to those of children who are 3-4 years old. For these children, the goal of language treatment is to close this gap to the extent possible. To accomplish this goal, therapists need to promote growth in the child's implicit language knowledge base across a range of communication skills. The treatment programs for these preschool-age children (ages 3-5) are diverse and often tailored to the particular needs of the child, based on the factors described earlier in this chapter. The factors that influence language treatment programs for preschool children with language disorders fall into four general areas: (1) treatment goals, (2) mode of teaching, (3) learning context, and (4) parameters of service delivery. These factors are summarized in Box 3-3 and described in greater detail in the subsections that follow.

BOX 3-3
Selected Examples of Child-Focused Elements of Language Treatment Programs for Preschool-Age Children

Treatment Goals

Vocabulary	• Words expressing cognitive states (think, know) (Rescorla et al., 2000) • Common verbs (Rescorla et al., 2000) • Time, place, and quantity terms (Owens, 2013)
Grammar	• General principle: target emerging grammatical forms (Fey et al., 2003) • Auxiliary verbs ("am," "will," etc.) (Paul and Norbury, 2012) • Tense (Rice et al., 2005) • Complex sentence forms, such as use of relative clauses (Schuele and Tolbert, 2001) • Presentation of variable lexical items along with the targeted grammatical structure to promote learning (Plante et al., 2014)
Pragmatics	• Continuation of on-topic conversation (Paul and Norbury, 2012) • Asking questions that consider the listener's perspective (Marton et al., 2005) • Use of verbal skills for conflict resolution (Marton et al., 2005)
Preliteracy	• Awareness of the sound composition of words (phonological awareness) (Justice and Ezell, 2000) • Concepts of print (Justice and Kaderavek, 2004) • Alphabetic knowledge (Lovelace and Stewart, 2007) • Knowledge of structures of stories (van Kleeck et al., 2006)

Mode of Teaching

Modeling	• Provide frequent examples of learning targets (Hemmeter and Kaiser, 1994; Leonard et al., 2004; Vasilyeva et al., 2006; Weismer and Murray-Branch, 1989)

Treatment goals Several principles govern the selection of treatment goals. First, the goals are based on evidence of aspects of communication that are known to be vulnerable in children with language disorders. Second, the goals are selected to enhance the child's ability to participate in social interactions and develop precursor skills for school entry. Third, although treatment goals for children with severe language disorders may be itemized

Comprehension	• Ask for verbal or nonverbal responses based on word, sentence, or story meaning (Byrne-Saricks, 1987)
Extensions	• Follow child's utterance with appropriate content that continues the conversation (Barnes et al., 1983; Cazden, 1965)
Expansions	• Clinician repeats what child says in a developmentally advanced form (Cleave et al., 2015; Proctor-Williams et al., 2001)
Recast	• Clinician repeats what child says in a developmentally advanced form (Cleave et al., 2015; Proctor-Williams et al., 2001)
Imitation	• Child is asked to imitate an utterance (Camarata et al., 1994; Connell, 1987; Connell and Stone, 1992)
Learning Context	
Clinician-directed	• Emphasis on high rates of stimulation and child responses, where clinician elicits language responses with little emphasis on true communication
Child-centered	• Emphasis on maintaining communication interactions and embedding teaching in the communication exchanges
Hybrid	• Combines control of the content and form of the talk by the clinician with a semi-natural communication exchange
Parameters of Service Delivery	
Dose of treatment	• Number of days per week and duration of sessions (Law and Conti-Ramsden, 2000; Schooling et al., 2010)
Agent of change	• Clinician versus parent (Fey et al., 1993, 1997)
Mode of participation	• Individual versus group (Boyle et al., 2007)
Treatment setting	• Center/clinic versus home (Schooling et al., 2010)

separately, they need to span comprehension, vocabulary, grammar, social communication/pragmatics, and preliteracy, and the treatment is likely to address several of these goals at once (Paul and Norbury, 2012). Finally, specific treatment goals will be based on the child's developmental readiness for learning. For instance, Fey and colleagues (2003) suggest targeting grammatical forms that are used at low frequencies and thus likely emerging in the child's system. Readiness also can be indicated by evidence that the child is able to use a language form or function when supported by adults (Schneider and Watkins, 1996).

Mode of teaching Two features are common to all of the teaching modes for preschool-age children with severe language disorders. First, an effort is made to increase the amount of language experience provided to the child. Learning theories in psychology often acknowledge that more trials in a learning task will result in better learning, and this principle also has been found to apply to language development (Hart and Risley, 1995; Huttenlocher et al., 1991; Matthews et al., 2005; Moerk, 1983). Second, an effort is made to enhance the saliency or prominence of the language target being taught to the child by increasing emphasis on or control over the placement of the target in the utterance (Dalal and Loeb, 2005; Weismer, 1997).

One instructional method, referred to as "modeling," draws on the social learning theory that emphasizes observational learning (Bandura, 1971). With this method, the child is provided an elevated number of exemplars of a language form. In some cases, this is done in the context of high-density exposures during focused treatment sessions, while in others, it is embedded in natural conversational interactions. In both kinds of settings, modeling has been found to result in gains in the targeted language forms (Leonard et al., 2004; Nye et al., 1987; Vasilyeva et al., 2006; Weismer and Murray-Branch, 1989).

As was noted earlier, talk that encompasses semantic extensions, recasts, and expansions is also often used in preschool programs where clinicians are the agent of change. Several preschool language intervention programs emphasizing responsive language have shown evidence of effectiveness (Bunce, 1991; Dale et al., 1996; Fey et al., 1993; Justice et al., 2008).

Common to all of the above teaching modes is the fact that the child is not taught directly to express the target language. In contrast, some treatment programs place a strong emphasis on a direct form of teaching through elicited imitation. In this case, the child is instructed to imitate a word or sentence and given feedback when he or she makes an imitative attempt. A substantial literature has shown that teaching through imitation can result in improved use of the targeted language forms (Camarata et al., 1994; Connell, 1987; Connell and Stone, 1992; Nye et al., 1987). Yet while imitation is clearly effective in teaching specific targeted behaviors, generalization beyond these targets is often limited.

In summary, an array of basic patterns of language interactions with children can be used to promote language growth. For example, Law and colleagues (2004, 2008) have performed meta-analyses on the effectiveness of language interventions and concluded that treatment programs are effective for improving vocabulary with a standardized mean difference of 0.89 and mixed evidence for improvement in expressive grammar. A recent meta-analysis on the effect of recasting on improvement in grammar found a mean standardized difference of 0.96 for gains in the targeted grammatical form measures and 0.76 for generalization to untreated grammatical forms (Cleave et al., 2015). The evidence is strongest for those methods that include responsive interactions, although directive language engagement, particularly in limited amounts, can also be effective. Most language intervention programs combine several of these methods, along with a general emphasis on overall increments in the frequency of language use.

Learning context Most language intervention programs for preschool children use multiple modes of teaching. When these modes are combined, they can result in different types of learning contexts that may be clinician-centered, child-centered, or a mix of the two. The clinician-centered context is one in which the emphasis is on high rates of listening and speaking the targeted language forms within a highly structured drill-and-practice setting. The clinician controls what is said and what the child does. Paul and Norbury (2012) note that this approach has been advocated by several clinical investigators on the grounds that children with language disorders need the structure and intensity of this learning context. In contrast with clinician-centered approaches are those that are child-centered, in which the emphasis is on preserving the qualities of natural adult–child interactions, and in particular the pragmatics of conversation. The child is allowed to lead the interaction and thus the content, while the clinician follows. The hybrid approach represents a middle ground. One prominent example is incidental teaching (Hart and Risley, 1975), in which the clinician arranges the play setting to provide for talk about the targets and motivations for talking. Interjected into the play are short intervals of focused teaching that involves more directive language. Many of these services are provided in school-based settings through IDEA.

Parameters of service delivery The ways in which speech and language services are provided vary along several parameters. One such parameter is the treatment "dose," including such variables as the duration of the treatment session, the number of sessions, and the spacing of treatment. Although one might expect that more treatment is likely to be more effective, the evidence in this regard is not clear (Schooling et al., 2010). Yoder and colleagues (2012) found that learner characteristics may interact with the influence of treatment dose and that dose effects are complex (Yoder et al., 2012).

Another important parameter of service delivery is the agent of change. For preschool children, the principal agent of change may be a speech-language clinician, a preschool teacher, or the child's parents. Comparisons of parents and clinicians as agents have shown that outcomes are largely comparable (Dale et al., 1996; Fey et al., 1993, 1997; Schooling et al., 2010). Outcomes also are comparable whether services are provided in groups or individually, and in centers and clinics or the children's homes (Schooling et al., 2010).

In summary, considerable evidence shows that clinical treatment for language disorders can improve preschool children's language abilities. However, the learning effects are greatest for those skills that are the target of intervention. The effects of treatment are less pronounced for those skills that reflect a widespread restructuring of the child's language system. As a result, the preschool child with a language disorder, particularly if the disorder is severe, is likely to continue to have the disorder by the time he or she enters school.

Treatment for Nonspeaking Preschool-Age Children

At the most extreme end of the continuum of severity of speech and language disorders are children who are nonspeaking. By 3 years of age, the absence of speech is indicative of some form of severe communication impairment (Whitman and Schwartz, 1985).

The speech of one-third to one-half of children with cerebral palsy is so limited that it is not functionally intelligible (Andersen et al., 2010; Himmelmann et al., 2013). Another group of children who fail to develop spoken communication are those with severe intellectual disability and/or autism. By 14 months of age, for example, most infants are able to draw the caregiver's attention to something by pointing and naming. This basic communication function is limited or absent in some children with severe intellectual disability or autism spectrum disorder. Provision of a basic functional communication system has been shown to reduce aggressive and self-injurious behavior in these children (Kurtz et al., 2003).

Such systems—termed alternative and augmentative communication systems—can be organized into two groups: those that depend on alternative body systems, such as gestures or facial expressions (unaided communication systems), and those that require some tool or equipment (aided systems) (Romski and Sevcik, 2005), ranging from a set of pictures or paper and pencil to computer-based speech-generating systems. For young children who are not literate, the most common options are those that do not require or use print. If such a child has good motor skills, an unaided system involving gesture or a picture-based system may be employed. A review of all of these systems is beyond the scope of this study, but given the focus of this report on young children with severe speech and language disorders, two systems used commonly with such children are described below.

One of the oldest alternative and augmentative communication systems entails the use of a set of pictures that are arranged on a board or placed on pages in a book (Beukelman and Mirenda, 2005). The pictures often represent basic messages that the child needs or wishes to express. For children with very limited motor abilities, the communication board can be placed on a tray attached to the child's wheelchair. As the child progresses in the use of the device, it is usually necessary to alter its content to include new messages. Furthermore, as the child's capabilities with language, print, and mobility change, other alternative and augmentative communication systems may be appropriate.

For some nonspeaking children, the absence of spoken communication is due to their lack of understanding of communication functions such as informing a listener about basic needs. Such children need to be introduced to rudimentary communication activities in the hope of not only improving their functional communication skills but also enabling their overall further progress. A common treatment program for this purpose is the picture exchange communication system (Bondy and Frost, 2001), in which the child is provided with pictures of desired objects and taught to use the pictures to request the objects from teachers or caregivers. Several studies have provided evidence that this treatment increases the number of communicative requests, although evidence that these skills generalize to other communication partners, to other communication functions, or to speech is limited at present (Flippin et al., 2010; Preston and Carter, 2009).

Preschool children who are nonspeaking because of poor language ability are likely to have lifelong needs for support, particularly if their deficits reflect severe receptive language disorders and/or other neurodevelopmental disorders. If such children develop any spoken communication skills, those skills may be quite limited. In contrast, if the basis of the communication problem is largely a limitation in speech production, and receptive language abilities are relatively unaffected, computer-based electronic communication systems are likely to be effective, and these children have a good chance of entering into regular education and mainstream society.

It is important to emphasize that for many children with severe deficits, the use of alternative and augmentative communication systems may not result in levels of communication found in typically developing children. However, if such a system can increase the child's ability to communicate five or six messages rather than one or two, the resulting gains for communicating with parents, teachers, and others may be substantial, and may prevent or resolve aggressive and self-injurious behaviors. Because of the heterogeneity in the etiology of those disorders that necessitate the use of such systems, as well as in the cognitive ability and speech and language level of affected children, much of the research on these interventions has a single-case (single-subject) design (Schlosser and Sigafoos, 2006). This literature indicates that children receiving these interventions improve in communication function, but with rare exceptions, they will not develop typical speaking ability and will continue to require alternative and augmentative systems as a primary means of communication.

Treatment for School-Age Children with Language Disorders

As noted earlier, language demands increase substantially as children move from the home to the school setting. Throughout the formal educational process, learning occurs through language and communication. In the classroom, the content of language children hear, and later read, is often new. Classroom language also is "decontextualized"; that is, it refers to events occurring in other times and places (Snow, 1991). Moreover, much of language in the classroom is no longer tailored or even directed to an individual child. In fact, in the primary grades, the majority of children in a classroom may not understand many of the important verbal concepts they encounter (Boehm, 1991). Thus, even children with mild language disorders enter school at a high risk for academic difficulty.

Children with severe language disorders have a particularly high risk of learning problems during the elementary years. As discussed in Chapter 2, children with severe and profound language disorders fall more than two standard deviations below the mean for their age group. Thus, a 6-year-old child may have language skills comparable to those of children 2 or more years younger. As a result, a large gap exists between the child's abilities and the array of language skills required to perform in school. As previously noted, speech and language treatments are not likely to resolve children's language difficulties completely, nor will they fully protect children from difficulties with school performance.

Researchers have recommended a curriculum-based model of treatment for school-age children with language disorders (ASHA, 1999; Simon, 1987; Wallach, 2008). In this model, treatment goals are aligned with the school curriculum, and learning priorities involve skills linked directly to reading, writing, and mathematics. IDEA also plays a role in this curriculum focus by emphasizing that school-based speech and language services should focus on those skills that affect the child's educational performance. The past two decades have seen an increased emphasis on incorporating speech and language services into the classroom whenever possible instead of removing children from their classrooms for treatment. Evidence concerning the relative effectiveness of classroom-based and pull-out services for children with language impairments is mixed (McGinty and Justice, 2006).

Curriculum-based treatment of speech and language disorders in school-age children emphasizes two related areas: (1) metalinguistics and (2) the language bases of reading and writing.

Metalinguistics

Reading and spelling require that a child think consciously about the sound composition of words and the meaning of words and whole narratives. This conscious knowledge of and talk about language itself is called *metalinguistics* (Bialystok and Ryan, 1985). One of the most common metalinguistic treatment targets for school-age children with language disorders has been *phonological awareness*, a form of metalinguistic skill having to do with understanding and awareness of the sound components of words. Learning to read involves the identification of these sound elements and their mapping onto letters and sequences of letters. A number of systematic training programs are available for improving children's phonological awareness (Adams et al., 1998; Blachman et al., 2000). In 2002, the National Reading Panel, commissioned by the U.S. Congress, identified 52 studies evaluating the effectiveness of phonological awareness training in improving reading and spelling (Ehri et al., 2001), concluding that its effect was moderate. A more recent literature review by Snowling and Hulme (2011) yielded similar findings.

Language Bases of Reading and Writing

Several decades of research on reading and writing has led to an understanding that these abilities are highly linked to spoken language abilities (Carroll and Snowling, 2004; Catts and Kamhi, 2005). A prominent model of reading comprehension by Hoover and Gough (1990) identifies two subcomponents that contribute to successful reading comprehension: word recognition and language comprehension. Oral language skills play an important role in each of these subprocesses, as shown in Figure 3-2. This figure, from Scarborough (2001), shows that children's word recognition entails phonological awareness, which is a common target of intervention for children with language disorders. In addition to being foundational for word reading, phonological awareness is important to spelling (Caravolas et al., 2001). Understanding what is read also involves much of the same language knowledge (vocabulary, grammar, sentence meanings, understanding of story structure, and verbal reasoning such as inferencing) as that involved in understanding what has been spoken. This knowledge is a focal point of school-based language intervention as well. Many of the methods used to promote grammatical skills in school-age children are the same as those described in the section on preschool language interventions, although the goals for grammatical development are more likely to involve use and, in particular, comprehension of complex sentences, such as those with relative clauses.

Mezynski (1983) argues for a strong correlation between vocabulary

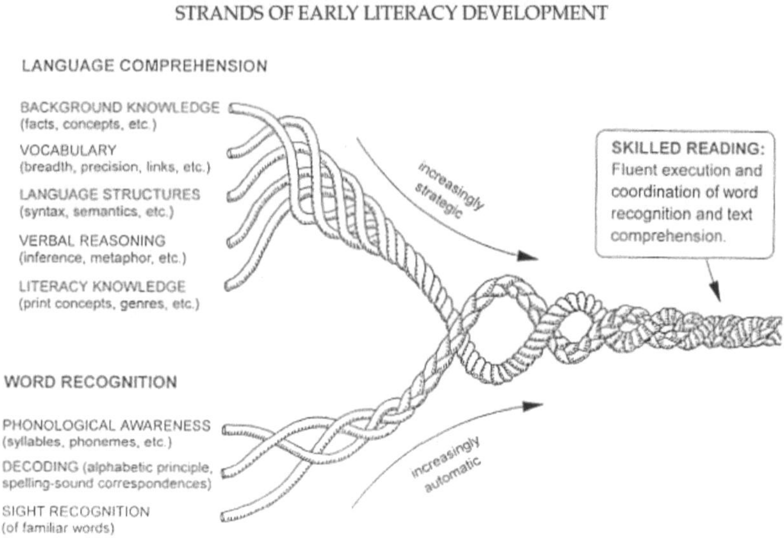

FIGURE 3-2 A depiction of the bases of reading development.
SOURCE: Used with permission by Guilford Press from the *Handbook of Early Literacy*, Figure 8.1, Scarborough's Rope, 2003.

and reading comprehension. Thus, a treatment program aimed at enhancing vocabulary could result in improvement in reading. More recently, Elleman and colleagues (2009) performed a meta-analysis of the literature on the effects of vocabulary intervention on reading comprehension. They found that children improved their reading comprehension only on measures that included the vocabulary they had been taught directly; their overall reading comprehension did not improve.

Other school-based treatment programs focus on the structure and content of stories and expository text (Nippold et al., 2008; Roth et al., 1996), inference making, and metalinguistic knowledge about participation in classroom communication. In general, considerable evidence indicates that such language interventions can result in improvements in the targeted abilities; it is less likely that these treatment effects generalize broadly to effect widespread gains in academic function.

Treatment for Speech Sound Disorders

As with language disorders, the severity of speech disorders can range from relatively mild to quite severe, up to and including a complete inability to speak. Broadly, intervention for speech disorders can be completed at two levels. Mild to moderate speech disorders (e.g., speaking with a lisp; deleting or distorting the final sounds in words; deleting sounds and consonant clusters; or substituting one sound for another, such as "w" for "r") often are treated with a focus on *speech production accuracy* for individual sounds (phonemes) (Bernthal et al., 2012). In more severe speech disorders, the focus of intervention may be on improving global *speech intelligibility*, wherein whole word production rather than individual phonemes is targeted (see Camarata, 2010; Camarata et al., 2006; Levy et al., 2012; McLeod, 2006). When overall speech intelligibility is extremely limited, intervention includes augmentative and alternative communication prostheses, discussed earlier (see Costantino and Bonati, 2014). Generally, primary approaches to behavioral treatment of speech disorders, regardless of level or theoretical underpinnings, include practice moving and coordinating movements of oral structures such as the lips, tongue, and soft palate to improve speech production (Williams et al., 2010).

Within the broad rubric of improving speech accuracy, there are a number of approaches, including articulation drill, motor learning, and phonological/lexical interventions. Examples of these approaches are briefly described below.

Articulation Drill and Motor Learning

Articulation drill approaches focused on motor placement and production of individual speech sounds (phonemes) often are a primary focus of intervention for speech disorders (McLeod and Bleile, 2004). In essence, a child is taught directly how to move and coordinate the articulatory mechanism for producing individual speech sounds (phonemes). For example, a child with a mild speech disorder who says the word "rabbit" as "wabbit" is incorrectly pronouncing the phoneme "r" as a "w." Intervention in this case would include direct instruction, motor practice, and drill on how to produce an "r" sound correctly. These drills often are completed on individual sounds in isolation as a preliminary step. After the child has learned to produce the phoneme correctly in isolation, syllabic productions are introduced (e.g., consonant-vowel syllables). Practice is then initiated until the target phoneme is produced correctly in this context as well. After the child has mastered production at the syllable level, word-level productions are initiated, with a transition to phrases and conversational speech to follow. This approach has long been a standard method in the field (Nemoy and Davis, 1954; Swift, 1918) and remains a core feature of intervention for speech disorders in children (Maas et al., 2014).

One key component of articulation drill is repeated motor practice of the tongue movements and coordination of the other articulators, such as lips and jaw, required for accurate pronunciation. Maas and colleagues

(2014) review motor learning approaches as applied to speech disorders in children. Although treatment goals often focus on individual speech sounds (phonemes), the authors note that motor practice principles can include syllables, words, and even phrases: "The possible types of targets are numerous and diverse, and include isolated speech movements, speech sounds, syllables, phonetically modified words, real words, nonsense words, and phrases/sentences" (p. 199). In addition to these targets, the authors observe that motor learning can also be applied to intonation and stress patterns needed for accurate speech production (see also Shriberg et al., 1997).

Other variations on articulation drill focus on phonemes but introduce specific targets with the goal of generating broader systems change in speech production. For example, Gierut (1990) argues that in maximal contrast articulation drill, speech intervention will be more efficient if selected phonemic contrasts differ in terms of place of articulation in the mouth (e.g., lips, alveolar ridge, soft palate, larynx), voicing (voiced as in "b" versus voiceless as in "p"), and manner (vowel-like, frication, and so on). Gierut's model predicts that training in very different speech sounds (e.g., "p" versus "r") will yield incidental learning of speech sounds with some of the features contained in the contrast (such as voicing and intermediate placement). Williams (2000) also hypothesizes that generalization will take place when training addresses contrasting speech targets, but that the generalization will be narrower than that proposed in maximal contrast treatment.

In a similar vein, some articulation drill intervention approaches focus on patterns of speech sound learning based on "phonological processes," which are patterns of speech sound production rooted in linguistic feature classifications (e.g., Chomsky and Halle, 1968). In this model, the focus of intervention is on highlighting specific linguistic features that account for systematic errors in disordered speech. For example, it is not uncommon for children with speech disorders to produce the sounds "f," "s," and "th" as "p," "t," and "t," respectively (saying *pea* for *fee*, *tee* for *see*, and *bat* for *bath*). These errors indicate that sounds that should be produced with a turbulent airflow (fricatives such as "f," "s," and "th") are instead being produced with complete occlusion of the oral cavity and an abrupt release (stops such as "p" and "t"). In phonological process intervention approaches, the substitution of stop consonants for fricative consonants is called "stopping" or "stopping of fricatives," so that intervention is designed to highlight correct production of entire sound classes, such as fricatives, when these are produced incorrectly by substituting speech sounds from another class (see Hodson and Paden, 1981; Ingram, 1981; Shriberg and Kwiatkowski, 1980). Interventions based on phonological process analysis continue to be included in current intervention studies (e.g., Dodd, 2013).

Phonological/Lexical Approaches

Although articulation drill can be applied to words or even phrases, these levels are often generalization targets after motor planning and/or articulation practice on individual speech sounds has been completed (see Camarata, 1993). A different approach to treating speech disorders is rooted in considering speech sounds within the context of word productions (see Storkel, 2004). These interventions are designed to improve word-level production rather than starting at the motor learning or individual phoneme level. Some approaches focused on lexical-phonological learning do not include motor practice or articulation drill. For example, Camarata (1993) found that responsive-interaction intervention based on transactional learning was associated with improved speech production. Similarly, Yoder and colleagues (2005) found that "broad target recasts" improved speech production in children with comorbid speech and language disorders. In addition, Crosbie and colleagues (2005) found that word-level speech production improved speech disorders in children. These latter studies show that both speech accuracy and speech intelligibility can be improved using lexical-transactional intervention.

Efficacy of Treatment for Speech Sound Disorders

A number of studies have found treatment to be associated with significant gains in speech accuracy and intelligibility (Almost and Rosenbaum, 1998; Baker and McCleod, 2011). However, there have been few long-term follow-up studies, and very few studies have been focused on children with severe speech disorders (Baker and McCleod, 2011). Similarly, in a review of the literature on speech intervention in mild to moderate speech disorders, Bernthal and colleagues (2012) conclude that "when comparing groups receiving intervention to those receiving no treatment, the intervention group consistently perform better than the no treatment groups on outcome assessment measures. Thus, it would appear that intervention for speech sound disorders does make a difference; however, additional information is needed regarding the effectiveness of specific treatment methods" (p. 270).

As noted, the literature on severe speech disorders, such as dysarthria and childhood apraxia of speech, is highly limited (Morgan and Vogel, 2008). Studies focus on populations such as children with Down syndrome and cerebral palsy as a means of evaluating treatment, and many of these studies are single-subject designs that provide evidence of individual short-term gains in speech intelligibility (as in Camarata et al., 2006). In general, randomized clinical trials that include children with severe speech disorders have been lacking. This is also the case for those children whose speech is so severely unintelligible that computerized speech devices are required. A recent meta-analysis of interventions using such devices (Gevarter et al., 2013) found evidence for improvement in specific skills targeted by the treatment and improvement in the use of the devices, but it is difficult to determine whether such interventions result in long-term improvement in speech intelligibility.

In summary, as with language disorders, a substantial literature indicates that short-term improvements are observed following intervention for speech disorders. A majority of these studies focus on the mild-to-moderate range of severity. Evidence with regard to severe speech disorders is much more limited, and a great deal of this evidence is focused on short-term proximal gains demonstrated using single-subject designs.

Treatment for Stuttering

A wide range of treatments have been developed for stuttering over the past century. These include psychological-psychodynamic approaches, operant conditioning-behavioral approaches, and technology applications such as delayed auditory feedback devices. In addition, a limited number of pharmacological treatments have been studied, yielding some evidence that medication can be effective in improving symptomology.

Broadly, the treatment literature indicates that individual symptoms of stuttering, such as repetitions, intonation patterns, and timing disruptions, can be improved with a variety of treatments. However, Nye and colleagues (2013) conducted a meta-analysis of the stuttering treatment literature and found limited evidence that therapy improves stuttering symptomology. The literature also indicates that recovery rates are higher in preschool than in school-age children, but longitudinal randomized trials comparing treatment with untreated recovery are needed. Stuttering in children whose dysfluencies persist into school age and into early adolescence is most resistant to treatment (Guitar, 2013).

PERSISTENCE OF PEDIATRIC SPEECH AND LANGUAGE DISORDERS IN CHILDREN

Over the past three decades, several longitudinal studies have examined the persistence of early speech and language delays during later preschool years and well into the school years.

Persistence of Early Speech and Language Delays

The question of persistence requires that the age of onset of speech and language disorders be considered. As discussed in Chapter 2, these disorders do not have a clear age of onset; rather, they emerge as a child begins to engage in spoken communication at around 2 years of age. This pattern of emergence results in a period of ambiguity with respect to when the diagnosis of a persistent disorder can be made. Early signs of delayed speech and language development become evident at approximately 2 years of age, when most children can understand and say a number of words. Several studies in the early 1990s analyzed parent reports of children's speech and language around this age. Parents were asked whether children who had very limited expressive language at around 2 years of age could be considered as having a persistent condition that warranted clinical intervention. Children in these studies who had very limited expressive language were categorized as "late talkers" (Paul, 1993; Rescorla and Schwartz, 1990; Thal, 1991; Weismer et al., 1994). Usually, to be considered a late talker, the child had to be free of other developmental or sensory disorders; thus, being a late talker was viewed as a possible early manifestation of primary language disorder. Even though the diagnosis often emphasized expressive vocabulary, many of these children also were found to have poor speech sound production, reduced language comprehension, limited use of word combinations, and limited use of nonverbal gestures and symbolic play (Desmarais et al., 2008). The investigators in these studies followed these late talkers longitudinally into the preschool years and in some cases into adolescence.

The language measures obtained during the preschool years for children who were late talkers as toddlers showed that, as a group, they continued to perform below their age mates on many language measures; however, their mean scores were also at the low end of the normal range (Dale and Hayiou-Thomas, 2013). Thus, there was evidence of improvement among at least a subgroup of these children. It should be noted that, although late-talking children may also display speech disorders, longitudinal studies of this group have not systematically assessed speech skills during follow-up. Children who are late talkers are more likely to continue to manifest language development at the lower end of the normal range, often lagging behind their same-age peers (Dollaghan, 2013; Thal et al., 2013).

An important feature of many of these studies is that the participants often were from socioeconomically advantaged homes. Paul and Weismer (2013) note that late talking can be viewed as one risk factor that, when combined with poverty, increases the risk that a child may have persistent problems. Many of the studies of late talkers also have identified other risk factors for persistence, such as poor language comprehension, limited engagement in communication, more severe language delay, and a family history of language and reading impairment (see also the discussion of risk factors in Chapter 2). Because most of the research on the persistence of late talking has focused on children with few other risk factors, further research is needed to determine the extent to which late talking in combination with other risk factors is predictive of the persistence of poor language skills.

Persistence of Language Disorders During the School Years

Although research on the persistence of early speech and language delay suggests that many children who are late to begin talking as toddlers show gains in language that eventually place them at the lower end of the normal range, a number of children who are late talkers as toddlers have persistent language disorders through the preschool years. Joining these children are those with normal language at 2 years of age who subsequently show declines in language skills (Ukoumunne et al., 2011) and those who also display speech disorders.

Several studies have assessed the long-term persistence of speech and language disorders among children who are at the end of the preschool years. Beitchman and colleagues (Johnson et al., 1999) followed a large sample of children with and without speech and language impairment at 5 years of age into adolescence and found that 71.4 percent had persisting language problems, compared with a rate of 5.5 percent in control children who had normal language in kindergarten. They also found that 10.9 percent of the speech-impaired group had persistent speech disorders at follow-up. These findings were similar to the statistically significant findings of Bishop and colleagues over a similar follow-up period: 90 percent of children with language impairment at 5 years of age continued to present with language impairment at 15 years of age (Stothard et al., 1998). However, an earlier study by Stark and Tallal (1988) found that only 21 percent of the 6-year-olds in their cohort continued to have specific language impairment by 10 years of age. A 28-year follow-up of early-school-age children with and without speech disorders (Felsenfeld et al., 1992) showed that performance on measures of both speech and expressive and receptive language in the speech-impaired group in adulthood was poorer than that of controls. Because the participants in this sample were initially identified using a speech measure only, their language ability at intake is unknown.

Subsequently, Tomblin and colleagues (2003) found that 51 percent of 6-year-old children who met criteria for language disorder continued to have impaired language 2 years later. A similar statistically significant rate of persistence (52 percent) was found 4 years later. Additional analyses of the language growth trajectories of these children with language impairment showed that they had very stable patterns of growth, and their language status at age 16 was highly predicted by their language status at age 6 (Tomblin et al., 2014a). Thus, although these children showed growth in language over the span of 10 years, there was little evidence of any recovery or resolution of their language impairment. In another recent examination of persistence of language impairment, Rice and Hoffman (2015) followed 519 children from age 2 to age 22 with regard to their vocabulary development. The authors found that children with language impairment had poorer rates of vocabulary growth than the controls throughout childhood. They found "minimal[ly], but statistically significant" male–female differences in this pattern of growth (Rice and Hoffman, 2015, p. 356). The results of these longitudinal studies strongly support the earlier conclusion drawn by Stothard and colleagues (1998) that "if a child's language difficulties are still present at age 5-6 prognosis is likely to be poor and the child will be at high risk of language, literacy, and educational difficulties throughout childhood and adolescence" (p. 417). This conclusion directly parallels what is seen in speech disorder. In a follow-up study of children with speech disorders, Shriberg and Kwiatkowski (1988) note that "findings indicate that a high percentage of children continued to have speech and language and other special educational needs as they neared middle school and beyond. Many children eventually required special class placements" (p. 144).

Persistence of Stuttering (Fluency Disorders)

As with mild to moderate speech disorders and mild to moderate language disorders, relatively minor dysfluencies of preschool children tend to resolve by the time children enter school or shortly thereafter. In a longitudinal study, for example, Kloth and colleagues (2000) found that 7 of 93 preschool children identified as at high risk for stuttering persisted as stutterers 6 years later. In contrast, in more severe cases and cases in which the onset of stuttering occurs later (i.e., after the child enters school), the disorder tends to persist and often is lifelong, although some improvement can be seen through the teenage years (Howell and Davis, 2011; Yairi and Ambrose, 1999).

Summary

In summary, children who present with poor speech and language ability are likely to show long-term patterns of poor speech and language development throughout childhood. If deficits occur in early childhood and are not severe, the child's language outcomes may progress into the broad range of typical development by the end of the preschool years. However, deficits are likely to persist in young children with severe deficits and in those with other risk factors, such as other developmental disorders and challenging family environments. High rates of persistence become much more likely for children whose language deficits remain at the end of the preschool years. Thus, the determination of a persisting language disorder in early childhood is at best provisional.

FINDINGS AND CONCLUSIONS

This chapter has reviewed the literature on current standards of care for speech and language disorders in children, which of these disorders are amenable to treatment and the typical time course required for this treatment, and the persistence of these disorders. Based on its review of the best available evidence, the committee reached the following findings and conclusions.

Findings

Treatment

3-1. Few treatments exist that can alter the underlying cause of a speech or language disorder.
3-2. Alternative and augmentative communication treatment can provide nonspeech alternatives to speech that lead to functional gains in communication.
3-3. Speech and language therapy during the preschool years focuses on the promotion of implicit learning of an abstract system of principles and symbols.
3-4. In accordance with policies and practice guidelines, speech-language intervention often is conducted in the home and/or classroom and incorporates communication needs within the family and the educational curriculum.
3-5. Evidence indicates that speech and language therapy results in gains in the skills and behaviors targeted by the therapy.

Persistence

3-6. Toddlers who are late talkers often make developmental gains; however, these gains may be less likely in children whose condition is severe and who have other neurodevelopmental and socioeconomic risk factors.
3-7. Children with language disorders at the age of 5 or 6 are likely to have persistent language problems throughout childhood.

Conclusions

3-1. Severe speech and language disorders are likely to persist throughout childhood.

3-2. Speech and language therapy does not substantially alter the course of these disorders and thus is not curative; however, it provides improved function in those areas that are targeted.

3-3. Although there is a large literature on treatment effects, data are lacking on the effect of treatment on more general quality-of-life outcomes, particularly among children with severe disorders and those living in poverty.

REFERENCES

Adams, M. J., B. R. Foorman, I. Lundberg, and T. Beeler. 1998. *Phonemic awareness in young children: A classroom curriculum*. Baltimore, MD: Paul H. Brookes Publishing Co.

Almost, D., and P. Rosenbaum. 1998. Effectiveness of speech intervention for phonological disorders: A randomized controlled trial. *Developmental Medicine and Child Neurology* 40(5):319-325.

Andersen, G., T. R. Mjøen, and T. Vik. 2010. Prevalence of speech problems and the use of augmentative and alternative communication in children with cerebral palsy: A registry-based study in Norway. *SIG 12 Perspectives on Augmentative and Alternative Communication* 19(1):12-20.

ASHA (American Speech-Language-Hearing Association). 1999. *The guidelines for the roles and responsibilities of the school-based speech-language pathologist*. Rockville, MD: ASHA.

ASHA. 2004. *Preferred practice patterns for the profession of speech-language pathology*. http://www.asha.org/policy/PP2004-00191.htm (accessed September 29, 2015).

ASHA. n.d. *Federal Medicaid requirements speech, language, and hearing benefits*. http://www.asha.org/practice/reimbursement/medicaid/medicaid_intro.htm (accessed October 26, 2015).

Baker, E., and S. McLeod, S. 2011. Evidence-based practice for children with speech sound disorders. Part 1: Narrative review. *Language, Speech, and Hearing Services in Schools* 42(2):102-139.

Bandura, A. 1971. *Psychological modeling*. New York: Lieber-Antherton.

Barnes, S., M. Gutfreund, D. Satterly, and G. Wells. 1983. Characteristics of adult speech which predicts children's language development. *Journal of Child Language* 10(1):65-84.

Bates, E. 1976. *Language and context. Studies in the acquisition of pragmatics*. New York: Academic Press.

Bates, E., and B. MacWhinney. 1987. Competition, variation, and language learning. In *Mechanisms of language acquisition*, edited by B. MacWhinney. Hillsdale, NJ: Lawrence Erlbaum Associates. Pp. 157-193.

Bernthal, J. E., N. W. Bankson, and P. Flipsen. 2012. *Articulation and phonological disorders: Speech sound disorders in children*. New York: Pearson Higher Education.

Beukelman, D., and P. Mirenda. 2005. *Augmentative and alternative communication*. Baltimore, MD: Paul H. Brookes Publishing Co.

Bialystok, E., and E. B. Ryan. 1985. Toward a definition of metalinguistic skill. *Merrill-Palmer Quarterly* 31(3):229-251.

Blachman, B. A., E. W. Ball, R. Black, and D. M. Tangel. 2000. *Road to the code: A phonological awareness program for young children*. Baltimore, MD: Paul H. Brookes Publishing Co.

Bock, K., and Z. M. Griffin. 2000. The persistence of structural priming: Transient activation or implicit learning? *Journal of Experimental Psychology: General* 129(2):177.

Boehm, A. 1991. Assessment of basic relational concepts. *The psychoeducational assessment of preschool children* (2nd ed.), edited by B. A. Bracken. Boston, MA: Allyn and Bacon. Pp. 86-106.

Bondy, A., and L. Frost. 2001. The picture exchange communication system. *Behavior Modification* 25(5):725-744.

Boyle, J., E. McCartney, J. Forbes, and A. O'Hare. 2007. A randomised controlled trial and economic evaluation of direct versus indirect and individual versus group modes of speech and language therapy for children with primary language impairment. *Health Technology Assessment (Winchester, England)* 11(25):iii-iv, xi-xii, 1-139.

Bradshaw, M. L., P. R. Hoffman, and J. A. Norris. 1998. Efficacy of expansions and cloze procedures in the development of interpretations by preschool children exhibiting delayed language development. *Language, Speech, and Hearing Services in Schools* 29(2):85-95.

Brookhouser, P. E., and M. P. Moeller. 1986. Choosing the appropriate habilitative track for the newly identified hearing-impaired child. *Annals of Otology, Rhinology & Laryngology* 95(1):51-59.

Brown, A., and R. A. Ferrara. 1999. Diagnosing zones of proximal development. In *Critical assessments: The zone of proximal development*, Vol. III, edited by P. Lloyd and L. Vygotsky. New York: Routledge. Pp. 225-256.

Brown, R., and U. Bellugi. 1964. Three processes in the child's acquisition of syntax. *Harvard Educational Review* 34(2):133-151.

Bunce, B. H. 1991. Referential communication skills: Guidelines for therapy. *Language, Speech, and Hearing Services in Schools* 22(1):296-301.

Byrne-Saricks, M. C. 1987. Treatment of language disorders in children: A review of experimental studies. In *Human communication and its disorders*, edited by H. Winitz. Norwood, NJ: Ablex Publishing Corp. Pp. 167-201.

Bzoch, K. R. 1997. *Communicative disorders related to cleft lip and palate*. Austin, TX: PRO-ED, Inc.

Camarata, S. M. 1993. The application of naturalistic conversation training to speech production in children with speech disabilities. *Journal of Applied Behavior Analysis* 26(2):173-182.

Camarata, S. M. 2010. Word based phonological intervention: Issues and evidence. In *Phonological intervention in children*, edited by L. Williams, S. McCloud, and R. McCauley. Baltimore, MD: Paul H. Brookes Publishing Co. Pp. 381-406.

Camarata, S. M., K. E. Nelson, and M. N. Camarata. 1994. Comparison of conversational-recasting and imitative procedures for training grammatical structures in children with specific language impairment. *Journal of Speech, Language, and Hearing Research* 37(6):1414-1423.

Camarata, S. M., P. Yoder, and M. N. Camarata. 2006. Simultaneous treatment of grammatical and speech-comprehensibility deficits in children with Down syndrome. *Down Syndrome Research and Practice* 11(1):9-17.

Caravolas, M., C. Hulme, and M. J. Snowling. 2001. The foundations of spelling ability: Evidence from a 3-year longitudinal study. *Journal of Memory and Language* 45(4):751-774.

Carroll, J. M., and M. J. Snowling. 2004. Language and phonological skills in children at high risk of reading difficulties. *Journal of Child Psychology and Psychiatry* 45(3):631-640.

Catts, H. W., and A. G. Kamhi. 2005. *The connections between language and reading disabilities.* Mahwah, NJ: Lawrence Erlbaum Associates.

Cazden, C. B. 1965. *Environmental assistance to the child's acquisition of grammar.* Cambridge, MA: Harvard University.

Chomsky, N. 1986. *Knowledge of language: Its nature origins and use.* Westport, CT: Greenwood Publishing Group.

Chomsky, N., and Halle, M. 1968. *The sound pattern of English.* Cambridge, MA: MIT Press.

Cleave, P. L., S. D. Becker, M. K. Curran, A. J. O. Van Horne, and M. E. Fey. 2015. The efficacy of recasts in language intervention: A systematic review and meta-analysis. *American Journal of Speech-Language Pathology* 24(2):237-255.

CMS (Centers for Medicare & Medicaid Services). n.d. *Early and periodic screening, diagnostic, and treatment.* http://www.medicaid.gov/Medicaid-CHIP-Program-Information/By-Topics/Benefits/Early-and-Periodic-Screening-Diagnostic-and-Treatment.html (accessed October 26, 2015).

Cohen, W., A. Hodson, A. O'Hare, J. Boyle, T. Durrani, E. McCartney, M. Mattey, L. Naftalin, and J. Watson. 2005. Effects of computer-based intervention through acoustically modified speech (Fast ForWord) in severe mixed receptive-expressive language impairment: Outcomes from a randomized controlled trial. *Journal of Speech, Language, and Hearing Research* 48(3):715-729.

Coleman, P. K., and K. H. Karraker. 2003. Maternal self-efficacy beliefs, competence in parenting, and toddlers' behavior and developmental status. *Infant Mental Health Journal* 24(2):126-148.

Connell, P. J. 1987. An effect of modeling and imitation teaching procedures on children with and without specific language impairment. *Journal of Speech Language and Hearing Research* 30(1):105-113.

Connell, P. J., and C. A. Stone. 1992. Morpheme learning of children with specific language impairment under controlled instructional conditions. *Journal of Speech and Hearing Research* 35(4):844-852.

Conway, C. M., A. Bauernschmidt, S. S. Huang, and D. B. Pisoni. 2010. Implicit statistical learning in language processing: Word predictability is the key. *Cognition* 114(3):356-371.

Costantino, M. A., and M. Bonati. 2014. A scoping review of interventions to supplement spoken communication for children with limited speech or language skills. *PLoS ONE* 9(3):e90744.

Crosbie, S., A. Holm, and B. Dodd. 2005. Intervention for children with severe speech disorder: A comparison of two approaches. *International Journal of Language & Communication Disorders* 40(4):467-491.

Cross, T. 1978. Mother's speech and its association with rate of linguistic development in young children. In *The development of communication*, edited by N. Waterso and C. Snow. Chichester, England: Wiley & Sons. Pp. 199-216.

Dalal, R. H., and D. F. Loeb. 2005. Imitative production of regular past tense-ed by English-speaking children with specific language impairment. *International Journal of Language & Communication Disorders* 40(1):67-82.

Dale, P. S., and M. E. Hayiou-Thomas. 2013. Outcomes for late talkers: A twin study. In *Late talkers: Language development, interventions and outcomes*, edited by P. S. Dale and L. Rescorla. Baltimore, MD: Paul H. Brookes Publishing Co. Pp. 241-257.

Dale, P. S., C. Crain-Thoreson, A. Notari-Syverson, and K. Cole. 1996. Parent-child book reading as an intervention technique for young children with language delays. *Topics in Early Childhood Special Education* 16(2):213-235.

Desmarais, C., A. Sylvestre, F. Meyer, I. Bairati, and N. Rouleau. 2008. Systematic review of the literature on characteristics of late-talking toddlers. *International Journal of Language & Communication Disorders/Royal College of Speech & Language Therapists* 43(4):361-389.

Dodd, B. 2013. *Differential diagnosis and treatment of children with speech disorder*. New York: John Wiley & Sons.

Dollaghan, C. 2013. Late talker as a clinical category. In *Late talkers: Language development, interventions and outcomes*, edited by L. Rescorla and P. S. Dale. Baltimore, MD: Paul H. Brookes Publishing Co. Pp. 91-112.

Dunst, C. J., C. M. Trivette, and D. W. Hamby. 2008. *Research synthesis and meta-analysis of studies of family-centered practices*. Asheville, NC: Winterberry Press.

Ehri, L. C., S. R. Nunes, D. M. Willows, B. V. Schuster, Z. Yaghoub-Zadeh, and T. Shanahan. 2001. Phonemic awareness instruction helps children learn to read: Evidence from the National Reading Panel's meta-analysis. *Reading Research Quarterly* 36(3):250-287.

Elleman, A. M., E. J. Lindo, P. Morphy, and D. L. Compton. 2009. The impact of vocabulary instruction on passage-level comprehension of school-age children: A meta-analysis. *Journal of Research on Educational Effectiveness* 2(1):1-44.

Felsenfeld, S., P. A. Broen, and M. McGue. 1992. A 28-year follow-up of adults with a history of moderate phonological disorder: Linguistic and personality results. *Journal of Speech and Hearing Research* 35(5):1114-1125.

Fey, M. E., P. L. Cleave, S. H. Long, and D. L. Hughes. 1993. Two approaches to the facilitation of grammar in children with language impairment: An experimental evaluation. *Journal of Speech, Language, and Hearing Research* 36(1):141-157.

Fey, M. E., P. L. Cleave, and S. H. Long. 1997. Two models of grammar facilitation in children with language impairments: Phase 2. *Journal of Speech, Language, and Hearing Research* 40(1):5-19.

Fey, M. E., T. E. Krulik, D. F. Loeb, and K. Proctor-Williams. 1999. Sentence recast use by parents of children with typical language and children with specific language impairment. *American Journal of Speech-Language Pathology* 8(3):273.

Fey, M. E., S. H. Long, and L. H. Finestack. 2003. Ten principles of grammar facilitation for children with specific language impairments. *American Journal of Speech-Language Pathology* 12(1):3-15.

Fey, M. E., S. F. Warren, M. Fairchild, S. Sokol, and P. J. Yoder. 2006. Early effects of responsivity education/prelinguistic milieu teaching for children with developmental delays and their parents. *Journal of Speech, Language, and Hearing Research* 49(3):526-547.

Finestack, L. H., and M. E. Fey. 2013. *Evidence-based language intervention approaches for young late talkers*. In *Late talkers: Language development, interventions, and outcomes*, edited by L. A. Rescorla and P. S. Dale. Baltimore, MD: Paul H. Brookes Publishing Co. Pp. 283-302.

Flippin, M., S. Reszka, and L. R. Watson. 2010. Effectiveness of the Picture Exchange Communication System (PECS) on communication and speech for children with autism spectrum disorders: A meta-analysis. *American Journal of Speech-Language Pathology* 19(2):178-195.

Gevarter, C., M. F. O'Reilly, L. Rojeski, N. Sammarco, R. Lang, G. E. Lancioni, and J. Sigafoos. 2013. Comparisons of intervention components within augmentative and alternative communication systems for individuals with developmental disabilities: A review of the literature. *Research in Developmental Disabilities* 34(12):4404-4414.

Gierut, J. A. 1990. Differential learning of phonological oppositions. *Journal of Speech, Language, and Hearing Research* 33(3):540-549.

Gillam, R. B., D. F. Loeb, L. M. Hoffman, T. Bohman, C. A. Champlin, L. Thibodeau, J. Widen, J. Brandel, and S. Friel-Patti. 2008. The efficacy of Fast ForWord language intervention in school-age children with language impairment: A randomized controlled trial. *Journal of Speech, Language, and Hearing Research* 51(1):97-119.

Girolametto, L., M. Verbey, and R. Tannock. 1994. Improving joint engagement in parent-child interaction: An intervention study. *Journal of Early Intervention* 18(2):155-167.

Girolametto, L., E. Weitzman, and J. Clements-Baartman. 1998. Vocabulary intervention for children with Down syndrome: Parent training using focused stimulation. *Infant-Toddler Intervention: The Transdisciplinary Journal* 8(2):109-125.

Goldfield, B. A. 1987. The contributions of child and caregiver to referential and expressive language. *Applied Psycholinguistics* 8(3):267-280.

Guitar, B. 2013. *Stuttering: An integrated approach to its nature and treatment.* Philadelphia, PA: Lippincott Williams & Wilkins.

Hadley, P. A. 2014. Approaching early grammatical intervention from a sentence-focused framework. *Language, Speech, and Hearing Services in Schools* 45(2):110-116.

Hardin-Jones, M. A., and D. L. Jones. 2005. Speech production of preschoolers with cleft palate. *The Cleft Palate-Craniofacial Journal* 42(1):7-13.

Hart, B., and T. R. Risley. 1975. Incidental teaching of language in the preschool. *Journal of Applied Behavior Analysis* 8(4):411-420.

Hart, B., and T. R. Risley. 1995. *Meaning differences in the everyday experiences of young American children.* Baltimore, MD: Paul H. Brookes Publishing Co.

Hemmeter, M. L., and A. P. Kaiser. 1994. Enhanced milieu teaching effects of parent-implemented language intervention. *Journal of Early Intervention* 18(3):269-289.

Himmelmann, K., K. Lindh, and M. J. C. Hidecker. 2013. Communication ability in cerebral palsy: A study from the CP register of western Sweden. *European Journal of Paediatric Neurology* 17(6):568-574.

Hodson, B. W., and E. P. Paden. 1981. Phonological processes which characterize unintelligible and intelligible speech in early childhood. *Journal of Speech and Hearing Disorders* 46(4):369-373.

Hoover, W. A., and P. B. Gough. 1990. The simple view of reading. *Reading and Writing* 2(2):127-160.

Howell, P., and S. Davis. 2011. Predicting persistence of and recovery from stuttering by the teenage years based on information gathered at age 8 years. *Journal of Developmental & Behavioral Pediatrics* 32(3):196-205.

Huttenlocher, J., W. Haight, A. Bryk, M. Seltzer, and T. Lyons. 1991. Early vocabulary growth: Relation to language input and gender. *Developmental Psychology* 27(2): 236-248.

Ingersoll, B., and K. Lalonde. 2010. The impact of object and gesture imitation training on language use in children with autism spectrum disorder. *Journal of Speech, Language, and Hearing Research* 53(4):1040-1051.

Ingram, D. 1981. *Procedures for the phonological analysis of children's language*, Vol. 2. Baltimore, MD: University Park Press.

Johnson, C. J., J. Beitchman, A. Young, M. D. Escobar, L. Atkinson, B. Wilson, E. B. Brownlie, L. Douglas, N. Taback, I. Lam, and M. Wang. 1999. Fourteen-year follow-up of children with and without speech/language impairments: Speech/language stability and outcomes. *Journal of Speech-Language-Hearing Research* 42(3):744-760.

Jones, T. L., and R. J. Prinz. 2005. Potential roles of parental self-efficacy in parent and child adjustment: A review. *Clinical Psychology Review* 25(3):341-363.

Justice, L. M., and H. K. Ezell. 2000. Enhancing children's print and word awareness through home-based parent intervention. *American Journal of Speech-Language Pathology* 9(3): 257-269.

Justice, L. M., and J. N. Kaderavek. 2004. Embedded-explicit emergent literacy intervention. I: Background and description of approach. *Language, Speech, and Hearing Services in Schools* 35(3):201-211.

Justice, L. M., A. Mashburn, K. L. Pence, and A. Wiggins. 2008. Experimental evaluation of a preschool language curriculum: Influence on children's expressive language skills. *Journal of Speech, Language, and Hearing Research* 51(4):983-1001.

Kasari, C., A. C. Gulsrud, C. Wong, S. Kwon, and J. Locke. 2010. Randomized controlled caregiver mediated joint engagement intervention for toddlers with autism. *Journal of Autism and Developmental Disorders* 40(9):1045-1056.

Kloth, S. A. M., F. W. Kraaimaat, P. Janssen, and G. J. Brutten. 2000. Persistence and remission of incipient stuttering among high-risk children. *Journal of Fluency Disorders* 24(4):253-265.

Kouri, T. A. 2005. Lexical training through modeling and elicitation procedures with late talkers who have specific language impairment and developmental delays. *Journal of Speech, Language, and Hearing Research* 48(1):157-171.

Kurtz, P. F., M. D. Chin, J. M. Huete, R. S. Tarbox, J. T. O'Connor, T. R. Paclawskyj, and K. S. Rush. 2003. Functional analysis and treatment of self-injurious behavior in young children: A summary of 30 cases. *Journal of Applied Behavior Analysis* 36(2):205-219.

Landry, S. H., K. E. Smith, C. L. Miller-Loncar, and P. R. Swank. 1997. Predicting cognitive-language and social growth curves from early maternal behaviors in children at varying degrees of biological risk. *Developmental Psychology* 33(6):1040.

Landry, S. H., K. E. Smith, P. R., Swank, and C. L. Miller-Loncar. 2000. Early maternal and child influences on children's later independent cognitive and social functioning. *Child Development* 71(2):358-375.

Landry, S. H., K. E. Smith, P. R. Swank, M. A. Assel, and S. Vellet. 2001. Does early responsive parenting have a special importance for children's development or is consistency across early childhood necessary? *Developmental Psychology* 37(3):387.

Landry, S. H., K. E. Smith, and P. R. Swank. 2006. Responsive parenting: Establishing early foundations for social, communication, and independent problem-solving skills. *Developmental Psychology* 42(4):627.

Law, J., and G. Conti-Ramsden. 2000. Treating children with speech and language impairments: Six hours of therapy is not enough. *British Medical Journal* 321(7266):908.

Law, J., Z. Garrett, and C. Nye. 2004. The efficacy of treatment for children with developmental speech and language delay/disorder: A meta-analysis. *Journal of Speech, Language, and Hearing Research* 47(4):924-943.

Law, J., Z. Garrett, and C. Nye. 2008. Speech and language therapy interventions for children with primary speech and language delay or disorder. *The Cochrane Collaboration* 1:1-62.

Leonard, L. B. 1981. Facilitating linguistic skills in children with specific language impairment. *Applied Psycholinguistics* 2:8118.

Leonard, L. B., R. G. Schwartz, K. Chapman, L. E. Rowan, P. A. Prelock, B. Terrell, A. L. Weiss, and C. Messick. 1982. Early lexical acquisition in children with specific language impairment. *Journal of Speech, Language, and Hearing Research* 25(4):554-564.

Leonard, L. B., S. M. Camarata, B. Brown, and M. N. Camarata. 2004. Tense and agreement in the speech of children with specific language impairment patterns of generalization through intervention. *Journal of Speech, Language, and Hearing Research* 47(6):1363-1379.

Levy, E. S., L. O. Ramig, and S. M. Camarata. 2012. The effects of two speech interventions on speech function in pediatric dysarthria. *Journal of Medical Speech-Language Pathology* 20(4):82-87.

Lonigan, C. J., and G. J. Whitehurst. 1998. Relative efficacy of parent and teacher involvement in a shared-reading intervention for preschool children from low-income backgrounds. *Early Childhood Research Quarterly* 13(2):263-290.

Lovelace, S., and S. R. Stewart. 2007. Increasing print awareness in preschoolers with language impairment using non-evocative print referencing. *Language, Speech, and Hearing Services in Schools* 38(1):16-30.

Maas, E., C. E. Gildersleeve-Neumann, K. J. Jakielski, and R. Stoeckel. 2014. Motor-based intervention protocols in treatment of childhood apraxia of speech (CAS). *Current Developmental Disorders Reports* 1(3):197-206.

Mahoney, G., A. Kaiser, L. Girolametto, J. MacDonald, C. Robinson, P. Safford, and D. Spiker. 1999. Parent education in early intervention: A call for a renewed focus. *Topics in Early Childhood Special Education* 19(3):131-140.

Marton, K., B. Abramoff, and S. Rosenzweig. 2005. Social cognition and language in children with specific language impairment (SLI). *Journal of Communication Disorders* 38(2):143-162.

Marulis, L. M., and S. B. Neuman. 2010. The effects of vocabulary intervention on young children's word learning: A meta-analysis. *Review of Educational Research* 80(3):300-335.

Matthews, D., E. Lieven, A. Theakston, and M. Tomasello. 2005. The role of frequency in the acquisition of English word order. *Cognitive Development* 20(1):121-136.

McGinty, A., and L. Justice. 2006. Classroom-based versus pullout interventions: A review of the experimental evidence. *EBP Briefs* 1(1):3-25.

McLeod, S. 2006. An holistic view of a child with unintelligible speech: Insights from the ICF and ICF-CY. *International Journal of Speech-Language Pathology* 8(3):293-315.

McLeod, S., and K. Bleile. 2004. The ICF: A framework for setting goals for children with speech impairment. *Child Language Teaching and Therapy* 20(3):199-219.

McWilliam, R. 1995. Integration of therapy and consultative special education: A continuum in early intervention. *Infants & Young Children* 7(4):29-38.

Mezynski, K. 1983. Issues concerning the acquisition of knowledge: Effects of vocabulary training on reading comprehension. *Review of Educational Research* 53(2):253-279.

Moerk, E. L. 1983. A behavioral analysis of controversial topics in first language acquisition: Reinforcements, corrections, modeling, input frequencies, and the three-term contingency pattern. *Journal of Psycholinguistic Research* 12(2):129-155.

Morgan, A. T., and A. P. Vogel. 2008. Intervention for childhood apraxia of speech. *The Cochrane Database of Systematic Reviews* 16(3).

Nelson, K., and J. Gruendel. 1986. *Event knowledge: Structure and function in development.* Mahwah, NJ: Lawrence Erlbaum Associates.

Nelson, K. E., G. Carskaddon, and J. D. Bonvillian. 1973. Syntax acquisition: Impact of experimental variation in adult verbal interaction with the child. *Child Development* 44(3):497-504.

Nelson, K. E., S. M. Camarata, J. Welsh, L. Butkovsky, and M. Camarata. 1996. Effects of imitative and conversational recasting treatment on the acquisition of grammar in children with specific language impairment and younger language-normal children. *Journal of Speech, Language, and Hearing Research* 39(4):850-859.

Nemoy, E., and S. Davis. 1954. *The correction of defective consonant sounds.* Magnolia, MA: The Expression Company.

Newport, E. L., and R. P. Meier. 1985. *The acquisition of American Sign Language.* Hillsdale, NJ: Lawrence Erlbaum Associates.

Niparko, J. K., E. A. Tobey, D. J. Thal, L. S. Eisenberg, N.-Y. Wang, A. L. Quittner, and N. E. Fink. 2010. Spoken language development in children following cochlear implantation. *Journal of the American Medical Association* 303(15):1498-1506.

Nippold, M. A., T. C. Mansfield, J. L. Billow, and J. B. Tomblin. 2008. Expository discourse in adolescents with language impairments: Examining syntactic developments. *American Journal of Speech-Language Pathology* 17:356-366.

Nye, C., S. H. Foster, and D. Seaman. 1987. Effectiveness of language intervention with the language/learning disabled. *Journal of Speech and Hearing Disorders* 52(4):348-357.

Nye, C., M. Vanryckeghem, J. B. Schwartz, C. Herder, H. M. Turner, and C. Howard. 2013. Behavioral stuttering interventions for children and adolescents: A systematic review and meta-analysis. *Journal of Speech, Language, and Hearing Research* 56(3):921-932.

Owens, Jr., R. E. 2013. *Language disorders: A functional approach to assessment and intervention.* New York: Pearson Higher Ed.

Paul, R. 1993. Patterns of development in late talkers: Preschool years. *Communication Disorders Quarterly* 15(1):7-14.

Paul, R., and C. Norbury. 2012. *Language disorders from infancy through adolescence: Listening, speaking, reading, writing, and communicating.* St. Louis, MO: Elsevier Mosby.

Paul, R., and S. E. Weismer. 2013. Late talking in contex: The clinicial implications of delayed language development. In *Late talkers: Language development, interventions and outcomes,* edited by P. S. Dale and L. Rescorla. Baltimore, MD: Paul H. Brookes Publishing Co. Pp. 203-218.

Peña, E. D., and R. Quinn. 2003. developing effective collaboration teams in speech-language pathology: A case study. *Communication Disorders Quarterly* 24(2):53-63.

Pinker, S. 1984. *Language learnability and language development.* Cambridge, MA: Harvard University Press.

Plante, E., T. Ogilvie, R. Vance, J. M. Aguilar, N. S. Dailey, C. Meyers, A. M. Lieser, and R. Burton. 2014. Variability in the language input to children enhances learning in a treatment context. *American Journal of Speech-Language Pathology* 23(4):530-545.

Preston, D., and M. Carter. 2009. A review of the efficacy of the picture exchange communication system intervention. *Journal of Autism and Developmental Disorders* 39(10): 1471-1486.

Proctor-Williams, K., M. E. Fey, and D. F. Loeb. 2001. Parental recasts and production of copulas and articles by children with specific language impairment and typical language. *American Journal of Speech-Language Pathology* 10(2):155-168.

Rescorla, L., and E. Schwartz. 1990. Outcome of toddlers with specific expressive language delay. *Applied Psycholinguistics* 11(4):393-407.

Rescorla, L., J. Mirak, and L. Singh. 2000. Vocabulary growth in late talkers: Lexical development from 2; 0 to 3; 0. *Journal of Child Language* 27(2):293-311.

Rice, M. L., and L. Hoffman. 2015. Predicting vocabulary growth in children with and without specific language impairment: a longitudinal study from 2; 6 to 21 years of age. *Journal of Speech, Language, and Hearing Research* 58(2):345-359.

Rice, M. L., S. F. Warren, and S. K. Betz. 2005. Language symptoms of developmental language disorders: An overview of autism, Down syndrome, fragile X, specific language impairment, and Williams syndrome. *Applied Psycholinguistics* 26(1):7-27.

Roberts, M. Y., and A. P. Kaiser. 2011. The effectiveness of parent-implemented language interventions: A meta-analysis. *American Journal of Speech-Language Pathology* 20(3): 180-199.

Robertson, S. B., and S. E. Weismer. 1999. Effects of treatment on linguistic and social skills in toddlers with delayed language development. *Journal of Speech, Language, and Hearing Research* 42(5):1234-1248.

Romski, M., and R. A. Sevcik. 2005. Augmentative communication and early intervention: Myths and realities. *Infants & Young Children* 18(3):174-185.

Roth, F. P., D. L. Speece, D. H. Cooper, and S. De La Paz. 1996. Unresolved mysteries: How do metalinguistic and narrative skills connect with early reading? *Journal of Special Education* 30(3):257-277.

Rowe, M. L. 2008. Child-directed speech: relation to socioeconomic status, knowledge of child development and child vocabulary skill. *Journal of Child Language* 35(1):185-205.

Rush, D. D., and M. L. Shelden. 2008. Tips and techniques for effective coaching interactions. *Brief Case* 1(2):1-4.

Scarborough, H. 2001. Connecting early language and literacy to later reading (dis)abilities: Evidence, theory, and practice. In *Handbook for research in early literacy*, edited by S. Neuman and D. Dickinson. New York: Guilford Press. Pp. 97-110.

Schank, R. C., and R. P. Ableson. 1977. *Scripts, plans, goals, and understanding*. Hillsdale, NJ: Lawrence Earlbaum Associates.

Schlosser, R. W., and J. Sigafoos. 2006. Augmentative and alternative communication interventions for persons with developmental disabilities: Narrative review of comparative single-subject experimental studies. *Research in Developmental Disabilities* 27(1):1-29.

Schneider, P., and R. V. Watkins. 1996. Applying Vygotskian developmental theory to language intervention. *Language, Speech, and Hearing Services in Schools* 27(2):157-170.

Schooling, T., R. Venediktov, and H. Leech. 2010. *Evidence-based systematic review: Effects of service delivery on the speech and language skills of children from birth to 5 years of age*. Rockville, MD: ASHA.

Schuele, C. M., and L. Tolbert. 2001. Omissions of obligatory relative markers in children with specific language impairment. *Clinical Linguistics & Phonetics* 15(4):257-274.

Shriberg, L. D., and J. Kwiatkowski. 1980. *Natural process analysis (NPA)*. Hoboken, NJ: John Wiley & Sons.

Shriberg, L. D., and J. Kwiatkowski. 1988. A follow-up study of children with phonologic disorders of unknown origin. *Journal of Speech & Hearing Disorders* 53(2):144-155.

Shriberg, L. D., D. M. Aram, and J. Kwiatkowski. 1997. Developmental Apraxia of Speech III. A Subtype Marked by Inappropriate Stress. *Journal of Speech, Language, and Hearing Research* 40(2):313-337.

Simon, C. S. 1987. Out of the broom closet and into the classroom: The emerging SLP. *Communication Disorders Quarterly* 11(1):41-66.

Snow, C. E. 1991. The theoretical basis for relationships between language and literacy in development. *Journal of Research in Childhood Education* 6(1):5-10.

Snowling, M. J., and C. Hulme. 2011. Evidence-based interventions for reading and language difficulties: Creating a virtuous circle. *British Journal of Educational Psychology* 81(1):1-23.

St Clair, M. C., P. Monaghan, and M. H. Christiansen. 2010. Learning grammatical categories from distributional cues: Flexible frames for language acquisition. *Cognition* 116(3):341-360.

Stark, R. E., and P. Tallal. 1988. *Language, speech, and reading disorders in children*. Boston, MA: Little, Brown and Co.

Storkel, H. L. 2004. The emerging lexicon of children with phonological delays: Phonotactic constraints and probability in acquisition. *Journal of Speech, Language, and Hearing Research* 47(5):1194-1212.

Stothard, S. E., M. J. Snowling, D. V. M. Bishop, B. B. Chipchase, and C. A. Kaplan. 1998. Language-impaired preschoolers: A follow-up into adolescence. *Journal of Speech Language and Hearing Research* 41(2):407-418.

Strong, G. K., C. J. Torgerson, D. Torgerson, and C. Hulme. 2011. A systematic meta-analytic review of evidence for the effectiveness of the "Fast ForWord" language intervention program. *Journal of Child Psychology and Psychiatry* 52(3):224-235.

Swift, W. 1918. *Speech defects in school age children.* Boston, MA: Houghton Mifflin Harcourt.

Szagun, G., and B. Stumper. 2012. Age or experience? The influence of age at implantation, social and linguistic environment on language development in children with cochlear implants. *Journal of Speech Language and Hearing Research* 55(6):1640-1654.

Tallal, P., S. L. Miller, G. Bedi, G. Byma, X. Wang, S. S. Nagarajan, C. Schreiner, W. M. Jenkins, and M. M. Merzenich. 1996. Language comprehension in language-learning impaired children improved with acoustically modified speech. *Science* 271(5245):81-84.

Tamis-LeMonda, C. S., M. H. Bornstein, L. Baumwell, and A. Melstein Damast. 1996. Responsive parenting in the second year: Specific influences on children's language and play. *Early Development and Parenting* 5(4):173-183.

Thal, D. 1991. Language and cognition in normal and late-talking toddlers. *Topics in Language Disorders* 11(4):33-42.

Thal, D., V. Marchman, and J. B. Tomblin. 2013. Late-talking toddlers: Characterization and prediction continued delay. In *Late talkers: Language development, interventions, and outcomes*, edited by P. S. Dale and L. Rescorla. Baltimore, MD: Paul H. Brookes Publishing Co. Pp. 169-202.

Tomblin, J. B., L. Spencer, S. Flock, R. Tyler, and B. Gantz. 1999. A comparison of language achievement in children with cochlear implants and children using hearing aids. *Journal of Speech Language and Hearing Research* 42(2):497-509.

Tomblin, J. B., X. Zhang, P. Buckwalter, and M. O'Brien. 2003. The stability of primary language disorder: Four years after kindergarten diagnosis. *Journal of Speech Language and Hearing Research* 46(6):1283-1296.

Tomblin, J. B., M. A. Nippold, and M. Fey. 2014a. The character and course of individual differences in spoken language. In *Understanding individual differences in language development across the school years*, edited by J. B. Tomblin and M. A. Nippold. New York: Psychological Press. Pp. 47-78.

Tomblin, J. B., J. J. Oleson, S. E. Ambrose, E. Walker, and M. Moeller. 2014b. The influence of hearing aids on the speech and language development of children with hearing loss. *JAMA Otolaryngology—Head & Neck Surgery* 140(5):403-409.

Trivette, C. M., C. J. Dunst, and D. W. Hamby. 2010. Influences of family-systems intervention practices on parent-child interactions and child development. *Topics in Early Childhood Special Education* 30(1):3-19.

Ukoumunne, O. C., M. Wake, J. Carlin, E. L. Bavin, J. Lum, J. Skeat, J. Williams, L. Conway, E. Cini, and S. Reilly. 2011. Profiles of language development in pre-school children: A longitudinal latent class analysis of data from the Early Language in Victoria Study. *Child: Care, Health and Development* 38(3):341-349.

U.S. Bureau of Labor Statistics. 2014. *Occupational outlook handbook.* http://www.bls.gov/ooh (accessed July 17, 2015).

van Kleeck, A., J. Vander Woude, and L. Hammett. 2006. Fostering literal and inferential language skills in Head Start preschoolers with language impairment using scripted book-sharing discussions. *American Journal of Speech-Language Pathology* 15(1):85-95.

Vasilyeva, M., J. Huttenlocher, and H. Waterfall. 2006. Effects of language intervention on syntactic skill levels in preschoolers. *Developmental Psychology* 42(1):164.

Wallach, G. P. 2008. *Language intervention for school-age students: Setting goals for academic success.* St. Louis, MO: Elsevier Health Sciences.

Warren, S. F., S. L. Bredin-Oja, M. Fairchild, L. H. Finestack, M. E. Fey, N. C. Brady, and R. J. McCauley. 2006. Responsivity education/prelinguistic milieu teaching. In *Treatment of language disorders in children*, edited by R. J. McCauley and M. D. Fey. Baltimore, MD: Paul H. Brookes Publishing Co. Pp. 47-75.

Warren, S. F., M. E. Fey, L. H. Finestack, N. C. Brady, S. L. Bredin-Oja, and K. K. Fleming. 2008. A randomized trial of longitudinal effects of low-intensity responsivity education/prelinguistic milieu teaching. *Journal of Speech, Language, and Hearing Research* 51(2):451-470.

Weismer, S. E. 1997. The role of stress in language processing and intervention. *Topics in Language Disorders* 17(4):41-52.

Weismer, S. E., and J. Murray-Branch. 1989. Modeling versus modeling plus evoked production training: A comparison of two language intervention methods. *Journal of Speech and Hearing Disorders* 54(2):269-281.

Weismer, S. E., J. Murray-Branch, and J. Miller. 1994. A prospective longitudinal study of language development in late talkers. *Journal of Speech and Hearing Research* 37(4): 852-867.

Whitehurst, G. J., D. S. Arnold, J. N. Epstein, A. L. Angell, M. Smith, and J. E. Fischel. 1994. A picture book reading intervention in day care and home for children from low-income families. *Developmental Psychology* 30(5):679.

Whitman, R. L., and E. R. Schwartz. 1985. The pediatrician's approach to the preschool child with language delay. *Clinical Pediatrics* 24(1):26-31.

Williams, A. L. 2000. Multiple oppositions theoretical foundations for an alternative contrastive intervention approach. *American Journal of Speech-Language Pathology* 9(4): 282-288.

Williams, A. L., S. McLeod, and R. J. McCauley. 2010. *Interventions for speech sound disorders in children*. Baltimore, MD: Paul H. Brookes Publishing Co.

Yairi, E., and N. G. Ambrose. 1999. Early childhood stuttering. I: Persistency and recovery rates. *Journal of Speech, Language, and Hearing Research* 42(5):1097-1112.

Yoder, P. J., and S. F. Warren. 1998. Maternal responsivity predicts the prelinguistic communication intervention that facilitates generalized intentional communication. *Journal of Speech, Language, and Hearing Research* 41(5):1207-1219.

Yoder, P. J., and S. F. Warren. 2001. Relative treatment effects of two prelinguistic communication interventions on language development in toddlers with developmental delays vary by maternal characteristics. *Journal of Speech, Language, and Hearing Research* 44(1):224-237.

Yoder, P. J., and S. F. Warren. 2002. Effects of prelinguistic milieu teaching and parent responsivity education on dyads involving children with intellectual disabilities. *Journal of Speech, Language, and Hearing Research* 45(6):1158-1174.

Yoder, P., S. Camarata, and E. Gardner. 2005. Treatment effects on speech intelligibility and length of utterance in children with specific language and intelligibility impairments. *Journal of Early Intervention* 28(1):34-49.

Yoder, P., M. E. Fey, and S. F. Warren. 2012. Studying the impact of intensity is important but complicated. *International Journal of Speech-Language Pathology* 14(5):410-413.

Zebrowski, P. M., and R. L. Schum. 1993. Counseling parents of children who stutter. *American Journal of Speech-Language Pathology* 2(2):65-73.

4

Supplemental Security Income for Children with Speech and Language Disorders

Preceding chapters address the role of speech and language in the health and development of children, factors associated with speech and language disorders and their impact (especially when the disorders are severe), the disorders' persistence, and approaches to and prospects for treatment. This chapter offers a programmatic context for the committee's task, which is to examine the intersection of speech and language disorders in children and the Supplemental Security Income (SSI) program. The chapter reviews the purpose of the SSI program for children, as well as how this purpose is accomplished through the program's design and operations. It also considers the application of this programmatic design and these operational features to children from low-income, resource-limited households with suspected speech and language disorders potentially severe enough to make them eligible for SSI benefits.

This committee was tasked with comparing trends in the prevalence and persistence of speech and language disorders among the general population of children under 18 and those who receive SSI. The purpose of this comparison is to provide the Social Security Administration (SSA) with insight into the extent to which the proportion of children receiving SSI benefits for speech and language disorders can be considered reasonable given (1) the proportion of children in the general population with such impairments, (2) the interaction between poverty and disability generally and poverty and speech and language disorders in particular, and (3) the SSI eligibility criteria and decision-making process. Therefore, understanding the SSI program design and process is integral to understanding the health characteristics of children who receive SSI benefits on the basis of speech and language disorders.

This chapter begins with an overview of the history of the SSI program for children. It then describes children served by the program and how eligibility is determined. Next, the chapter reviews the program's eligibility and determination process, including the speech and language-related criteria that apply when children's eligibility is evaluated and the SSA's process for that evaluation, as well as the number of child SSI recipients that results from this process. The chapter also summarizes the committee's approach to the use and interpretation of SSI administrative data. The final section presents the committee's findings and conclusions.

HISTORY OF THE SUPPLEMENTAL SECURITY INCOME PROGRAM FOR CHILDREN[1]

Created by the Social Security Amendments of 1972 (Public Law 92-603), the SSI program came into effect in 1974 and was developed to replace disparate state-based benefit programs for the needy aged, blind, and disabled population. The program was intended to provide a supplemental form of income support to particularly disadvantaged households. Administered by the SSA, the program provides monthly payments to persons who meet its eligibility standards. SSI recipients include children whose health conditions or disabilities are severe enough to meet the program's disability eligibility criteria and whose family income and assets do not exceed limits imposed by the SSA (Fremstad and Vallas, 2012). In December 2014, nearly 1.3 million children were receiving SSI payments (SSA, 2015b).

The administration of the SSI program is complex—the product of the legislation itself, its implementing regulations, and important judicial decisions. Understanding how the program has evolved over the past 40 years is essential to understanding disability trends observed among children participating in the program. Understanding the program's evolution in turn requires disentangling the standards and procedures under the statute and its implementing regulations. The following subsections provide a brief overview; a more detailed version of the program's history can be found in the recent report *Mental Disorders and Disabilities Among Low-Income Children* (NASEM, 2015).

When signed into law by President Nixon in 1972, the children's SSI program had a simple aim: "Disabled children living in low-income

[1] Much of this section on the history of the SSI program was adapted from the concurrent study on mental disorders in children, *Mental Disorders and Disabilities Among Low-Income Children* (NASEM, 2015).

households are among the most disadvantaged of all Americans and are deserving of special assistance. . . . Poor children with disabilities should be eligible for SSI benefits because their needs are often greater than non-disabled children" (U.S. House of Representatives, 1971).

SSI eligibility standards for children have evolved in three distinct phases. The first phase extended from program implementation in 1974 to 1990. The second phase began in 1990 with the U.S. Supreme Court's decision in *Sullivan v. Zebley*[2] and lasted until the third phase. That phase began with the 1996 passage of the Personal Responsibility and Work Opportunity Reconciliation Act,[3] which narrowed the definition of disability for children. Each phase is described in turn below.

SSI Childhood Disability Eligibility Standards from 1974 to 1990

From 1974 to 1990, the Social Security Act set a "comparable severity standard" for determining children's eligibility for benefits. Specifically, the statute allowed eligibility "in the case of a child under the age of 18, if he suffers from any medically determinable physical or mental impairment of comparable severity . . . to one that would result in disability in an adult." In its initial interpretation and application of this standard, the SSA used an approach that was significantly narrower than that used for adults. In the case of adults, a determination of disability is based on a "five-step test."[4] This test begins by assessing (1) whether the adult is engaged in substantial gainful activity and (2) whether the adult's disability can be expected to last at least 1 year (the durational standard) or result in death. If both of these conditions are met, then in the third step, the SSA determines whether the claimant's impairment either "matches or is equal to" one of the listed medical impairments in the SSA's Listing of Impairments[5]—or "Listings"—for adults. If so, the adult is determined to qualify for SSI benefits. If not, then in the fourth and fifth steps, the SSA evaluates "whether the claimant can do his own past work or any other work that exists in the national economy."[6]

In the period between implementation of the program and the *Zebley* court decision in 1990, children's eligibility determinations underwent only the first three steps used for adults (i.e., a review of substantial gainful

---

[2] *Sullivan v. Zebley*, 493 U.S. 521 (1990).

[3] Personal Responsibility and Work Opportunity Reconciliation Act, Public Law 104-193 (104th Congress).

[4] The disability determination process for adults continues to include the "five-step test"; see http://www.ssa.gov/policy/docs/rsnotes/rsn2013-01.html (accessed September 30, 2015).

[5] The Listing of Impairments was issued by the SSA and used to identify medical conditions for purposes of determining disability (see the glossary of terms in Appendix A).

[6] 493 U.S. at 523-524.

activity, the minimum duration requirement, and meeting or equaling one of the Listings). In other words, the eligibility determination process for children was an abbreviated[7] version of the adult test, lacking the fourth and fifth steps because they addressed employment-related questions that did not apply to most children. Therefore, if a child did not satisfy the third step of the test—that is, did not have an impairment that either matched or medically equaled a listed impairment for adults—benefits would be denied. There then would be "no further inquiry,"[8] even though the level of disability required to meet or equal a Listing was higher than the statutory requirement for degree of disability.

Sullivan v. Zebley and Its Impact (1990-1996)

In 1990, the U.S. Supreme Court decided *Sullivan v. Zebley*, a landmark case originally filed in 1983. This case challenged the legality of the SSA's implementation of the SSI children's program. The plaintiffs argued that by failing to include an assessment of function in the determination of children's eligibility, the SSA's standards and procedures contravened the terms of the SSI statute itself. The plaintiffs' argument was based on the fact that although the law specified that a child would qualify for benefits if "he suffers from any . . . impairment of comparable severity to one that would render an adult unable to engage in any substantial gainful activity,"[9] the SSA had failed to ensure equal treatment by its failure to develop a functional test for children. "In plain words, the . . . provisions mean that a child is entitled to benefits if his impairment is as severe as one that would prevent an adult from working."[10]

The Supreme Court ruled in *Zebley* that the SSA's Listings-only policy for determining children's disability status was inconsistent with the program's "comparable severity" standard. The Court asserted that for children, the "Secretary explicitly has set the medical criteria defining the listed impairments at a higher level of severity than the statutory standard."[11] According to the Court, this omission amounted to a violation of the law because "the Listings obviously do not cover all illnesses and abnormalities that actually can be disabling."[12] Indeed, the Court noted that the 1979 rules themselves made clear that the Listings did not offer a complete description of children's disability, since they stated that "the Listing criteria

[7] 493 U.S. at 523-524.
[8] 493 U.S. at 526.
[9] 493 U.S. at 526.
[10] 493 U.S. at 529.
[11] 529 U.S. at 530.
[12] 529 U.S. at 530.

are intended to identify the more commonly occurring impairments."[13] Furthermore, the Court pointed out that even those medical conditions covered in the SSA's Listings use definitions that exceed the level of severity specified in the law itself. As a result, the inability to meet or equal the standards of the Listings had the potential to exclude claimants with impairments severe enough to preclude *substantial* gainful activity but not severe enough to prevent *any* gainful activity.[14] The Court determined that the SSA's approach excluded not only claimants whose impairments "actually" precluded work but also those "who have unlisted impairments, or [a] combination of impairments, that do not fulfill all of the criteria for any one listed impairment."[15] For these reasons, the "child-disability regulations are simply inconsistent with the statutory standard of 'comparable severity.'"[16] Holding that the SSA's standard was "manifestly contrary to the statute" because it lacked an individualized functional assessment, the Court's decision led to a new approach to determining disability in children.

In implementing *Zebley*, the SSA issued new regulations that provided for an individual functional assessment for children. This assessment used a severity rating scale to evaluate a child's day-to-day functioning across six domains.[17] It evaluated whether a child's impairments "substantially" reduced his or her ability to function "independently, appropriately, and effectively in an age-appropriate manner."[18] This functional assessment expanded how children who met the program's financial eligibility standards could be determined to have a qualifying disability.

Following *Zebley*'s implementation, a child's eligibility might continue to turn on a finding that the applicant had an impairment that met or equaled a Listing and that such impairment could be expected to last for at least 12 months or result in death. Alternatively, and consistent with the determination process used for adults, a child's eligibility could rest on a determination that one or more impairments substantially reduced age-appropriate, independent, and effective functioning. In mid- to late 1994, the SSA introduced an impairment code for speech and language disorders, which is discussed in detail in the following subsection.[19]

The adoption of the functional disability test in *Zebley*'s wake, coupled with new impairment codes and revised Listings for mental disorders that took effect in 1990, had an upward impact on SSI eligibility and enrollment for children and adolescents. Furthermore, as initial application approvals

---

[13] 529 U.S. at 530.
[14] 491 U.S. at 534.
[15] 491 U.S. at 534.
[16] 491 U.S. at 536.
[17] 58 Fed. Reg. 47532 (September 9, 1993).
[18] 20 C.F.R. § 416.924(a) (1993).
[19] Personal communication, J. Firmin, Social Security Administration, June 24, 2015.

grew, the total number of SSI child beneficiaries also grew. Between 1991 and 1996, SSI child beneficiaries increased from 397,000 to 955,000 (Tambornino et al., 2015).

As noted previously, duration of disability is integral to the statutory eligibility test, whose durational standard is intended to identify children and adults who are not just temporarily disabled but whose disabilities can be expected to last a long time. Thus, children whose impairments are expected to subside or diminish will not be found eligible for benefits.

Childhood Disability Eligibility Standards: 1996 to the Present

The Personal Responsibility and Work Opportunity Reconciliation Act (PRWORA) made sweeping changes to the nation's welfare program. While the centerpiece of this legislation was abolishing Aid to Families with Dependent Children (AFDC) and creating Temporary Assistance to Needy Families (TANF), the law also established new eligibility restrictions[20] applicable to SSI benefits. Of relevance to the present study, the act revised the definition of disability in children by effectively tightening the functional standard. The new statutory standard, which remains in effect today, specified that a child under 18 is considered disabled for SSI benefit purposes if she or he has a "medically determinable physical or mental impairment that results in marked and severe functional limitations"[21] and that can be expected to last for a continuous 12-month period or result in death. This terminology narrowed the earlier *Zebley* standard that was based on whether an impairment "substantially limited" age-appropriate development. At the same time, the law maintained the recognition that a finding of disability could rest on a functional impact finding. The 1996 amendments further specified that "notwithstanding [a finding of an impairment causing marked and severe functional limitations], no individual under the age of 18 who engages in substantial gainful activity (determined in accordance with regulations . . .) may be considered to be disabled."[22] The amendments also ordered changes to the medical criteria for evaluating mental and emotional disorders and ordered a "discontinuance" of the individualized functional assessment that was in effect at the time of enactment.[23] In addition, the act revised the medical improvement review standard for children under 18 to include a determination, through periodic reviews, of whether a child

[20] Public Law 104-193, Title II, Subtitle A (§ 200).
[21] 42 U.S.C. § 1382c, as amended by PRWORA § 211(a).
[22] Id. § 211(a).
[23] Id. § 211(b).

receiving SSI benefits had an "impairment or combination of impairments [that] no longer results in marked and severe functional limitations."[24]

The SSA implemented the SSI children's amendments of the PRWORA through regulations published in 2000[25] that eliminated its post-*Zebley* individualized functional assessment test and implemented the law's more restrictive "marked and severe functional limitations" standard. As revised, the rules significantly narrowed the functional basis of children's SSI eligibility by establishing a three-step sequential evaluation process, discussed below. After the act was passed, the number of new child SSI beneficiary awards temporarily declined. This occurred in response to both the stricter disability definition and concomitant changes to the children's eligibility determination process (Tambornino et al., 2015). In a 2002 assessment commissioned by the SSA, it was estimated that by 2001, the revised regulations had led to a 19 percent reduction in the total number of child and young adult SSI recipients (Rogowski et al., 2002). After the 1996 act was passed, mandated reevaluations led to the termination of SSI payments for more than 90,000 children in 1997 (Coe and Rutledge, 2013). Nevertheless, SSI awards for children with mental disorders—which include speech and language disorders—began rising again after 1997 (SSA, 2006b). Changes over time in the prevalence of speech and language disorders among the general population and in SSI program participation are discussed in detail in Chapter 5.

SSI ELIGIBILITY AND THE ELIGIBILITY DETERMINATION PROCESS

The purpose of the SSI program is to provide cash assistance to individuals with limited income and resources who are age 65 or older, blind (any age), or disabled (any age). In 33 states and the District of Columbia, SSI eligibility also confers Medicaid eligibility, although many children with disabilities may qualify for Medicaid based on family income alone. The value of the income transfer that SSI provides to families is modest because to qualify for benefits, families must have limited means. The modest payment amount is illustrated by the fact that in 2010, nearly one-third of families that received the children's SSI benefit continued to have total family income below the federal poverty level (FPL) (Bailey and Hemmeter, 2014).

At the same time, however, the value of the children's SSI benefit is substantial for many families. Bailey and Hemmeter (2014) estimate that if families that received children's SSI benefits had not done so, 58.0 percent (n = 692,696) would have had incomes below 100 percent of the FPL (see

---

[24] Id. § 211(c), amending 42 U.S.C. § 1382(a)(4).

[25] 65 Fed. Reg. 54747 (September 11, 2000).

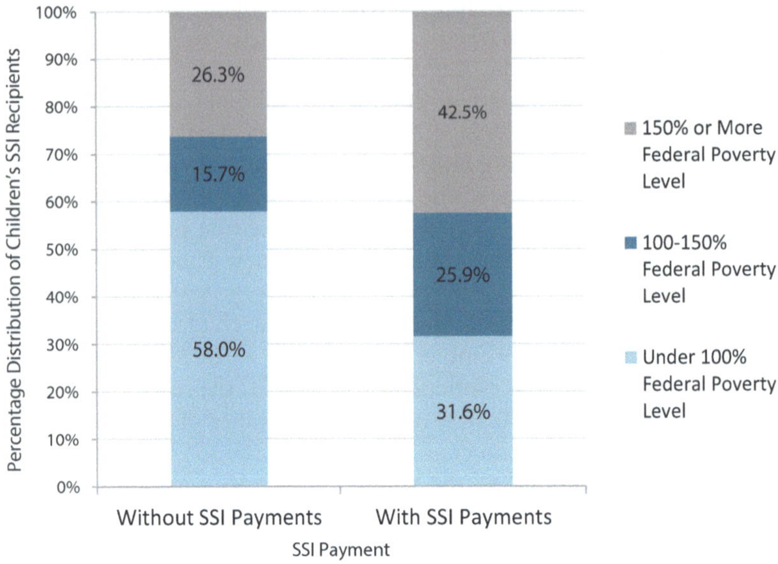

FIGURE 4-1 Percentage distribution of child SSI recipients, by family income relative to the federal poverty level, with and without SSI payments, September-December 2010.
NOTES: In 2010, the federal poverty level for a family of four was $22,050 (HHS, 2015b). The sample size is 1,193,848. Totals do not necessarily equal the sum of rounded components.
SOURCE: Bailey and Hemmeter, 2014.

Figure 4-1). In other words, SSI payments raised family income above the FPL for more than a quarter of families with child SSI beneficiaries (58.0 percent minus 31.6 percent).[26] Still, economic vulnerability remains notable for these families. Bailey and Hemmeter (2014) found that approximately 58.0 percent (31.6 percent plus 25.9 percent) of families receiving children's SSI benefits continued to have incomes below 150 percent of the FPL,[27] even after accounting for receipt of the benefit.

---

[26] The federal poverty level (FPL) is set by the U.S. Department of Health and Human Services and varies by the number of people living in the household. In 2015, the FPL for a family of four was $24,250 in the 48 contiguous states, and slightly higher in Alaska and Hawaii ($30,320 and $27,890, respectively) (HHS, 2015a).

[27] Poverty researchers typically identify 200 percent of the FPL as the income threshold for adequate subsistence (Boushey et al., 2001).

The Narrow Focus of the Children's SSI Program

From its origins, the SSI program was structured to assist only low-income children and adults with severe disabilities that could be expected to persist over a long period of time or result in death. Although the 1996 amendments preserved the functional test for children's eligibility determinations, they also set as a standard that children must have "marked and severe" disabilities to qualify for the program. As a result, the SSI eligibility determination process evaluates the extent to which physical and mental health conditions are sufficiently severe to impair children's ability to function. A fundamental aspect of functioning ability is communication through speech and language, as described in previous chapters.

As a legal entitlement to cash welfare assistance that is based on income and disability, the SSI program, as a matter of law, is significantly more restrictive in defining disability relative to other disability programs. Other programs that provide educational, social, or health services to children with disabilities and activity limitations are less stringent.

By contrast, as discussed in Chapter 5, a far greater universe of children could qualify as "children with special health care needs"[28] for state services furnished under the Title V Maternal and Child Health Block Grant program. (The actual range of those services varies from state to state, as evidenced by state program performance data collected by the Health Resources and Services Administration [HRSA], the federal agency that administers Title V.[29]) For Title V policy-making and program purposes, the concept of children with special health care needs encompasses not only the narrow group of children who qualify for SSI assistance[30] but also a far broader group identified in statute[31] and further defined by HRSA as children "who have or are at increased risk for a chronic physical, developmental, behavioral, or emotional condition and who also require health and related services of a type or amount beyond that required by children generally" (McPherson et al., 1998). As discussed at greater length in Chapter 5, this broader definition of children with special health care needs produces far higher population estimates; government data show that 15.1 percent of all children—a far greater proportion than that represented by the SSI children's disability program—can be considered "children with special health care needs" (HHS et al., 2013).

Similarly, the SSI disability standard for children is much narrower than the standard for determining eligibility for services under the Individuals

---

[28] 42 U.S.C. § 701 et seq.

[29] See https://mchdata.hrsa.gov/tvisreports/Snapshot/SnapShotMenu.aspx (accessed September 30, 2015).

[30] 42 U.S.C. § 701(a)(1).

[31] 42 U.S.C. § 701(a)(1).

with Disabilities Education Act (IDEA). This law was originally enacted in 1975 to ensure that students with disabilities would have access to a free and appropriate public education. The act explicitly identifies speech and language impairments as a type of disability and defines them as "a communication disorder, such as stuttering, impaired articulation, a language impairment, or a voice impairment, that adversely affects a child's educational performance."[32] In contrast to the SSI program, IDEA has no financial eligibility tests, nor does it have severity tests with duration requirements. A child will not receive SSI if his or her impairment is expected to improve; however, IDEA provides special education services to children with speech or language impairment regardless of whether the condition is expected to improve. The total number of children receiving IDEA services in the 2012-2013 time period stood at 6.4 million (U.S. Department of Education, 2015), about four times the total number of children entitled to SSI benefits during that time period.

Determining SSI Eligibility for Children

For a child to receive SSI benefits, two basic conditions must be met: (1) the child must meet criteria for citizenship or alien status, residency, work, income, and resources; and (2) the child must be found to have a severe impairment that meets the statutory and regulatory standards for disability. State agencies that are fully funded by the federal government and work under the guidance and rules of the SSA are responsible for making disability determinations (SSA, 2007).

The process for becoming eligible for child SSI benefits begins when an individual files an application with the SSA. The determination process (which the SSA terms the "adjudication process") proceeds through multiple steps, as illustrated in Figure 4-2. Each step in the process is discussed in detail below. It should be noted that while this report describes the adjudication process as proceeding through four steps, the SSA formally describes it as a three-step process, but with Step 3 having two parts—Step 3a and Step 3b. The Step 3 discussed in this report is the same as the SSA's Step 3a, while Step 4 is the same as the SSA's Step 3b.

Step 1: Work, Income, and Resources

Determination of employment status and financial eligibility is the first step in the determination of a child's eligibility for SSI disability benefits. The work, income, and resource eligibility criteria must be met prior to any evaluation of disability.

[32] 34 C.F.R. § 300(8).

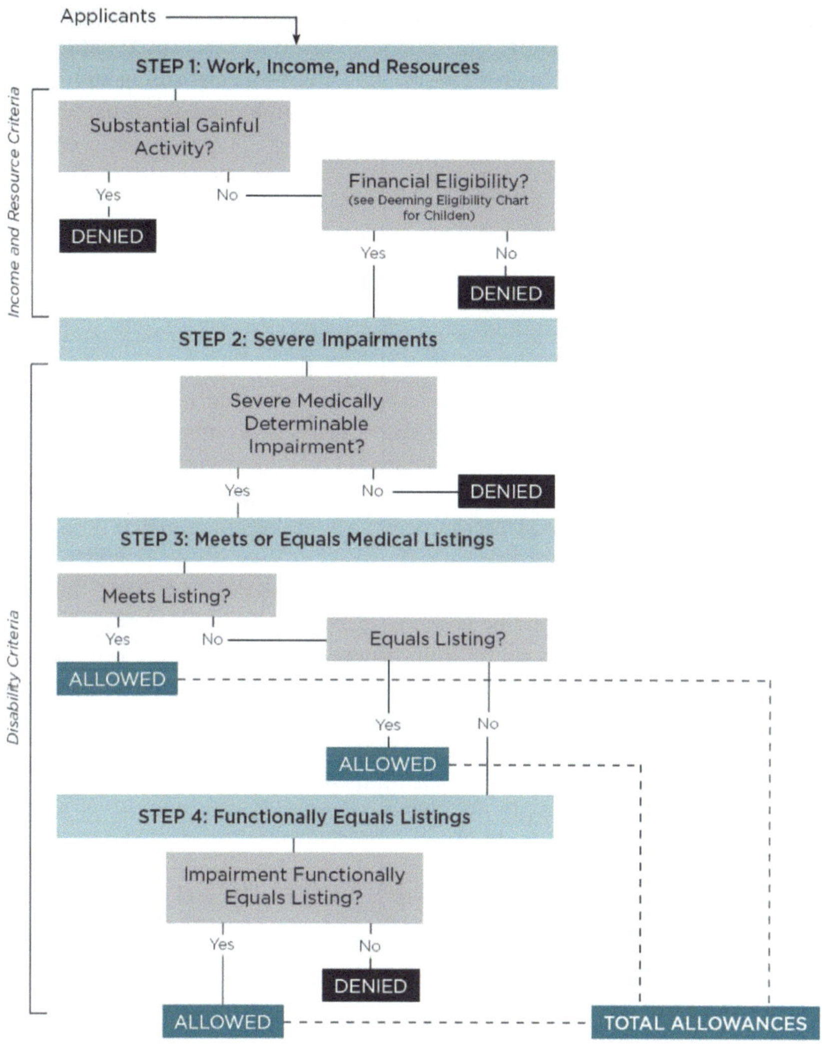

FIGURE 4-2 For purposes of this report, the SSI eligibility determination process for children.
SOURCE: Wixon and Strand, 2013.

Once an application for child SSI benefits has been filed, the SSA field office first determines whether the child is engaged in substantial gainful activity (SGA). SGA[33] is defined as work that involves performing significant and productive physical or mental duties and that is done (or intended) for pay or profit (SSA, 2014a). If a child engages in SGA, the claim is denied. If a child is not employed, the field office proceeds to evaluate financial eligibility based on the child's income and the parents' and stepparents' income and resources (Wixon and Strand, 2013).

Until a child attains age 18, a portion of his or her parents' and stepparents' income is used to determine financial eligibility through a complex process known as deeming. A certain portion of the parents' and stepparents' income and resources is "deemed" to be available to the child as a member of the household and therefore counted toward eligibility. Some types of parental income and resources are deemed, and others are not. Income that is not deemed includes TANF, pensions from the U.S. Department of Veterans Affairs, general assistance, foster care payments for an ineligible child, and income used to make court-ordered support payments (SSA, 2014d).

If the employment, income, and resources criteria are met, the case proceeds to Step 2. It should be noted that, because of the deeming process, the SSI income eligibility criteria do not necessarily predict the household's poverty level. After deeming exclusions have been applied, children eligible for SSI may come from households with incomes above 100 percent of the FPL. In 2014, three-quarters of children receiving SSI benefits were in households with incomes below 200 percent of the FPL, without taking into account the income from the SSI benefit (Bailey and Hemmeter, 2014).

Step 2: Medically Determinable Impairment, Severity, and Duration

In Step 2, the Disability Determination Services examiner evaluates whether an applicant has a "severe medically determinable impairment" as required by the Social Security Act and as defined by statute and in the Code of Federal Regulations (SSA, 2011). If not, the claim is denied. The SSA defines a medically determinable physical or mental impairment as an impairment that results "from anatomical, physiological, or psychological abnormalities which can be shown by medically acceptable clinical and laboratory diagnostic techniques" (SSA, 2013a). Such an impairment must be established by medical evidence that includes symptoms, signs, and

[33] The monthly SGA amount for nonblind disabled individuals for 2015 is the amount for 2000 multiplied by the ratio of the national average wage index for 2013 to that for 1998, or if larger the amount for 2014 ($1,070). If the amount so calculated is not a multiple of $10, it is rounded to the nearest multiple of $10 (SSA, n.d.).

laboratory findings (SSA, 2013a). Furthermore, the medical evidence cannot turn on parental communications or observations; instead, it must come from an SSA-approved list of medical sources, which includes licensed physicians and, in the case of speech and language disorders, speech-language pathologists (SSA, 2013a). Information supplied by parents and caregivers is relevant, but by itself is an insufficient basis for a determination of disability. If there is insufficient medical evidence to support a finding of a medically determinable impairment, the claim is denied.

Applications also are denied if the applicant's impairment is not considered severe. The SSA defines a nonsevere impairment as an impairment or combination of impairments that does not "cause more than a minimal limitation in the individual's ability to function in an age-appropriate manner" (SSA, 2014b). Applications are denied as well if the applicant's impairment is not expected to cause death or has neither lasted 12 months nor can be expected to last for a continuous period of 12 months or more (SSA, 2000). If the Disability Determination Services examiner finds that the claimant has a severe, medically determinable impairment, the claim proceeds to Step 3.

Step 3: The Medical Listings

In Step 3, the Disability Determination Services examiner performs a medical screen to determine whether the child has one or more severe impairments that either "meet" or "medically equal" the criteria in the SSA's Listing of Impairments (Wixon and Strand, 2013). The relevant definitions are as follows:

- *Meets a Listing*—If the evidence in a case establishes that all of the criteria required by one of the Listings, along with the duration requirement, are met, the claimant's impairment meets that specific Listing (SSA, 2013b).
- *Medically equals a Listing*—If a claimant's impairment is not found to meet the exact criteria of a specific Listing, the claimant can still be found eligible if the impairment is at least equal in severity and duration to the criteria for any listed impairment, as established by the relevant evidence in the claimant's case record (SSA, 2013b).

If a child's impairment "meets" or "medically equals" a Listing, benefits are awarded. Otherwise, the claim proceeds to Step 4.

Step 4: Functional Equivalence

In Step 4, the Disability Determination Services examiner evaluates whether the impairment functionally equals the Listings—that is, whether the child's impairment is of Listing-level severity, which means it must result in "marked" limitations in two domains of functioning or "extreme" limitation in one domain (Wixon and Strand, 2013). The SSA evaluates functional equivalency from both a qualitative and a quantitative perspective, and the regulations on this point are extensive.

From a *qualitative* perspective, the SSA considers an impairment to be "extreme" if it interferes "very seriously" with a child's ability to independently initiate, sustain, or complete age-appropriate activities. The interactive and cumulative effects of functional limitations are evaluated using all available evidence. The SSA considers an impairment to be "marked" if it "seriously" interferes with age-appropriate function. Thus, eligibility is denied for impairments that do not interfere either very seriously or seriously with age-appropriate functioning. As in the case of impairments that "meet or equal" the Listing for a particular impairment, the evidence on which a functional determination must rest is comprehensive. The evidence includes data and information drawn from a variety of professional sources, including clinical, educational, and social and rehabilitative programs serving children; parental reports and observations cannot form the sole evidentiary basis for a finding that an impairment is severe based on function.

From a *quantitative* perspective, the SSA considers an impairment to be "extreme" if a child registers a valid score that is at least three standard deviations from the mean on a comprehensive standardized test designed to measure functioning in any one of the six functional domains (see below) *and* if the child's day-to-day functioning in domain-related activities is consistent with that score. The SSA considers a child to have a "marked" limitation if the child's standardized score for each domain falls between two and three standard deviations from the mean, and this score is reflected in the child's day-to-day functioning. For children under age 3, an extreme limitation is one that causes function at a level typical for one-half of the child's chronological age, while a marked limitation is one that causes function at a level typical for between one-half and two-thirds of the child's chronological age. In a sample of 1,000 children, only about 1 would be expected to meet this standard for a extreme limitation; only 2 in 100 would be expected to meet this standard for a marked limitation. These definitions of extreme and marked limitations are comparable to and in some cases more stringent than standards for identifying children aged birth to 3 years eligible for early intervention under IDEA Part C based on developmental delays (U.S. Department of Education, 2011; see also Rosenberg et al., 2013).

On balance, whether they are measured quantitatively or qualitatively, impairments tied to function must be extreme or marked to support a finding of SSI eligibility. Furthermore, the core requirement is that the child's condition must be at least marked and severe. This standard places SSI eligibility criteria on a more limited plane than that used to qualify children for services for children with special health care needs under either IDEA or Title V.

Six activity domains As noted above, when determining functional equivalence, the SSA considers a child's function in six activity domains. These domains are broad areas of functioning that encompass activities children can and cannot perform at home, at school, and in the community compared with children of the same age who do not have impairments (IOM, 2010). Information concerning functioning in the six domains is collected from medical sources, parents, teachers, and others who can describe functioning at home, in childcare, at school, and in the community (SSA, 2015a). The SSA also may request a consultative exam if the medical evidence provided is inadequate (SSA, 2015a).

The first domain, "acquiring and using information," refers to how well a child can acquire or learn and then use information (SSA, 2015a). An example of limited functioning in acquiring and using information is having difficulty remembering things learned in school the previous day (SSA, 2015a).

The second domain, "attending and completing tasks," describes how well a child can focus and maintain attention throughout and finish activities (SSA, 2015a). A child with limited functioning in this domain is repeatedly distracted from activities (SSA, 2015a).

The third domain, "interacting and relating with others," encompasses how well a child can "initiate and sustain emotional connections with others, develop and use language of the community, cooperate with others, comply with rules, respond to criticism, and respect and take care of possessions of others" (SSA, 2015a). When a child is unable to form close friendships, he or she is limited in interacting and relating with others (SSA, 2015a).

The fourth domain, "moving about and manipulating objects," describes gross and fine motor skills that include a child's ability to move from one place to another and to move and manipulate things. Difficulty climbing up and down stairs is an example of limitation in this domain (SSA, 2015a).

The fifth domain, "caring for yourself," refers to how well a child can maintain a healthy emotional and physical state by ensuring that physical and emotional wants and needs are met; coping with stress and environmental changes; and taking care of his or her health, possessions, and living area (SSA, 2015a). A child with limitations in this domain may not dress or bathe him- or herself appropriately when age is taken into account (SSA, 2015a).

The sixth domain, "health and physical well-being," describes the "cumulative physical effects of physical or mental impairments and their associated treatments and therapies on functioning" (SSA, 2015a). A child who has frequent seizures related to his or her impairment will have a limitation in this domain (SSA, 2015a).

In this evaluation stage, the rules are replete with age-specific examples that describe language and communication skills, given the significance of speech and language to child development. For example, one of the specific factors the SSA considers is a child's ability to "develop and use the language of" the community to which he or she belongs.[34] In another example, the SSA identifies the ability to "use words instead of actions to express yourself" in the case of preschool children.[35] Difficulty in "communicating with others; e.g., in using verbal and nonverbal skills to express yourself, carrying on a conversation, or in asking others for assistance" is similarly considered evidence when the interaction function is evaluated.[36]

Marked and extreme limitations As noted, to functionally equal the Listings, a child's impairment must result in "marked" limitation in two domains or "extreme" limitation in one domain (SSA, 2014c). When deciding whether a child has a marked or extreme limitation, the SSA considers functional limitations due to the child's impairment and their interactive and cumulative effects (SSA, 2014c). Relevant information in the child's case record, such as signs, symptoms, laboratory findings, and parental and teacher descriptions of function, are used to determine functioning (SSA, 2014c). Medical evidence such as formal testing also is used to provide developmental and functional information, and the standard scores from the formal tests along with the standard deviations of scores are used together with the information obtained regarding functioning to determine whether a child exhibits marked or extreme limitation in a domain (SSA, 2014c).

Marked limitation When a child has a marked limitation, his or her impairment interferes seriously with the ability to independently initiate, sustain, or complete activities (SSA, 2014c). A marked limitation can be described as "more than moderate" but "less than extreme" (SSA, 2014c). The impairment can affect day-to-day functioning by seriously limiting only one activity, or the impairment's interactive and cumulative effects can limit

[34] 20 C.F.R. § 416.926(e).
[35] 20 C.F.R. § 416.926(e).
[36] 20 C.F.R. § 416.926(e).

several activities (SSA, 2014c). For children of any age, marked limitation is determined if a valid score on a comprehensive standardized test designed to measure ability or functioning in a domain is two standard deviations or more but less than three standard deviations below the mean (SSA, 2014c). The test should be designed to measure ability or functioning in that particular domain, and the child's day-to-day functioning in domain-related activities should be consistent with the score (SSA, 2014c). For children who have not yet reached age 3 and cannot be tested, a marked limitation is determined if they function at a level that is more than one-half but still less than two-thirds of that typical for their chronological age (SSA, 2014c). To meet the definition of marked limitation, comprehensive standardized test scores must be between two and three standard deviations below the mean (SSA, 2014c).

Extreme limitation A child is determined to have an extreme limitation when the impairment interferes very seriously with the ability to independently initiate, sustain, or complete activities (SSA, 2014c). An extreme limitation also is described as "more than marked" (SSA, 2014c). The impairment can affect day-to-day functioning by very seriously limiting only one activity, or its interactive and cumulative effects can limit several activities (SSA, 2014c). As mentioned above, comprehensive standardized test scores are used for determining impairment that can be considered an extreme limitation (SSA, 2014c). A valid score for an extreme limitation is three standard deviations or more below the mean (SSA, 2014c). Children who have not yet attained age 3 are considered to have an extreme limitation if functioning at a level one-half of that typical for their chronological age or less (SSA, 2014c). Benefits are awarded if it is found that a child's impairment results in limitations that functionally equal those of the Listings; otherwise, the application for benefits is denied.

The Appeals Process

A claimant has the right to appeal a determination, decision, or dismissal after any step of the disability determination process and can present additional evidence to support his or her case or appoint a representative to do so (Morton, 2014). The appeals process encompasses three levels of administrative review within the SSA before the case can be appealed to the U.S. court system (Morton, 2014). These three levels are reconsideration, an evidentiary hearing before an administrative law judge, and an appeal to a special appeals board.

Suspensions and Terminations

A recipient's benefit payments are suspended or terminated when he or she is no longer eligible for benefits. Suspension of benefit payments occurs when a recipient is found to no longer be eligible for a number of reasons, including having excess income or resources, whereabouts being unknown, residing in a Medicaid facility or public institution, or no longer being disabled. Suspensions can last up to 12 months after suspension. Payments can be reinstated if, within 12 months after a recipient's payments are suspended, the recipient's circumstances revert to being consistent with the eligibility criteria. Termination of SSI benefits occurs when a recipient is ineligible for 12 consecutive months; a terminated recipient cannot receive disability benefit payments without submitting a new application. Termination can occur when a recipient dies or after 12 consecutive months of suspension.

Continuing Disability Reviews

Continuing disability reviews are performed periodically to determine whether SSI recipients (including children) continue to qualify for benefits (SSA, 1986). The frequency of such reviews depends on whether the impairment is expected to improve and whether the disability is considered permanent (SSA, 2006a). For impairments that are expected to improve, continuing disability reviews are required at 6- to 18-month intervals following the most recent decision (SSA, 2006a). When a disability is not considered permanent but a medical improvement in the impairment cannot be predicted, a continuing disability review should be conducted at least once every 3 years (SSA, 2006a). When a disability is considered permanent, a continuing disability review should be conducted no less than once every 7 years and no more than once every 5 years (SSA, 2006a).

The U.S. Government Accountability Office (GAO, 2012) has reported that, because of resource constraints and competing workload priorities, SSA has not performed continuing disability reviews at these prescribed intervals. The GAO found that the number of reviews had decreased by 70 percent between 2000 and 2011 and that as of August 1, 2011, the SSA was experiencing a backlog of about 435,000 child SSI recipients with mental disorders who had not yet received a prescribed continuing disability review. For many of these children, medical improvement was neither expected nor possible. In response to these GAO findings, the SSA noted that it had conducted fewer reviews for children than required by law because of funding constraints and competing demands for reviews for adults (GAO, 2012).

TABLE 4-1 Childhood Listing Impairment Codes for Speech and Language Disorders

Listing	Diagnostic Category Label	Impairment Code
112.12	Speech and Language Impairment	3153
111.09	Loss of Voice (Communication Impairment)	7840

NOTE: Impairment codes are based on the *International Classification of Diseases, Ninth Revision, Clinical Modification* (SSA, 2013c).

APPLICATION OF THE SSI DISABILITY CRITERIA TO CHILDREN WITH SPEECH AND LANGUAGE DISORDERS

In addition to understanding the overall SSI adjudication process, it is important to understand how specific disorders are evaluated. This is especially true for speech and language disorders in children for which there are impairment codes but no specific Listings. This section provides greater detail on how children with speech and language impairments are determined to be medically eligible for SSI.

Eligibility for SSI for Children with a Speech or a Language Disorder

The impairment codes for childhood speech and language disorders used for the SSA's disability evaluation are "speech and language impairment" (3153)[37] and "loss of voice" (communication impairment) (7840) (see Table 4-1).[38] These codes are included in Part B of the Listing of Impairments, which contains additional medical criteria that apply only to the evaluation of impairments in children under age 18. As noted earlier, the criteria in the Listings are incorporated into the SSA's multistep evaluation process. From this point forward, when the committee refers to children with speech and language disorders within the SSI program, it is referring to children with one of these two primary impairments.

Evaluating Speech and Language Disorders in Children

The process for identifying children with speech and language disorders who are eligible for SSI benefits is consistent with the multidimensional,

[37] SSI impairment codes are based on the *International Classification of Diseases, Ninth Revision, Clinical Modification* (SSA, 2013c).

[38] The SSA added the impairment code 3153 for speech and language impairment in mid- to late 1994 (personal communication, J. Firmin, Social Security Administration, June 24, 2015). The SSA has used impairment code 7840 for loss of voice since the 1980s (personal communication, J. Firmin, Social Security Administration, June 24, 2015).

multimethod, and multisource perspective evident in current professional practices. Specifically, as described above, children are assessed across multiple domains to determine the presence and severity of impairments in any individual areas, as well as the combined and interacting effects of these impairments on day-to-day functioning. Likewise, children's case records include multiple forms of evidence concerning impairment and functioning (e.g., test scores, classroom records, progress in intervention), with no single piece of evidence being considered in isolation. Finally, information from parents, caregivers, and others with direct knowledge of children's daily functioning in age-appropriate environments and activities (e.g., Child Function Report Forms [SSA 3375-3379], Teacher Questionnaire Form [SSA 5565]) also is used to ensure that formal and criterion-referenced scores in the case record are consistent with levels of functioning in typical settings. The descriptions of "marked" and "extreme" limitations that are used to identify impairments sufficiently severe to functionally equal the Listings also are consistent with professional practice in interpreting norm- and criterion-referenced tests of speech and language.

The following subsections provide individual case examples as well as information gleaned from a review of a random sample of case files to illustrate the types of evidence used to determine eligibility for SSI and the characteristics of children who are allowed or denied eligibility on the basis of speech and language disorders.

Case Examples of Speech and Language Impairments

Although a number of medical Listings and impairment codes concern conditions that are strongly associated with speech and/or language impairments (such as autism and attention deficit hyperactivity disorder), speech and language delays often occur in the absence of known medical or other causes (see Chapter 2). According to the SSA, approximately 80 percent of allowed cases involving a primary impairment of speech and language impairment (code 3153) do not meet or medically equal a Listing, but are allowed using functional equivalence rules.[39] These cases include speech and language impairments with both known causes and unknown causes. As discussed earlier in this chapter, a functional equivalence determination requires extensive documentation, using various types of evidence, of a child's abilities across six functional domains and relative to the child's chronological age. A child must then exhibit speech and language impairments that are two to three standard deviations off the norm for a child of that age.

The following are case examples from the SSA for primary impairment

[39] 20 C.F.R. § 416.926(a).

code 3153, speech and language impairment. These examples illustrate the types of evidence used to determine eligibility and the characteristics of children who are allowed or denied eligibility. The SSA provided two case examples of 4-year-old children with primary speech impairments who applied for SSI. One child was found to meet the functional equivalence standard and was awarded benefits; the other did not meet the standard and was denied benefits.

Allowed Case: 4-Year-Old Male

This child's file included clinical evaluation records related to occupational therapy, physical therapy, speech and language therapy, and psychological testing, as well as an early-intervention individual family service plan prepared pursuant to IDEA concerning the child's developmental, fine motor, expressive language, and speech delays. However, only the evidence regarding his delayed speech met the functional equivalence standard. Specifically, a speech-language pathology evaluation noted severe speech delays and stated that the child's speech was intelligible to others only 25 percent of the time, despite the fact that by age 4, speech intelligibility at or near 100 percent is expected. Consistent with this evidence, the child's caregiver, who completed Form SSA-3377, described abnormal speech patterns and noted that despite being with him all day, the caregiver still found his speech very difficult to understand. As noted in the age-specific examples for the domain of "interacting and relating with others," children aged 3-6 are expected to "use words instead of actions to express yourself," to "relate to caregivers with increasing independence, choose your own friends, and play cooperatively with other children . . . without continual adult supervision," and "initiate and participate in conversations . . . speaking clearly enough that both familiar and unfamiliar listeners can understand what you say most of the time" (SSA, 2015a). The subject child's inability to speak intelligibly represented an extreme limitation in this domain (see Table 4-2); he was given a primary diagnosis of speech and language

TABLE 4-2 Allowed Case: Functional Domain Summary

Domain	Rating
Acquiring and using information	Less than marked limitation
Attending and completing tasks	Less than marked limitation
Interacting and relating with others	**Extreme limitation**
Moving and manipulating objects	No limitation
Caring for self	Less than marked limitation
Health and physical well-being	No limitation

SOURCE: Unpublished dataset provided by the Social Security Administration.

impairment (code 3153), with medical evidence insufficient to establish a secondary diagnosis (code 6490).

Denied Case: 4-Year-Old Female

This case file contained several types of evidence regarding the child's speech, including clinical reports and results of a standardized speech articulation test. A speech-language pathologist reported that the child was receiving one session of speech therapy per week. At the time of the report, the child's speech was intelligible 75 percent of the time, with speech errors remaining in only a few sounds. In addition, the child was reported to have obtained a standard score of 112 (slightly above the expected mean of 100) on a standardized speech articulation test approximately 3 months earlier. The child's language, speech fluency, and voice characteristics were described as age-appropriate, and her speech impairment was described as not interfering with her academic progress.

Other evidence in the file was inconsistent with the results of a telephone interview with the child's mother, who reported that the child could rarely be understood by anyone other than the mother because of a "bad stutter." The mother also indicated that others often asked the child to repeat herself because they could not understand her speech.

In this case, the child's speech deficits, although sufficiently severe to warrant treatment, were not rated as causing an extreme functional limitation in the domain of "interacting and relating with others" relative to peers her age (see Table 4-3). She was assigned a primary impairment of speech and language impairment (code 3153), with medical evidence insufficient to establish a secondary diagnosis (code 6490), and her claim was denied.

TABLE 4-3 Denied Case: Functional Domain Summary

Domain	Rating
Acquiring and using information	No limitation
Attending and completing tasks	No limitation
Interacting and relating with others	Less than marked limitation
Moving and manipulating objects	No limitation
Caring for self	No limitation
Health and physical well-being	No limitation

SOURCE: Unpublished dataset provided by the Social Security Administration.

Summary of Review of the SSA Case Files

As part of its charge, the committee was asked to "identify the kinds of care documented or reported to be received" by children with speech and language disorders who are enrolled in the SSI program. To shed light on this question, the committee reviewed a random sample of case files for children who receive SSI benefits based on primary speech and language disorders.[40] The results of this review provide additional insight into the underlying health characteristics of such children, as well as the types of evidence the SSA considers as part of the disability determination process.

Appendix C describes the methods used to select the 152 cases reviewed by the committee, all of which contain an initial allowance based on a primary speech and language impairment (code 3153) and any secondary impairment code. Because the review involved children determined to be entitled to SSI benefits, all of the cases met the SSI financial eligibility criteria, described earlier in this chapter. According to the SSA, 20 percent of children with speech and language disorders who receive SSI benefits are initially allowed because their condition "meets or medically equals" a Listing, while 80 percent are allowed because their condition "functionally equals" the Listings. The committee thus asked the SSA to select case files such that 20 percent were allowed on the basis of meeting or equaling the Listings and the remaining 80 percent on the basis of functional equivalence to the Listings. Finally, the group of files to be reviewed was further limited to case files for individuals under age 18. Although the case files reviewed cannot be considered representative of the entire SSI child population with speech and language disorders, the review provides evidence that is consistent with evidence from other sources considered by the committee.

The median age of the children in the sample of case files at the time of their application was 4 years, and the majority of children were between 6 months and 7 years of age (n = 134).[41] The young age at which the children in this sample applied for SSI benefits is consistent with the evidence presented in Chapter 2 regarding the age at which speech and language disorders are typically identified. The sample of case files also included more boys than girls (108 and 44, respectively). As noted in Chapters 2 and 5, this breakdown is consistent with epidemiologic reports on the sex distribution of children with speech and language disorders.

The case review also offered insight into the characteristics of the children in this sample. For example, the impairment code for speech and language disorders includes multiple underlying conditions: articulation/phonological disorders, language disorders, voice disorders, and fluency

[40] Cases were randomly selected by a manual process whereby the SSA staff selected records that are approximately equally distributed based on Social Security numbers.

[41] Two of the case files were excluded because of errors in the date of birth listed.

disorder (stuttering). Language disorders were pervasive in the sample; 145 of the 152 cases exhibited these problems. Many of the children with language disorders (n = 78) also had articulation/phonology disorders.

The committee observed a range of secondary impairment codes within the sample of case files. Among the children whose disorder met or equaled a Listing, all were assigned a secondary impairment code; among those whose eligibility was determined on the basis of functional equivalence to a Listing, the majority were assigned a secondary impairment code (n = 124). Figure 4-3 shows that these secondary impairment codes were primarily learning disorder (n = 21), "autistic disorder" (n = 19), intellectual disability (n = 11), and attention deficit hyperactivity disorder (n = 11). Figure 4-3 thus shows that the most common secondary impairment codes recorded in the sample of case files are for those conditions that, as noted in Chapter 2,

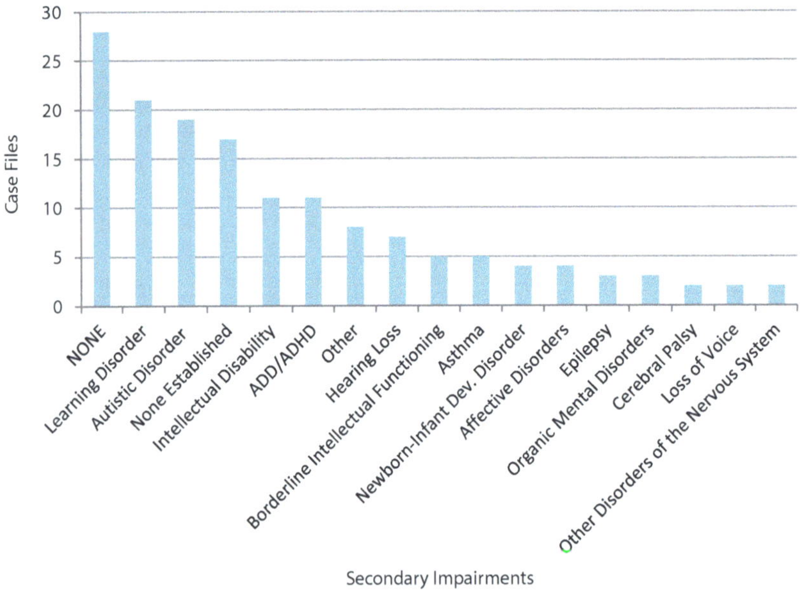

FIGURE 4-3 Secondary impairments for children with the primary impairment code for speech and language disorders within the random sample of cases reviewed.
NOTES: "Other" encompasses those conditions with only one case, such as "other congenital anomalies" and "other cerebral degenerations." The sample size is 152 case files. ADD = attention deficit disorder; ADHD = attention deficit hyperactivity disorder.
SOURCE: Unpublished dataset provided by the Social Security Administration.

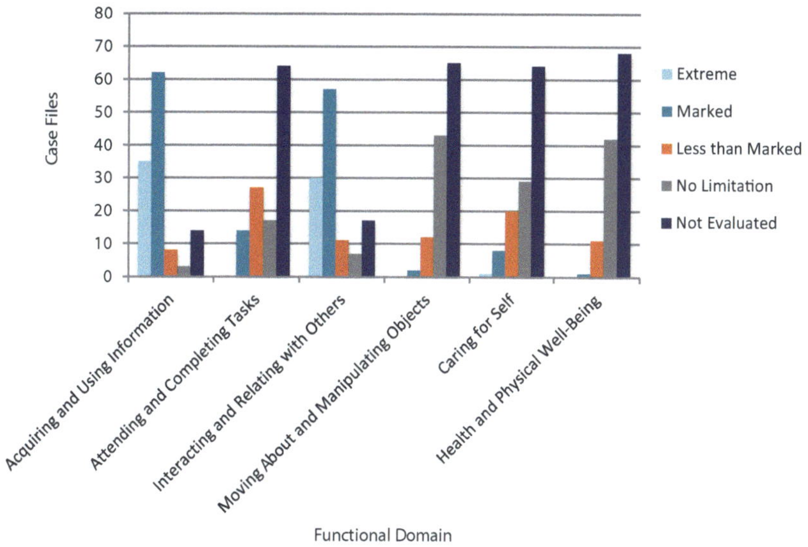

FIGURE 4-4 Functional limitations documented in case files reviewed, by functional domain.
NOTE: The sample size is 152 case files.
SOURCE: Unpublished dataset provided by the Social Security Administration.

frequently co-occur within the general population of children with speech and language disorders.

As discussed earlier in this chapter, age-appropriate functioning across six domains is central to an SSI child eligibility determination based on functional status. All but two of the case files in the random sample reviewed included a function report form completed by a parent or guardian. Figure 4-4 shows each functional domain, with the documented levels of severity within each domain. The committee observed that children in the sample of case files had extreme or marked functional limitations in the domains most likely to be affected by a severe inability to communicate, including "acquiring and using information" and "interacting and relating to others." By contrast, in the functional domains that are associated with physical health and functioning, the children in the sample showed no limitation or were not evaluated. Among the children in the sample whose eligibility was based on functional equivalency, 98 had an extreme or marked functional limitation in the domain of "acquiring and using information," while 88 had an extreme or a marked functional limitation in the domain of "interacting and relating with others."

The case review also shed light on the types of evidence used by the SSA in making eligibility determinations. Because the evidence is derived overwhelmingly from diagnostic, evaluation, and treatment information, the cases also helped the committee understand the types of treatment that the children in the sample were documented or reported as having received and the extent to which such diagnostic and evaluation services reflect the professional standards described in Chapters 2 and 3. For example, Chapter 2 describes the standardized tests typically used to diagnose speech and language disorders in children. Of the cases in the sample reviewed, 143 included evidence of standardized testing. Three case files that lacked information regarding standardized testing included diagnostic evidence derived from nonstandardized ratings and measurements, as well as spontaneous language samples, evidence that is often used to make diagnoses of speech and language disorders in children. Finally, nearly all of the case files in the sample included information from speech-language pathologists regarding the child's speech and language status, and more than half contained developmental screening reports from a pediatrician. In all, only two of all of the cases reviewed lacked the type of specialized, objective clinical and evaluative data one would expect to find in a case based on functional equivalency.

As discussed in Chapter 3, standard practice for children with extreme or marked speech and language disorders is to provide some form of speech and/or language treatment to reduce severity and improve functioning. Nearly two-thirds of the case files in the sample included evidence of IDEA participation, either through an Individualized Family Services Plan, in the case of children from birth to 3 years of age, or an Individualized Education Plan, in the case of children ages 3 to 21. The presence of an IDEA-related case document in the file indicates that at the time of the initial application, the majority of the children in the sample already were receiving IDEA services. Furthermore, as Table 4-4 shows, the majority of the children in

TABLE 4-4 Relationship Between Receipt of Speech-Language Therapy and IDEA Services Documented in the Case Files Reviewed

Speech-Language Therapy Documented in File	Individualized Education Plan or Individual Family Service Plan in File	
	Yes	No
Yes	68	33
Uncertain	14	13
No	12	12

NOTE: The sample size is 152 case files.
SOURCE: Unpublished dataset provided by the Social Security Administration.

the sample already were receiving at least some speech-language therapy; among children already receiving speech-language therapy, most were receiving IDEA services more generally.

Taken together, the information provided by the case file review suggests that the sample of children with speech and language disorders was similar in age and gender distribution to children in the general population. Children in the sample could also be expected to experience marked or extreme functional limitations of the type that would be expected to arise from severe speech and language disorders. Secondary impairments, when documented, are consistent with secondary impairments among the general population of children with speech and language disorders. Finally, evidence of evaluation and treatment documented or reported to have been received in the case files is consistent with professional standards. While this information cannot be considered representative of, or generalized to, the entire SSI child disability population with primary speech and language disorders, it does provide additional insight into children who receive SSI benefits for these disorders.

THE SSI DETERMINATION PROCESS AND THE NUMBER OF CHILD SSI RECIPIENTS

The SSI determination process evaluates the financial and medical eligibility of children who apply for SSI disability benefits. The number of participants and changes in the proportion of children with disabilities who participate in the program are a direct product of this process. For speech and language disorders, program participation comprises the number of children with these disorders who apply for benefits and are subsequently allowed by the SSI determination process.

Figure 4-5 conceptualizes the process and context of SSI program participation. As noted previously, an allowance is a finding that a child who applied for disability benefits is eligible based on both the financial and the disability criteria. Therefore, the total number of allowances is the total number of new cases within any given period of time. Because nearly all allowances result in an applicant's becoming an SSI benefit recipient, the term "recipients" denotes the current number of children receiving SSI benefits. Finally, once a child becomes an SSI recipient, he or she will continue to receive benefits until eligibility is suspended or terminated. Therefore, the number of child SSI recipients at any given point in time is a function of the number of allowances, terminations, suspensions, and reentries of suspended individuals.

Generally, the number of child SSI beneficiaries includes children who presently meet the medical eligibility criteria, whose families currently meet the financial eligibility criteria, and who have applied for benefits. However,

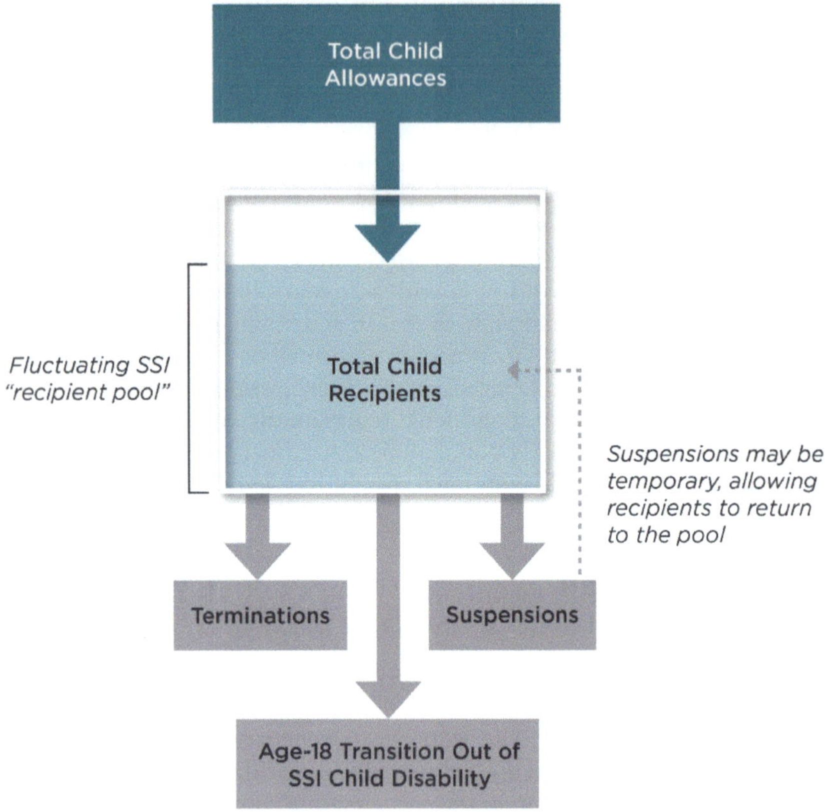

FIGURE 4-5 Relationship of allowances, recipients, terminations, and suspensions in the SSI child disability program.

some recipients may no longer meet the medical eligibility criteria, but have not (yet) been terminated because they have not been reevaluated.

The total number of child SSI recipients fluctuates depending on the number of allowances, terminations, suspensions, and suspension reentries over time. Overall growth in the population of children would be expected to contribute some growth in the program as well. Based on the statutory requirements for both duration and condition severity, one would expect the number of children allowed (found eligible for the program) in 1 year to exceed the number who exited the program (excluding age-18 transitions out of the SSI child disability program). One would also expect allowances to be affected by macroeconomic conditions. During a period of economic expansion, as family income increases and joblessness decreases, one would

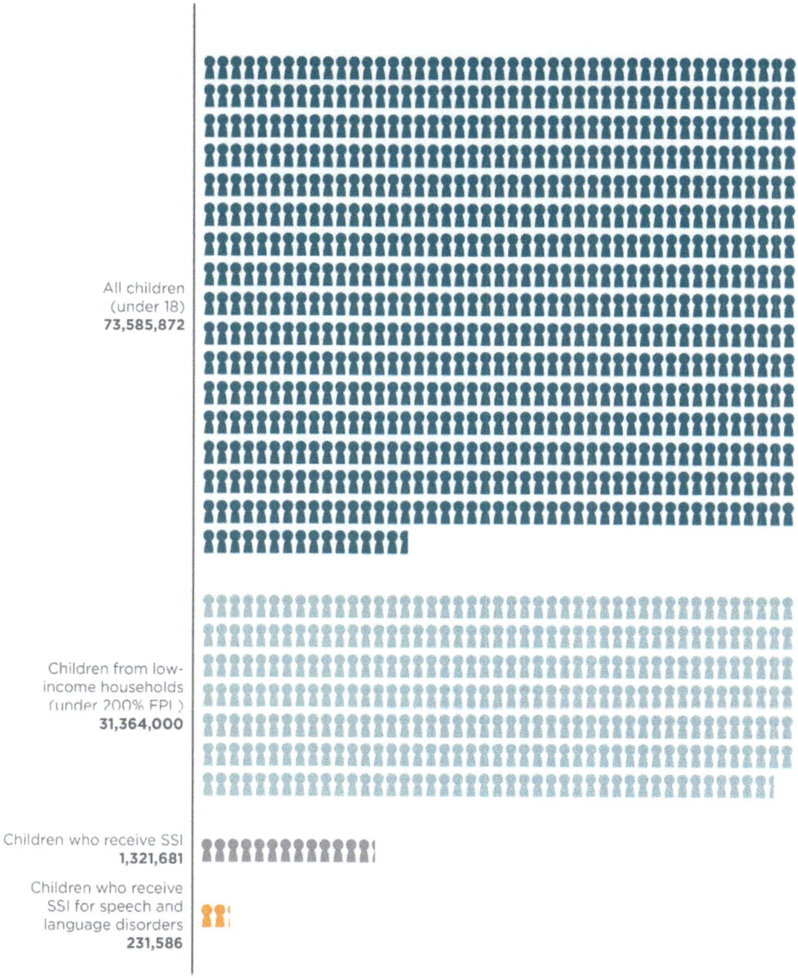

FIGURE 4-6 The number of children receiving SSI for speech and language disorders (which includes impairment codes 3153 and 7840) is a small subpopulation of children in the general U.S. population.
NOTES: FPL = federal poverty level; SSI = Supplemental Security Income. All data are from 2013. Scale = 1 symbol to 100,000 children. The Current Population Survey table creator was used to generate numbers of children in families with incomes below 200 percent of the federal poverty level. Parameters used to generate the numbers include get count of: persons in poverty universe (everyone except unrelated individuals under 15); years: 2004 to 2013; census 2010 weights; row variable: age; column variable: income-to-poverty ratio; and customized formatting: income-to-poverty ratio cutoff of 200 percent. These populations are not mutually exclusive.
SOURCES: SSA, 2014e; U.S. Census Bureau, 2014, 2015; unpublished dataset provided by the Social Security Administration.

expect fewer children to meet the SSA's financial eligibility criteria. By contrast, during periods of economic downturn—for example, during the recent U.S. recession—more children would meet the program's financial eligibility criteria as a result of relatively higher unemployment.

Figure 4-6 shows how SSI recipients with speech and language disorders are a small subpopulation of all U.S. children. Approximately 0.31 percent[42] of U.S. children receive SSI benefits for speech and language disorders (U.S. Census Bureau, 2014).

In addition to changes in macroeconomic conditions, the expanded use of diagnostic and treatment services has helped identify more children with disabilities (Houtrow et al., 2014). Efforts to raise awareness of developmental disabilities may increase the number of children who are identified as medically eligible for SSI as well. For example, the SSA Office of Disability supported an interdisciplinary case assessment project with the Association of University Centers on Disabilities to train Disability Determination Services adjudicators (SSA, 2002). According to the case assessment findings from the first 3 years (through 2001), the collaboration helped adjudicators ascertain previously unidentified language issues, which affected whether children, across all age categories, qualified for initial or continued benefits (SSA, 2002). Thus, better identification of speech and language disorders may increase the number of children who are identified as medically eligible for SSI.

FINDINGS AND CONCLUSIONS

This chapter has reviewed the SSI program for children, how it has changed over time, and how those changes have shaped the population of children receiving SSI benefits for speech and language disorders. The committee's review of the relevant statutes and regulations was supplemented by individual case examples, as well as a review of a random sample of SSI case files. Based on its review of the best available evidence, the committee formulated the following findings and conclusions.

Findings

4-1. To qualify for the SSI program, children and their families must meet a number of eligibility standards that are designed to restrict the program to children with severe conditions and those whose families have low incomes and very limited resources.

[42] The percentage 0.31 was calculated by dividing total child recipients of SSI for speech and language disorders by the total population of U.S. children in 2013.

4-2. The SSI program is designed to assist the families of children whose conditions are severe and for whom the persistence of severity is expected, as measured by duration over time.

4-3. An analysis of the impact of SSI revealed that children's SSI benefits raised family income above the FPL by 26.4 percent for families with child SSI beneficiaries. However, 58.0 percent of families receiving children's SSI benefits continued to have income below 150 percent of the FPL, even after accounting for receipt of the benefit.

4-4. More children receive services under IDEA and the Title V Program for Children with Special Health Care Needs—which are designed to identify children with substantial disability-related needs for health and educational services—than receive SSI. Neither of these programs uses a "marked or extreme" standard for disability, and neither has financial eligibility regulations.

4-5. To qualify for SSI benefits, children must meet a complex and detailed set of financial-related, work-related, and disability-related eligibility criteria. The evidence required to document severity of disability is extensive and rests on clinical and educational data and information, as well as information gleaned from professionals and standardized testing. Parental observations and reports alone are an insufficient basis for a finding of disability.

4-6. The SSA's standard for marked or extreme impairment requires that children display a degree of disability that places them at least two and three standard deviations, respectively, below normal age-appropriate functional levels.

4-7. To determine the severity of speech and language disorders in children, the SSA employs the results of professionally administered assessments and also takes into account other clinical evidence that would be consistent with severe speech and language disorders.

Conclusions

4-1. SSI is a safety net for severely disabled children whose conditions are expected to persist over time and who live in low-income, resource-limited families.

4-2. Children of families with low incomes are more likely than the general population to have disabilities, including speech and language disorders. The SSI program is designed to award benefits to the most severely impaired children from low-income, resource-limited families. Currently, 0.31 percent of U.S. children receive SSI benefits for speech and language disorders.

4-3. The disability standard for SSI (at least two to three standard deviations below normal age-appropriate functional levels) places a child far below his or her same-age peers in function and is well beyond the severity of a clinical diagnosis for speech and language disorders.

4-4. SSI benefits have the effect of lifting some children and their families out of poverty.

REFERENCES

Bailey, M. S., and J. Hemmeter. 2014. *Characteristics of noninstitutionalized DI and SSI program participants, 2010 update.* www.ssa.gov/policy/docs/rsnotes/rsn2014-02.html (accessed July 10, 2015).

Boushey, H., C. Brocht, B. Gundersen, and J. Bernstein. 2001. *Hardships in America: The real story of working families.* Washington, DC: Economic Policy Institute.

Coe, N. B., and M. S. Rutledge. 2013. *What is the long-term impact of Zebley on adult and child outcomes?* Center for Retirement Research and Boston College Working Paper No. 2013-3. http://crr.bc.edu/wp-content/uploads/2013/01/wp_2013-3-508.pdf (accessed July 7, 2015).

Fremstad, S., and R. Vallas. 2012. *Supplemental Security Income for children with disabilities.* Washington, DC: National Academy of Social Insurance.

GAO (U.S. Government Accountability Office). 2012. *Supplemental Security Income: Better management oversight needed for children's benefits.* GAO-12-497. http://purl.fdlp.gov/GPO/gpo25551 (accessed July 7, 2015).

HHS (U.S. Department of Health and Human Services). 2015a. *2015 poverty guidelines.* http://aspe.hhs.gov/2015-poverty-guidelines (accessed September 14, 2015).

HHS. 2015b. *Prior HHS poverty guidelines and* Federal Register *references.* http://aspe.hhs.gov/prior-hhs-poverty-guidelines-and-federal-register-references (accessed September 1, 2015).

HHS, HRSA (Health Resources and Services Administration), and MCHB (Maternal and Child Health Bureau). 2013. *The National Survey of Children with Special Health Care Needs chartbook 2009-2010.* Rockville, MD: HHS.

Houtrow, A. J., K. Larson, L. M. Olson, P. W. Newacheck, and N. Halfon. 2014. Changing trends of childhood disability, 2001-2011. *Pediatrics* 134(3):530-538.

IOM (Institute of Medicine). 2010. *HIV and disability: Updating the social security listings.* Washington, DC: The National Academies Press.

McPherson, M., P. Arango, H. Fox, C. Lauver, M. McManus, P. Newacheck, J. Perrin, J. Shonkoff, and B. Strickland. 1998. A new definition of children with special health care needs. *Pediatrics* 102(1):137-140.

Morton, W. R. 2014. *Primer on disability benefits: Social Security Disability Insurance (SSDI) and Supplemental Security Income (SSI).* http://fas.org/sgp/crs/misc/RL32279.pdf (accessed August 31, 2015).

NASEM (National Academies of Sciences, Engineering, and Medicine). 2015. *Mental disorders and disabilities among low-income children.* Washington, DC: The National Academies Press.

Rogowski, J., L. Karoly, J. Klerman, M. Inkelas, M. Rowe, and R. Hirscher. 2002. *Final report for policy evaluation of the effect of the 1996 welfare reform legislation on SSI benefits for disabled children.* Santa Monica, CA: RAND.

Rosenberg, S. A., C. C. Robinson, E. F. Shaw, and M. C. Ellison. 2013. Part C early intervention for infants and toddlers: Percentage eligible versus served. *Pediatrics* 131(1):38-46.

SSA (Social Security Administration). 1986. *Code of Federal Regulations 416.989: We may conduct a review to find out whether you continue to be disabled.* www.socialsecurity.gov/OP_Home/cfr20/416/416-0989.htm (accessed August 15, 2014).

SSA. 2000. *Code of Federal Regulations 416.906: Basic definition of disability for children.* www.socialsecurity.gov/OP_Home/cfr20/416/416-0906.htm (accessed September 1, 2015).

SSA. 2002. *SSA/AUCD Case Assessment project: Findings from first three years (1998-2001).* Disability Determinations Services administrators' letter no. 596. Silver Spring, MD: Association of University Centers on Disabilities. http://www.aucd.org/template/index.cfm (accessed November 10, 2015).

SSA. 2006a. *Code of Federal Regulations 416.990: When and how often we will conduct a continuing disability review.* www.socialsecurity.gov/OP_Home/cfr20/416/416-0990.htm (accessed August 15, 2014).

SSA. 2006b. *Trends in the Social Security and Supplemental Security Income disability programs.* Publication no. 13-11831. Washington, DC: SSA.

SSA. 2007. *Code of Federal Regulations 416.903: Who makes disability and blindness determinations.* www.socialsecurity.gov/OP_Home/cfr20/416/416-0903.htm (accessed August 15, 2014).

SSA. 2011. *Code of Federal Regulations 416.924: How we determine disability for children.* www.socialsecurity.gov/OP_Home/cfr20/416/416-0924.htm (accessed August 15, 2014).

SSA. 2013a. *DI 25205.005: Evidence of a medically determinable impairment.* https://secure.ssa.gov/poms.nsf/lnx/0425205005 (accessed January 30, 2015).

SSA. 2013b. *POMS DI 22001.020: Impairment(s) meets or medically equals a listing.* https://secure.ssa.gov/poms.nsf/lnx/0422001020 (accessed July 7, 2015).

SSA. 2013c. SSI annual statistical report, 2013. www.ssa.gov/policy/docs/statcomps/ssi_asr/2013/glossary.html (accessed November 16, 2015).

SSA. 2014a. *Code of Federal Regulations 416.972: What we mean by substantial gainful activity.* www.ssa.gov/OP_Home/cfr20/416/416-0972.htm (accessed August 15, 2014).

SSA. 2014b. *DI 26510.045: Completing item 22 (regulation basis code) on the SSA-831.* https://secure.ssa.gov/poms.nsf/lnx/0426510045 (accessed February 2, 2015).

SSA. 2014c. *Program operations manual system (POMS): DI 25225.020: How we define "marked" and "extreme" limitations (Section 416.926a(e)).* https://secure.ssa.gov/poms.nsf/lnx/0425225020 (accessed December 30, 2014).

SSA. 2014d. *Spotlight on deeming parental income and resources—2014 edition.* www.socialsecurity.gov/ssi/spotlights/spot-deeming.htm (accessed December 29, 2014).

SSA. 2014e. *SSI monthly statistics: Table 2: SSI federally administered payments recipients by eligibility category and age, 2004-2013.* www.ssa.gov/policy/docs/statcomps/ssi_monthly/index.html (accessed May 8, 2015).

SSA. 2015a. *Code of Federal Regulations 416.926a: Functional equivalence for children.* www.ssa.gov/OP_Home/cfr20/416/416-0926a.htm (accessed February 2, 2015).

SSA. 2015b. *SSI monthly statistics: Table 2: Recipients, by eligibility category and age, July 2014-July 2015.* http://www.ssa.gov/policy/docs/statcomps/ssi_monthly/2015-07/table02.html (accessed September 17, 2015).

SSA. n.d. *Determinations of substantial gainful activity (SGA).* www.socialsecurity.gov/oact/cola/sgadet.html (accessed August 11, 2015).

Tambornino, J., G. Crouse, and P. Winston. 2015. *National trends in the child SSI program.* http://aspe.hhs.gov/hsp/15/ChildSSI/rb_ChildSSI.pdf (accessed April 21, 2015).

U.S. Census Bureau. 2014. *Total population by child and adult populations.* http://datacenter.kidscount.org/data/tables/99-total-population-by-child-and-adult-populations?loc=1&loct=1#detailed/1/any/false/35,18,17,16,15/39,41/416,417 (accessed November 14, 2014).

U.S. Census Bureau. 2015. *CPS table creator.* www.census.gov/cps/data/cpstablecrea tor.html (accessed July 13, 2015).

U.S. Department of Education. 2011. Early intervention program for infants and toddlers with disabilities: Assistance to states for the education of children with disabilities. Final rule and proposed rule 34 CFR Part 303. *Federal Register* 76:188.

U.S. Department of Education. 2015. *Children and youth with disabilities.* http://nces.ed.gov/programs/coe/indicator_cgg.asp (accessed September 2, 2015).

U.S. House of Representatives. 1971. *Social Security Amendments of 1971: Report of the Ways and Means Committee on H.R. 1.* H. Report No. 92-251, pp. 146-148.

Wixon, B., and A. Strand. 2013. *Identifying SSA's sequential disability determination steps using administrative data.* Research and statistics note no. 2013-01. http://www.ssa.gov/policy/docs/rsnotes/rsn2013-01.html (accessed July 7, 2015).

5

Comparison of Trends in Childhood Speech and Language Disorders in the General Population and the Supplemental Security Income Program Population

One of the key aims of this report is to "identify trends in the prevalence of speech and language disorders in children and assess factors that influence these trends" among both the general population and children receiving Supplemental Security Income (SSI) on the basis of speech and language disorders (see the committee's statement of task in Box 1-1 in Chapter 1). To achieve this aim, this chapter builds on the discussion of speech and language disorders in children and their prevalence in Chapter 2, the persistence of these disorders in Chapter 3, and the structure of the SSI program for children with these disorders in Chapter 4.

To develop an overview of trends in the prevalence of speech and language disorders, the committee reviewed available research and datasets that include information on these disorders in children over the past decade. As is described in detail later in this chapter, available datasets have significant limitations, resulting in some limits on the extent to which trends in the prevalence of these disorders can be described with precision. Nevertheless, available research and datasets make it possible to draw evidence-based conclusions related to some basic issues concerning these trends—in particular, those issues that may directly impact the nature and size of the population of children receiving SSI benefits based on having these disorders. It was also possible to draw conclusions about gaps in knowledge that need to be addressed to provide more precise information about the prevalence of speech and language disorders among both the general population of children and those receiving SSI benefits on the basis of having these disorders.

This chapter begins by reviewing the data sources used by the committee to gather information on trends in the prevalence of childhood speech and language disorders. It then presents this information (1) for the general population, (2) according to demographic and other characteristics, (3) for the SSI population, and (4) for Medicaid beneficiaries. Next is a discussion of the strengths and limitations of the data available for examining these prevalence trends. The final section contains the committee's findings and conclusions.

DATA SOURCES

The committee used three different types of data to address the aim of this chapter: clinical data from small treatment studies, population data from large national surveys, and administrative or service data from large federal programs. Detailed information on the strengths and limitations of these data sources is provided later in the chapter.

Clinical data come from published research studies conducted with clinical or treatment populations. They provide detailed information about each study subject; depending on the study, this may include information on diagnosis, the course of the disorder over time, and/or treatment. Clinical studies typically share the characteristic of the child's speech or language disorder having been diagnosed by a professional (as opposed to reported by a parent or a guardian).

Population data from large national surveys provide less detailed information on each participant relative to clinical studies. However, information from national surveys is more representative of the populations of children from which respondents to the survey are drawn (e.g., all children living in the United States). Population data from national surveys typically are based on parent or guardian identification of speech and language disorders in children, and clinical corroboration of the condition or treatment received by the child is rare.

Finally, *administrative* or *service data* describe the population of children who receive services through large federal programs such as the Individuals with Disabilities Education Act (IDEA) (special education services) or Medicaid (health insurance). By definition, information derived from administrative data is representative only of the children who qualify to receive services under these programs and therefore does not reflect the characteristics of children in the general U.S. population.

For purposes of this chapter, *trends* are defined as changes in prevalence over time, with *prevalence* being the proportion of a population with a speech or language disorder. To describe trends in speech and language disorders among children in the general U.S. population, the committee considered a number of national datasets, reviewed later in this section and described in greater detail in Appendix B. In addition, during its two public workshops, the committee solicited expert testimony that provided informed perspectives on the availability, content, and value of these national data. The committee determined that no single dataset or small set of data sources can provide definitive population estimates of the prevalence of speech and language disorders among U.S. children. Where data that can be used for this purpose do exist, their utility is limited by the problems discussed later in this chapter.

To examine trends in the number of speech and language disorders among children receiving SSI benefits, the committee used data from the Social Security Administration (SSA). Except where noted otherwise, these data were extracted for the years 2004 through 2014 from the SSA 831 file. Data related to poverty level and population size were retrieved from the U.S. Census Bureau for the years 2004 to 2013. Suspension and termination data were retrieved from SSI annual statistical reports for the years 2004 to 2013.

Trend data to which the committee had access, however, are best described as serial cross-sections because they do not follow individual children over time. Instead, these serial cross-sections provide snapshots over time. The committee pieced these snapshots together to provide rough estimates of changes in prevalence among populations of beneficiaries (in the case of administrative data) or respondents (in the case of population survey data) over successive years. Because children observed in 1 year may not be the same as those observed in another year, the composition of these populations changed over time. Consequently, these data cannot be used to describe the natural history of speech and language disorders over time. (This topic—the persistence of speech and language disorders following treatment—is covered in Chapter 3.) Not only may changes in population composition over time affect rates of observed prevalence, but changes in the SSA program procedures, changes in eligibility and determination guidelines (as described in Chapter 4), and economic conditions also may influence changes in the rate of identification of speech and language disorders within a given population of children at a given point in time. For these reasons, precise conclusions about trends cannot be drawn. The same caveats apply to changes in the gender distribution of children identified as having speech and language disorders.

The committee derived information on comorbidities (i.e., other co-occurring disorders) among children with speech and language disorders from an analysis of Medicaid claims data from 20 states, performed by a team at Rutgers University under contract to the Institute of Medicine. These data provide a snapshot of comorbid disorders occurring among a subset of child Medicaid recipients with speech and language disorders who received treatment in the preceding year. The analysis examined rates of speech and language disorders among children who were Medicaid enrollees. It also yielded information on the subset of children who were eligible for Medicaid because of their participation in the SSI disability program. Medicaid claims are generated as a result of a treatment encounter between a child and his or her health care provider. To be captured in this Medicaid dataset, the child must have been eligible for Medicaid and to have obtained some sort of treatment or health care service. Furthermore, a child in the Medicaid dataset would be identified as having a speech or language disorder only if a diagnosis of such a disorder were listed on an insurance claim during the child's Medicaid-covered encounter. Not all children with speech and language disorders are Medicaid beneficiaries; not all children with these disorders seek or obtain treatment; and not all children with these disorders will have their condition correctly coded during their health care visit.

Just as the Medicaid population does not include all children with speech and language disorders, the SSI population with childhood disabilities does not include all children with speech and language disorders or even all children with disabilities. The eligibility and determination process required to qualify for the SSI program produces a beneficiary population that is very different from the general population of children with speech and language disorders in the United States (see Chapter 4). As discussed in Chapter 4, children with these disorders are eligible for SSI benefits only if their disorder is "marked" or "extreme" and they come from a family with low income. This profile reflects the intent of the SSI program—to support the most vulnerable and severely impaired children. For this reason, trends in the prevalence of speech and language disorders within the SSI population and the general U.S. population are not comparable.

As noted earlier, the committee relied upon large national surveys and administrative or service data sources to identify trends in prevalence of childhood speech and language disorders. Generally, any nationally representative survey was considered if it used questions or other methods to ascertain whether a child had such a disorder. For example, data from the National Survey of Children with Special Health Care Needs and the National Survey of Children's Health are reported here because both surveys include questions about speech and language disorders. On the other hand, some national surveys were excluded because they lack such questions. Two prominent examples are the Medical Expenditure Panel Survey and the National Health and Nutrition Examination Survey. While these surveys collect extensive information on health and do include questions related to disabilities and chronic illnesses, neither asks any questions about speech and language disorders in children.

Notably, the data sources the committee used to estimate trends in prevalence are heterogeneous in their approach to ascertaining speech and language disorders and in the populations they include. For example, the

Survey of Income and Program Participation includes two salient questions that can be used to identify children with these disorders: the first asks whether the child has any difficulty having speech understood, and the second asks whether "speech problems" were identified as the condition that caused the child to have difficulty with activities of daily living. The National Survey of Children's Health, by contrast, posed the question: "Has a doctor or other health care provider ever told you that [child's name] had stuttering, stammering, or other speech problems?" (DRC, 2012b). Clearly, these are different ways of ascertaining whether a child has a speech disorder. When surveys rely solely on parental reports of a condition, the responses may be inaccurate. Conversely, surveys that ask about a doctor's opinion may underestimate the prevalence of speech and language disorders among children who do not come to the attention of a medical provider. All national surveys that do not include clinical corroboration (i.e., direct assessment of the child as an integral part of the study) present this potential problem.

With respect to administrative or service data, such as Medicaid claims data, these data do not provide an accurate estimate of the prevalence of a given condition. Instead, these data can be used to understand the number and characteristics of children who receive services from a specific program (e.g., special education, Title V, SSI). Medicaid claims data, for example, typically are analyzed to understand utilization and costs of health care services among Medicaid participants.

Table 5-1 provides an overview of the surveys and sources of administrative/service data the committee used. The variety of approaches to determining speech and language disorders is evident in this table. For surveys, the second column of the table lists the question(s) used by each to identify these disorders. The table also shows that none of the survey datasets can be used to determine the severity of the child's condition, and very limited information is available for two of the datasets on what treatment an individual child received. Furthermore, as discussed earlier, individual children cannot be studied over time in any of these datasets. While the Survey of Income and Program Participation is longitudinal, and participants can be studied over time, disability questions are asked only once. It is also important to emphasize that, with few exceptions (e.g., the National Survey of Children with Special Health Care Needs and the National Health Interview Survey—Voice, Speech, and Language Supplement), the surveys focus on speech problems and do not ask *explicitly* about language disorders, such as comprehension difficulties. This omission could result in an underestimate of the number of respondents with such disorders. Note that in the following discussion of data from these sources, use of the terms "speech," "language," and "speech and language" reflects the wording of the questions included in each survey.

TABLE 5-1 Overview of Data Sources with Information on Children with Speech and Language Disorders

Population Data	Indicator of Speech and Language Disorders	Is Condition Severity Measured?	Can Children Be Studied Over Time?	Is Information Available on Treatment?
National Health Interview Survey	During the past 12 months, has [child] had any of the following conditions? (Response list includes stuttering and stammering.) *-AND-* How long [has child] had a speech problem?	No	No	No
National Health Interview Survey—Voice, Speech, and Language Supplement	Numerous survey questions related to "speech problems,"including: Did a health or education professional EVER tell you a diagnosis or reason for [child's name] voice, swallowing, speech, or language problem? *-AND-* At what age did [child] FIRST begin to have any speech problems?	Yes	No	Yes
National Survey of Children with Special Health Care Needs	Compared to other children the same age, would you say [he/she] experiences a lot, a little, or no difficulty speaking, communicating, or being understood?	No	No	Yes
National Survey of Children's Health	Has a doctor or other health care provider ever told you that [child] had . . . stuttering, stammering, or other speech problems?	No	No	No
Survey of Income and Program Participation	Any difficulty having speech understood? *-AND-* "Speech problems" was identified as condition causing child to have difficulty with activities of daily living.	No	No (disability questions are asked only in one topical module)	No

Administrative/Service Data	Indicator of Speech and Language Disorder	Is Condition Severity Measured?	Can Children Be Studied Over Time?	Is Information Available on Treatment?
Individuals with Disabilities Education Act (IDEA) child count data	Percentage of children reported by local education agencies as having a primary disability of "speech or language impairment"	No	No	No
Medicaid claims data	ICD-9* diagnostic codes for developmental speech disorders (315.3) or deafness (389), expressive language disorder (315.31), mixed receptive-expressive language disorder (315.32), speech and language developmental delay due to hearing loss (315.34), childhood onset fluency disorder (315.35), other developmental speech or language disorder (315.39), speech and language deficit unspecified (438.10), other speech and language deficits (438.19), and other speech disturbance (784.59); speech and language disorders also must be coded based on their underlying cause, if any	No severity codes for developmental speech disorders or deafness	Yes	Yes
SSA data	Impairment codes for "speech and language impairment" (3153) or "loss of voice-communication impairment" (7840) on SSA Form 831	Yes	No	No

* ICD-9 refers to the *International Classification of Diseases, Ninth Revision, Clinical Modification*.
SOURCES: CDC, 2015; DRC, 2012b,c.

With respect to administrative/service datasets, Table 5-1 shows the indicator of speech and language disorders provided by each. As with the survey datasets, the table also shows whether the severity of the child's condition and any treatment received can be determined, and whether children with these disorders can be studied over time.

National Health Interview Survey

The National Health Interview Survey is a cross-sectional survey based on personal household interviews. It serves as the principal source of information on the health of the civilian noninstitutionalized population of the United States and is administered by the National Center for Health Statistics (CDC, 2012a). Its purposes include monitoring trends in illness and disability and tracking progress toward the achievement of national health objectives, and it enables analysis of these data by many demographic and socioeconomic characteristics (CDC, 2012a).

The National Health Interview Survey is an ongoing survey that has been conducted continuously since 1957, with substantial content revision every 10-15 years (CDC, 2012a). Apart from major revisions, its questions remain largely unchanged from year to year, allowing trend analyses over multiple years (CDC, 2012a). The survey, with a sample size of approximately 35,000 households containing about 87,500 persons, collects limited information on all individuals in a household (CDC, 2012a). For each household, one sample adult and one sample child (if present) are randomly selected, and additional information on health status is collected in the Sample Child Core and Sample Adult Core questionnaires (CDC, 2012a). This additional information encompasses numerous disabling and health conditions, health care services, and health behaviors (CDC, 2012a).

The value of the National Health Interview Survey in the context of this study is that the sample is representative of all U.S. civilian households, and the data collected facilitate examining relationships among many health variables. A key shortcoming of this survey for purposes of this study is its limited ability to identify children with speech and language disorders. The salient questions ask about whether the child "had any stuttering or stammering" during the past 12 months or has a "speech problem [that] causes limitation" and if so, whether the speech problem was chronic (CDC, 2015). In addition, the data are reported by an adult living in the household who is knowledgeable about the child, but include no corroborating information from clinical assessment. Because the sample varies from year to year, longitudinal monitoring is not possible, but trend data on stuttering/stammering or speech problems can be derived.

National Health Interview Survey—Voice, Speech, and Language Supplement

To gather additional information on speech and language impairments, the National Center for Health Statistics fielded a supplement to the National Health Interview Survey in 2012. The National Health Interview Survey—Voice, Speech, and Language Supplement is a one-time survey that was conducted using data collection methods similar to those used for the National Health Interview Survey to identify children aged 3-17 years with reported problems with voice, swallowing, speech, or language during the past 12 months (Black et al., 2015). The sample size was 13,275 children, 7.7 percent of whom had such problems according to parent or guardian reports—5.0 percent speech problems and 3.3 percent language problems[1] (Black et al., 2015). Among younger children (aged 3-10) with voice, speech, language, or swallowing problems, one-third had multiple such problems, compared with about one-quarter among older children (aged 11-17) (Black et al., 2015).

The Voice, Speech, and Language Supplement provides information on prevalence, causes, age of onset, problem severity, receipt of intervention services, and other (comorbid) conditions (Hoffman, 2015). Its greatest shortcoming for present purposes is its one-time occurrence; the relatively small sample size, which limits disaggregation in analyses; the inclusion of all levels of severity, from mild to severe; and the fact that all of the data are based on parent or guardian reports, with no direct clinical assessment or corroboration to confirm the presence of a speech or language disorder.

National Survey of Children with Special Health Care Needs

The National Survey of Children with Special Health Care Needs was a national cross-sectional telephone survey administered by the National Center for Health Statistics. Its purpose was to gather information on the health and functional status of children with special health care needs, including their physical, emotional, and behavioral health; their health care access; their service utilization and its quality; and the impact of chronic conditions on their family (DRC, 2012c). This survey was fielded three times, with data being collected on children with speech and language disorders in the 2005-2006 and 2009-2010 iterations; no questions about etiology or diagnoses were asked in the 2001 survey.

The survey used a five-question special health care needs screener, developed by the Maternal and Child Health Bureau, to identify a minimum

[1] Some of the survey respondents reported that children had both speech and language disorders.

of 750 children with special health care needs in each state (CDC, 2014a). The screener asked about (1) use of medication prescribed by a doctor; (2) more use of medical care, mental health, or educational services than is usual for children of the same age; (3) being limited or prevented in any way from doing things most children of the same age can do; (4) receipt of special therapy, such as physical, occupational, or speech therapy; and (5) any kind of emotional, developmental, or behavioral problem for which the child needed or received treatment or counseling (Blumberg, 2015). To qualify as a child with a special health care need, at least one of these questions had to be answered affirmatively because of a medical or other health condition that had or was expected to have a duration of at least 12 months (Blumberg, 2015).

The data from this survey allow for analyses at the national, state, and regional levels. The 2005-2006 and 2009-2010 surveys each screened more than 370,000 households to identify more than 40,000 children with special health care needs (CDC, 2014a). The value of this survey for present purposes is that it provides information on a much larger sample of children with special health care needs relative to other surveys. The data are representative of noninstitutionalized children with special health care needs in each state.

At the same time, however, these data have several shortcomings in the context of this study. First, the screener questions did not include a question about speech or language disorders; speech and language questions were asked only for children screened into the survey by the screener questions. As a result, data from this survey do not allow for a direct assessment of prevalence, although prevalence can be estimated. A study commissioned by the SSA in 2001-2002 found that about 10 percent of child SSI recipients had been missed by the special needs screener, and of those who had been missed, 53 percent had intellectual disability; 8 percent had speech disturbances; 4 percent had other specific learning difficulties; 4 percent had attention deficit hyperactivity disorder/attention deficit disorder; and the rest had a wide range of physical, cognitive, and behavioral conditions (Ireys et al., 2004). Second, like all the other surveys described here, this survey provides no clinical corroboration of a child's condition; all information is based on parent or guardian reports. Third, the survey did not collect detailed information about speech therapy or other service utilization, the etiology of the speech or language impairment, the child's age at the time of diagnosis, receipt of social welfare benefits, or measures of poverty or family well-being. Fourth, all levels of severity, from mild to severe, were included and cannot be disaggregated. Finally, because the survey was cross-sectional, no information is available about individual children's conditions over time.

National Survey of Children's Health

The National Survey of Children's Health was a cross-sectional telephone survey administered by the National Center for Health Statistics. Its purpose was to gather information on multiple, intersecting aspects of children's lives, including physical and mental health status and functioning; access to care; and the child's family, neighborhood, and social context (DRC, 2012a). The survey, fielded in 2007 and 2011, collected data on children with and without disabilities or other special health care needs. Both the 2007 and 2011 surveys included more than 90,000 children who were representative of all noninstitutionalized U.S. children (CDC, 2013a).

This survey has key shortcomings in the context of this study. First, it collected no information about receipt of SSI benefits, nor did it collect detailed information about speech therapy or other service utilization, etiology, age at time of child's diagnosis, receipt of social welfare benefits, or measures of poverty or family well-being. Second, all the information collected is based on parent or guardian reports, with no clinical corroboration of a child's condition. Finally, the survey's serial cross-sectional nature does not allow for measuring or monitoring specific children's conditions or status over time.

Survey of Income and Program Participation

The Survey of Income and Program Participation is a longitudinal telephone panel survey administered by the U.S. Census Bureau. It collects data related to sources and amounts of various types of income and assets, labor force participation, participation in and eligibility for social welfare programs, and general demographic characteristics. Its purpose is to enable assessment of the effectiveness of existing federal, state, and local programs and to provide accurate statistics on the distribution of income and measures of economic well-being in the United States (U.S. Census Bureau, 2015b). This survey has been fielded annually since the late 1970s (U.S. Census Bureau, 2015b). Its design is a continuous series of national panels with sample sizes ranging from approximately 14,000 to 52,000 households (U.S. Census Bureau, 2015b). The 2008 survey included approximately 15,000 children in 9,000 households (NBER, 2015). During the time frame of interest to this study (i.e., the past decade), sampled households participated in a panel for 2 years, and data were collected on each member of the household. Core questions were asked several times, allowing for some monitoring over time, and topical questions were asked in selected waves.

This survey provides detailed data on income and assets, receipt of social welfare benefits, and material hardship (U.S. Census Bureau, 2015b).

However, it has key shortcomings in the context of this study. First, it collects no information about speech therapy or other service utilization, etiology, or age of child's diagnosis. Second, it provides no direct clinical assessment data to confirm a child's condition; all information is provided by parents or guardians. Third, because many questions and the survey format have changed over the years, multiyear comparisons are often problematic. Fourth, even though the survey is longitudinal, questions about disability status are asked only once, and it is not possible to measure or monitor children's disability status over time. Finally, the survey collects information about disabilities only for children who are 6 years of age and older.

Individuals with Disabilities Education Act (IDEA) Child Count Data

IDEA child count data are administrative data collected and reported annually. Each state reports the number of children receiving special education services funded in part by federal monies from IDEA Part B (ages 3-21) or Part C (ages birth through 2 years) (U.S. Department of Education, 2014). In 2012-2013, approximately 6.4 million children received special education services (U.S. Department of Education, 2015).

The value of IDEA data is that the program is designed to serve all children aged 0-21 in the United States who are eligible to participate; eligibility for services is based on information derived from a variety of instruments used to evaluate the child; and assessments should display no bias with respect to the student's racial, cultural, or linguistic background or disabilities. The results of these assessments are used by a multidisciplinary team to determine whether children have disabilities.

While all children with disabilities are legally entitled to receive IDEA services, the child count data may underrepresent the true prevalence of conditions because the data are based only on those children for whom parents agreed to receive publicly funded services, and the data quality may be affected by the multiple reporting entities. Variability in the number of recipients across states and school districts suggests that eligibility criteria and service delivery processes vary considerably. A significant shortcoming in the context of this study is that the condition reported in the child count data is only the primary disability used in making the service eligibility determination. Therefore, a child may have a speech or language disorder but be counted under a different eligibility category (e.g., autism, learning disability, hearing impairment), which can result in an underestimate of the prevalence of speech and language disorders. Nonetheless, these data do provide valuable information about trends in the percentage of children whose primary disability is determined to be a speech or language impairment, obtained from a multifaceted assessment that was evaluated by a multidisciplinary team.

The next section provides information about the prevalence of speech and language disorders in the general population of U.S. children derived from national survey data, including the National Survey of Children's Health, the National Survey of Children with Special Health Care Needs, and the National Health Interview Survey—Voice, Speech, and Language Supplement. Further details on all of these surveys is provided in Appendix B.

TRENDS IN THE PREVALENCE OF CHILDHOOD SPEECH AND LANGUAGE DISORDERS IN THE GENERAL POPULATION

Chapter 2 includes *clinical data* on the overall prevalence of childhood speech and language disorders in the general U.S. population. In this section, *population data* are used to estimate trends—or changes over time—in the prevalence of these disorders in the general population. A subsequent section presents estimates of trends in the child SSI program population based on administrative or service data.

Estimates of the prevalence of childhood speech and language disorders in the general population vary depending on the survey data that are used. Figures 5-1 and 5-2 show the proportion of noninstitutionalized children with speech and language disorders in the general population derived from two datasets: the 2005-2006 and 2009-2010 National Survey of Children with Special Health Care Needs (see Figure 5-1) and the 2007 and 2011 National Survey of Children's Health (see Figure 5-2). In an effort to have comparable data points (similar periods in time from two different surveys) the committee used data from the two National Surveys of Children with Special Health Care Needs that included speech and language disorders and the two closest years in which the National Survey of Children's Health was fielded.

To derive estimates of trends in prevalence in the general U.S. population, the committee used weighted percentages from the National Survey of Children's Health and the National Survey of Children with Special Health Care Needs. (See Appendix D for a detailed description of the methods used to calculate estimates of trends in prevalence from the national survey data.) For the National Survey of Children's Health, the result was an estimated 26 percent increase from 2007 to 2011 (from 3.8 to 4.8 percent or from 2,697 to 3,916), with relatively equivalent increases noted in children of different racial or ethnic identities (CDC, 2013b,c) (see Figure 5-2). For the 2005-2006 and 2009-2010 National Survey of Children with Special Health Care Needs, the committee multiplied the weighted percentage of children with speech problems in each year (using the survey weights recommended by the National Center for Health Statistics) by the percentage

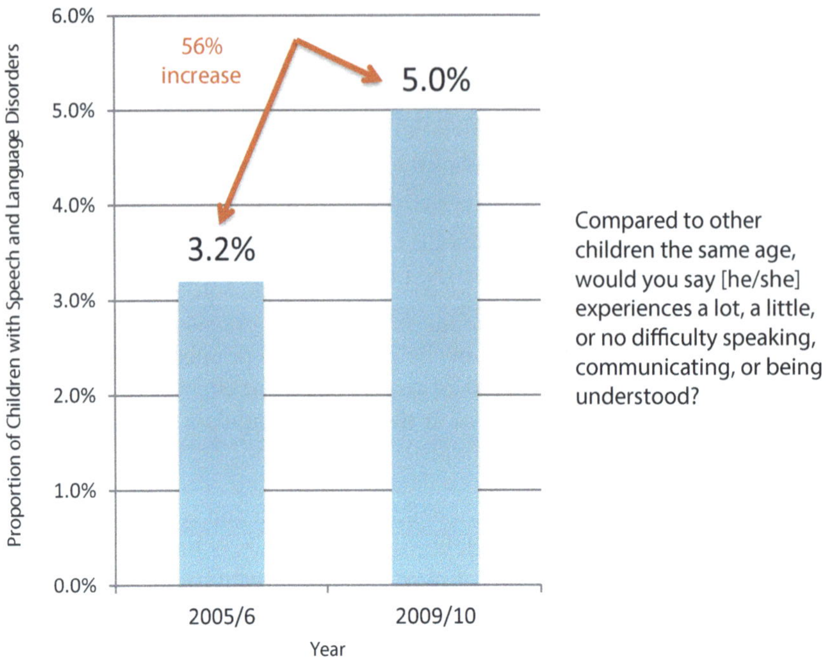

FIGURE 5-1 Proportion of children with speech and language disorders in the general U.S. population based on the 2005-2006 and 2009-2010 National Survey of Children with Special Health Care Needs.
NOTE: The sample size in 2005-2006 is 38,296. The sample size in 2009-2010 is 39,747.

of children with special health care needs in the larger population.[2] The percentages of children with speech problems for 2005-2006 and 2009-2010 were 23 percent and 33 percent, respectively (CDC, 2007, 2012b, 2014b,c). In 2005-2006 and 2009-2010, the percentages of children with special health care needs were 13.9 percent and 15.1 percent, respectively (HHS, 2013; HHS et al., 2008). The result was an estimated 56 percent increase in prevalence from 3.2 to 5.0 percent (from 8,435 to 11,936) from 2005-2006 to 2009-2010 (see Figure 5-1). Together, these prevalence estimates indicate that the proportion of children in the general U.S. population with speech and language disorders increased from 3.2 percent in 2005-2006 to 4.8 percent in 2011 (CDC, 2007, 2013c, 2014b; HHS et al., 2008). The

[2] In 2009-2010, the percentage of children with special health care needs in the larger population was 15.1 percent (HHS, 2013).

committee notes that this is an approximate estimate, based on parent and guardian reports, that includes all levels of severity of speech and language disorders as measured by the questions used in the respective surveys.

Not shown in Figures 5-1 and 5-2 is the National Health Interview Survey's single question on stuttering. Responses to this question suggest a slight but gradual increase from 2000 through 2012, particularly among the younger age groups (3-11), and more stable rates for children aged 12-17.

To derive an estimated range for the overall prevalence of reported speech and language problems of any severity, the committee used estimates based on clinical data (see Chapter 2) and the population data described above. The result was an estimated overall prevalence of speech and language disorders of 3-16 percent of the general U.S. population aged birth through 21 years.

Administrative data from IDEA suggest that, relative to their proportion of the general U.S. population (2-15 percent for those aged birth-21, as

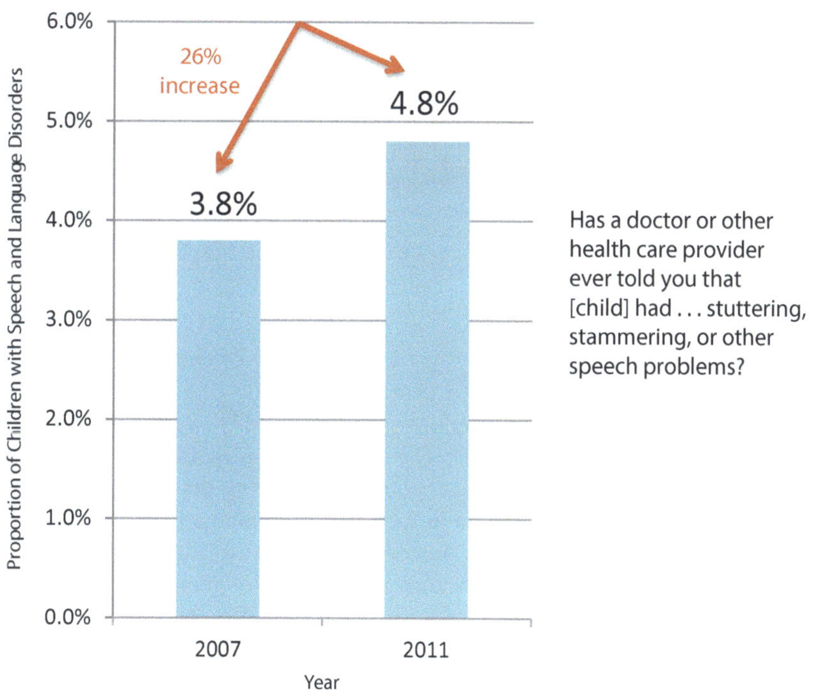

FIGURE 5-2 Proportion of children with speech and language disorders in the general U.S. population based on the 2007 and 2011 National Survey of Children's Health.

NOTE: The sample size in 2007 is 81,955. The sample size in 2011 is 85,581.

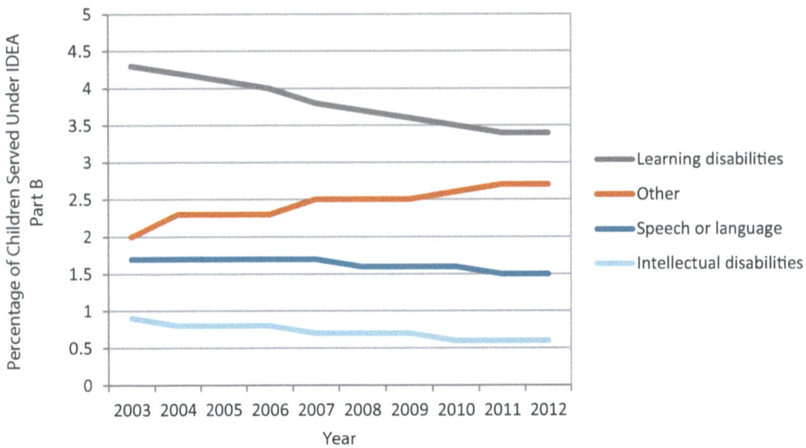

FIGURE 5-3 Percentage of the general U.S. population of children aged 6-21 years served under IDEA Part B, by year and disability category, fall 2003 through fall 2012.
NOTE: According to the U.S. Department of Education, percentage was calculated by dividing the number of students ages 6 through 21 served under IDEA, Part B, in the disability category in the year by the estimated U.S. resident population ages 6 through 21 for that year, then multiplying the result by 100. The numbers of students served under IDEA Part B are included in Appendix C.
SOURCE: U.S. Department of Education, 2014.

reported above), a substantially smaller percentage of children who receive special education services have a primary condition of speech and/or language impairment (1.5-1.7 percent of those aged 6-21) (see Figure 5-3) (U.S. Department of Education, 2014). The smaller percentages for the IDEA dataset are also consistent with other sources indicating that only about two-thirds of children reported to have speech and language problems received intervention services during the preceding year (Bainbridge, 2015; Black et al., 2015). Some of the children with speech and language impairments in IDEA data also likely have more serious impairments than children in the survey datasets described above. With respect to trends in prevalence, IDEA data stand in contrast to the survey data reported above, indicating that the prevalence of speech and language disorders among children receiving IDEA services remained steady from 2003 to 2012.

Why the prevalence of speech and language disorders as measured by the National Survey of Children's Health and the National Survey of

Children with Special Health Care Needs has increased over time is unclear. However, analyses of similar increases among children with autism spectrum disorder and attention deficit hyperactivity disorder may provide some insight. The available epidemiologic literature shows a consistent increase in the prevalence of these latter two conditions over time (Newschaffer et al., 2005; Visser et al., 2010). Factors identified as causes for these increases include increased awareness of developmental disorders due to media attention and advocacy, increased availability of early intervention and special education services, changes in access and practices that are leading to children being identified as having a developmental disorder at a higher frequency, changes in the definition of certain conditions (e.g., autism spectrum disorder), and an increase in the assignment of co-occurring diagnoses among children with developmental disorders (NASEM, 2015). Although there have been no similar studies of the epidemiology of speech and language disorders, the committee believes the available evidence suggests that the same factors have contributed to the increasing prevalence of these disorders.

VARIATIONS IN THE PREVALENCE OF SPEECH AND LANGUAGE DISORDERS BY DEMOGRAPHIC AND OTHER CHARACTERISTICS

This section summarizes the available evidence on variations in the prevalence of childhood speech and language disorders by the following characteristics: age, gender, race/ethnicity, socioeconomic status, and comorbidities.

Age

The available evidence indicates that speech and language disorders are highly variable with age.

Age of Children with Speech and Language Disorders

Across national population surveys, the percentage of children with reported speech and language disorders is generally higher among younger children; these disorders are most common among children aged 3-6 years (11.0 percent), followed by those aged 7-10 years (9.3 percent), and their reported prevalence is lowest among children in their teens (4.9 percent) (see Table 5-2 and the discussion of persistence in Chapter 3) (Bainbridge, 2015; Black et al., 2015).

IDEA child count data show that the percentage of children with speech or language impairments is considerably higher in the younger age group

TABLE 5-2 National Health Interview Survey—Voice, Speech, Language Supplement: Prevalence of Speech and Language Disorders, by Age

Age Group	Prevalence (%)
3-6 years	11.0
7-10 years	9.3
11-17 years	4.9

NOTE: The prevalence estimates for children aged 3-6 and 7-10 are significantly different from that for children aged 11-17 years ($p < 0.05$).
SOURCE: Black et al., 2015.

of 3-5 years (44.7 percent) than in the older age group of 6-21 years (18.2 percent) (see Figure 5-4) (U.S. Department of Education, 2014).

Age of Onset

As noted in Chapter 1, age of onset of speech and language disorders is difficult to pinpoint, although it is likely to be early in the child's life. Available data on these disorders are more likely to reflect age of identification than age of onset. Identification of speech and language disorders requires that children be of an age when speech is typically present, and disruptions or delays in speech become evident. Data from the National Health Interview Survey—Voice, Speech, and Language Supplement indicate that these disorders are identified in the overwhelming majority of children by age 6. More than half of speech problems are identified in the first 2 years of the child's life, and almost one-third between 3 and 5 years of age.

Gender

Data sources consistently document sex differences in speech and language disorders, with boys demonstrating speech and language problems approximately twice as frequently as girls (see also Chapter 2). Data from the National Health Interview Survey (2000-2012) indicate that about 69 percent of children identified with stuttering and stammering problems are boys, compared with 31 percent for girls (Bainbridge, 2015). The National Health Interview Survey—Voice, Speech, and Language Supplement shows the prevalence of voice, speech, swallowing, or language problems to be 4.3 percent of all boys versus 2.2 percent of all girls (Hoffman, 2015). Finally, data from the National Survey of Children with Special Health Care Needs indicate that 67 percent of all children with a great deal of difficulty with speech are boys (Blumberg, 2015).

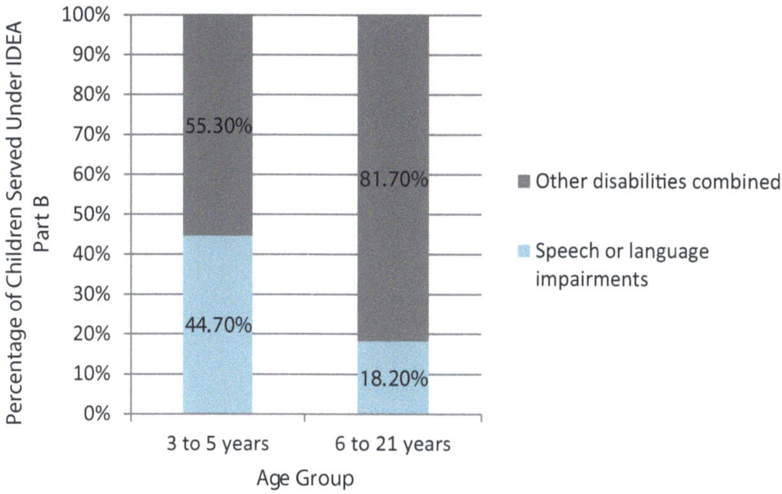

FIGURE 5-4 Percentage of children served under IDEA Part B by age group: Fall 2012.
NOTE: In the age group 3-5 years, the "other disabilities combined" category includes developmental delay, autism, deafness-blindness, emotional disturbance, hearing impairments, intellectual disabilities, multiple disabilities, orthopedic impairments, other health impairments, specific learning disabilities, traumatic brain injury, and visual impairments. In the age group 6-21 years, the "other disabilities combined" category includes specific learning disabilities, other health impairments, autism, intellectual disabilities, emotional disturbance, deafness-blindness, developmental delay, hearing impairments, multiple disabilities, orthopedic impairments, traumatic brain injury, and visual impairments.
SOURCE: U.S. Department of Education, 2014.

Race/Ethnicity

Figure 5-5 shows the weighted racial and ethnic composition of children with speech and language disorders, using data from the 2007 and 2011 National Survey of Children's Health (CDC, 2013b,c). In addition to depicting the proportion of children with speech and language disorders by race and Hispanic ethnicity, the figure shows the reported increase in each group over time. As is evident, the percentage of children reported to have speech and language disorders increased over time within each racial or ethnic group.

Figure 5-6 shows the prevalence of speech and language disorders in children by race/ethnicity based on the National Health Interview Survey—Voice, Speech, and Language Supplement. Although not statistically

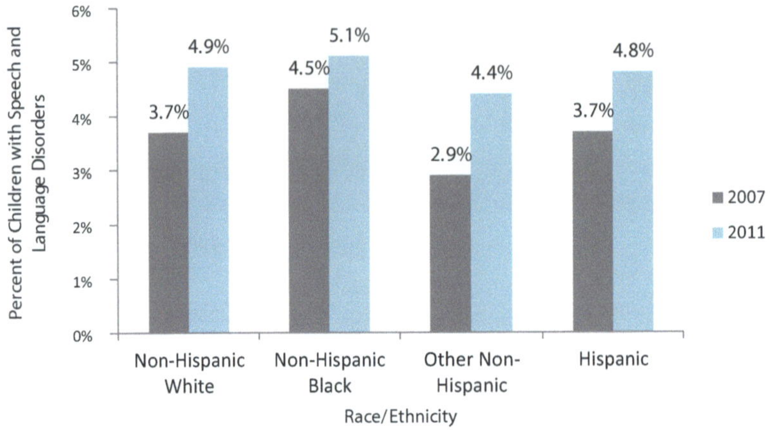

FIGURE 5-5 Prevalence of speech and language disorders by race/ethnicity among children aged 0-17 years based on the 2007 and 2011 National Survey of Children's Health.
NOTE: The sample size is 81,955 in 2007 and 85,581 in 2011.

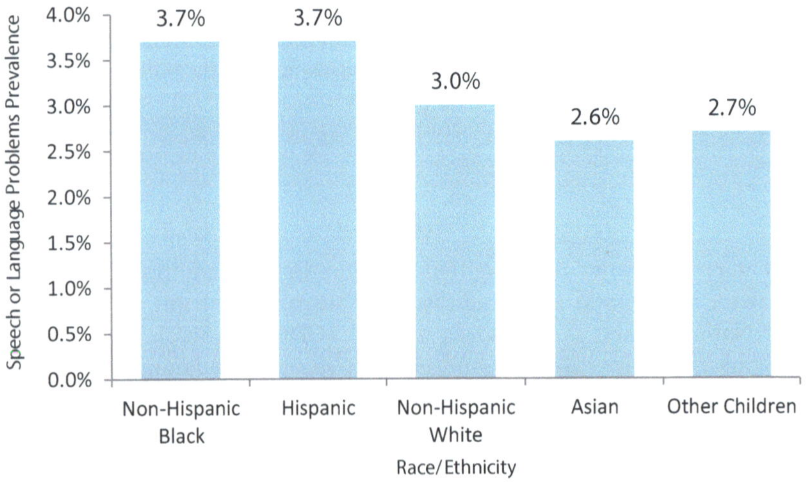

FIGURE 5-6 Prevalence of speech and language disorders among children aged 3-17 years based on the National Health Interview Survey—Voice, Speech, and Language Supplement.

significant, this survey showed higher rates for non-Hispanic black (3.7 percent) and Hispanic (3.7 percent) children compared with non-Hispanic white (3.0 percent), Asian (2.6 percent), and other (2.7 percent) children (Hoffman, 2015).

In summary, the committee found no apparent racial or ethnic differences in the prevalence of speech and language disorders based on the surveys it reviewed. The surveys show slight variability across racial/ethnic groups, but the findings are not statistically significant.

Socioeconomic Status

A greater proportion of children with speech and language disorders than of children without such disorders are in families that live in poverty or have low incomes. Low income here means total income below 200 percent of the federal poverty level (FPL) (Boushey et al., 2001; National Center for Children in Poverty, 2013). The FPL varies by household size. In 2015, for a family of four living in the 48 contiguous United States, it was $24,250 (HHS, 2015a). Thus, for example, a family of four with income below 200 percent of that number ($48,500) would be defined as having low income. In 2013, approximately 44 percent of U.S. children lived in low-income households (National Center for Children in Poverty, 2013). Figures 5-7 and 5-8 show data from the Survey of Income and Program Participation indicating that children with speech and language disorders are more likely than other children to live in poor or low-income households (26 versus 21 percent and 28 versus 23 percent, respectively) (NBER, 2015).

The National Survey of Children with Special Health Care Needs, 2009-2010, yields similar findings, showing that relative to all children with special health care needs, those with any speech and language problems were more likely to live in poverty (30.8 versus 22.2 percent) or in low-income households (24.0 versus 21.8 percent) and less likely to live at 400 percent of the FPL or above (19.5 versus 27.5 percent) (Blumberg, 2015). This finding was even more marked for children with the most severe speech and language disorders who lived in poverty (33.4 versus 22.2 percent) or in low-income households (23.0 versus 21.8 percent); these children also were less likely to live well above the poverty level (18.3 versus 27.5 percent) (Blumberg, 2015). In data from the National Health Interview Survey—Voice, Speech, and Language Supplement (2012), the prevalence of communication problems decreased from 5.4 percent in children living below the FPL to 1.9 percent for children in families at five times the poverty level (Hoffman, 2015).

Families with low incomes often face material deprivation. Figure 5-9 shows 2010 data from the Survey of Income and Program Participation indicating that households that experience various types of material hardship

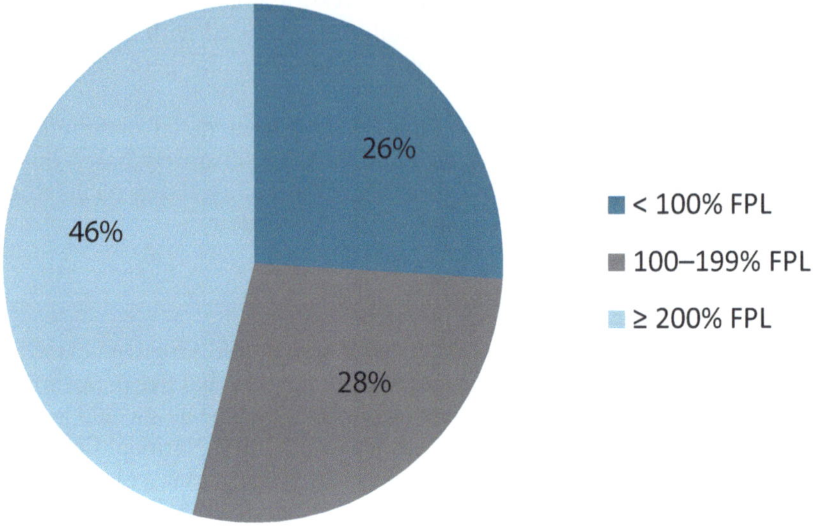

FIGURE 5-7 Children aged 6-17 with speech and language disorders, by family income relative to the federal poverty level (FPL).
NOTE: The sample size is 277.
SOURCE: 2010 Survey of Income and Program Participation.

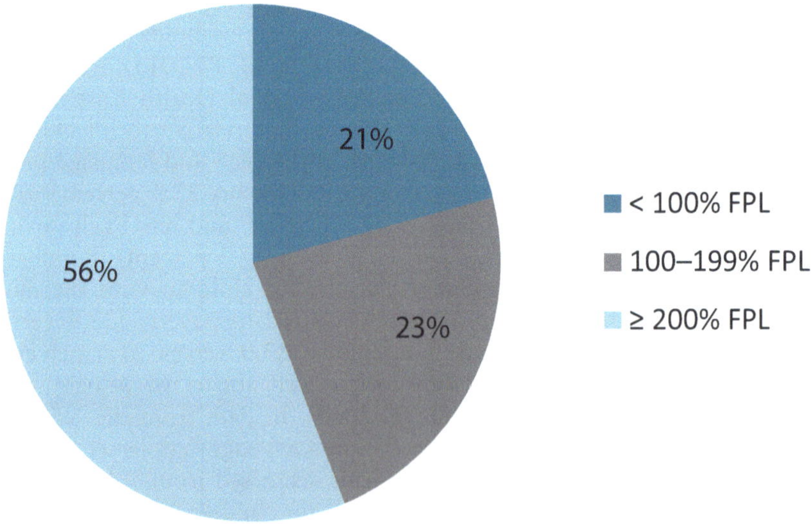

FIGURE 5-8 Children aged 6-17 without speech and language disorders, by family income relative to the federal poverty level (FPL).
NOTE: The sample size is 14,507.
SOURCE: 2010 Survey of Income and Program Participation.

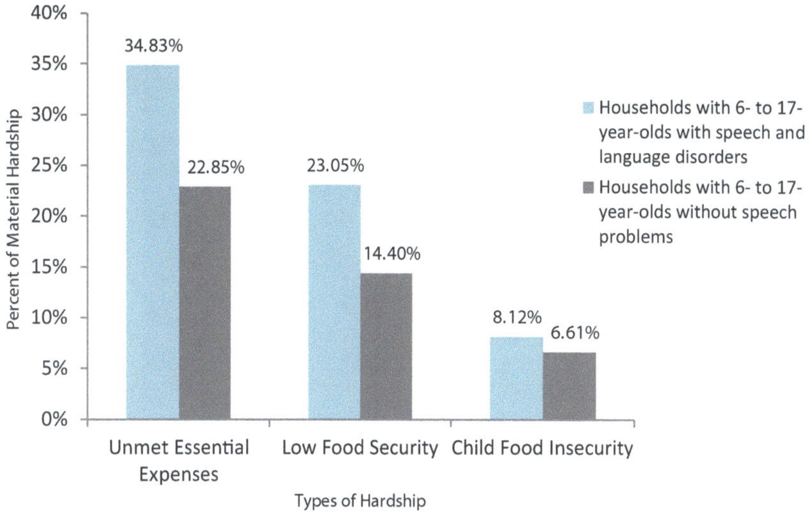

FIGURE 5-9 Material hardship among families with and without children with speech and language disorders.
NOTE: The sample size of children with speech and language disorders is 277 and without speech and language disorders is 14,507.
SOURCE: 2010 Survey of Income and Program Participation.

are more likely than households that do not experience such hardship to have children with speech and language disorders (NBER, 2015).

Food insecurity is defined as insufficient access to adequate food, which occurs as a result of limited financial and other resources (Coleman-Jensen et al., 2013). In the case of household food insecurity, many parents forego their own meals so they can feed their children. Child food insecurity (illustrated in Figure 5-9), a situation in which children have insufficient food, is rarer. Figure 5-9 shows that both household food insecurity and child food insecurity are higher among households with children with speech and language disorders than among other households (e.g., 8 percent versus 7 percent for child food insecurity) (NBER, 2015). The third indicator of hardship is the inability to meet necessary household expenses (e.g., rent, utilities), which shows a similar pattern.

With respect to health service utilization of children with speech and language disorders, having insurance is generally considered a prerequisite for receiving appropriate care when it is needed (HHS, n.d.). According to data from the 2011 National Survey of Children's Health, just 4 percent of children with speech problems were uninsured (CDC, 2013c). Of the

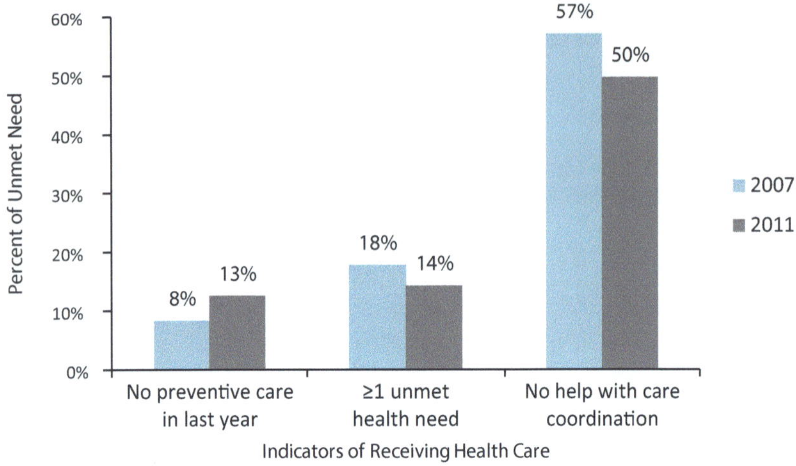

FIGURE 5-10 Unmet health care needs for children with speech problems.
NOTE: In 2007, the sample sizes for no preventive care in past year, ≥ 1 unmet health need, and no help with care coordination are 2,469, 2,487, and 980, respectively. In 2011, the respective sample sizes are 3,529, 3,548, and 1,410.
SOURCE: 2007 and 2011 National Survey of Children's Health.

remainder, 44 percent had public insurance (Medicaid, TriCare, or the State Children's Health Insurance Program), and 53 percent had private insurance (CDC, 2013c). Yet despite having nearly universal levels of insurance, children with speech or language disorders experienced significant barriers to receiving needed health care services. Figure 5-10 illustrates the relatively high rates of unmet need for these children in terms of three common indicators of receiving health care (CDC, 2013b,c). The rates of unmet need for care were relatively stable from 2007 to 2011.

Comorbidities

As discussed in Chapter 2, children with speech and language disorders have a high likelihood of experiencing other problems as well. Based on the 2000-2012 National Health Interview Survey, more than 40 percent of children with speech and language disorders experience such comorbidities as developmental delay[3] (32 percent), autism (12 percent), or intellectual

[3] Developmental delay refers to physical, cognitive, communication, social or emotional, or adaptive developmental milestones that are not reached by a child at the expected times.

disability (10 percent) (Bainbridge, 2015). Data from the National Health Interview Survey—Voice, Speech, and Language Supplement indicate that intellectual disability is the most common comorbidity, representing 52 percent of all comorbidities, followed by developmental delay (27.6 percent), seizures (26.4 percent), and attention deficit hyperactivity disorder (10.4 percent) (Hoffman, 2015). What cannot be ascertained from these data is the frequency with which children experience speech and language disorders as comorbidities of other disorders or primary diagnoses.

TRENDS IN CHILDHOOD SPEECH AND LANGUAGE DISORDERS IN THE SUPPLEMENTAL SECURITY INCOME POPULATION

In analyzing trends in childhood speech and language disorders in the SSI population, the committee included any child who was allowed based on code 3153 (speech and language impairment) or 7840 (loss of voice [communication impairment]) from SSA Form 831. From this point forward, unless otherwise noted, the discussion of children with speech and language disorders who receive SSI benefits encompasses those with these two primary impairments.

It is also important to remember that the SSA's eligibility and determination process requires that children have a "marked" or "extreme" impairment, as described in Chapter 4. Because the datasets used in estimating the prevalence of speech and language disorders in the general U.S. population impose no such severity restrictions, definitive comparisons between the two populations are not possible. Impairments determined through the SSA process can be either primary—where the child's chief presenting problem is a speech or language impairment—or secondary—where the child has been determined to have another impairment for which a speech or language impairment is a comorbidity or a secondary impairment. As described in detail in Chapter 2, speech and language impairments are commonly associated with a variety of other developmental disorders, including disorders that may themselves result in a child's qualifying for SSI benefits (e.g., autism spectrum disorder, attention deficit hyperactivity disorder, intellectual disability). The remainder of this section presents information regarding

- the number of children qualifying for (i.e., allowances) and receiving (i.e., recipients) SSI benefits for speech and language disorders as a primary condition;
- the frequency with which other impairments (i.e., conditions) identified in the SSA eligibility and determination process are comorbid with primary speech or language disorders;

- the number of children for whom speech and language disorders are secondary impairments, and the comorbidity of other primary impairments among these children;
- the reasons that children who receive SSI benefits exit from the program (i.e., are suspended or terminated); and
- the concentration of the lowest-income children within the SSI program resulting from suspensions and terminations related to income and resources.

Note that in the figures that follow, the number of *recipients* represents the total number of children receiving SSI benefits in a given federal fiscal year, and includes children under 18 years of age who qualified in previous years and were still eligible. *Allowances*, on the other hand, represent the new cases of children who became eligible for SSI benefits in that year. Because the number of newly eligible children is smaller than the total number of current beneficiaries, the number of allowances for a given year will always be lower than the number of recipients. As discussed previously, recipients of SSI benefits for speech and language disorders must have "marked" or "extreme" disorders to qualify for SSI benefits, and the vast majority of these children are not expected to recover from or be cured of those disorders. Thus, the majority of these children will continue to qualify for SSI benefits until they are age 18 unless their eligibility status changes for another reason (e.g., family income and/or resources increase to the point that the child no longer qualifies; the child dies; or some other event occurs that affects a relatively small number of children, such as moving out of the United States, failing to complete paperwork, or moving into a residential institution).

Trends in Initial Allowances and Total Number of Recipients for Primary Speech and Language Impairments

The committee worked to identify and understand the trends over time in the total number of SSI recipients for primary speech and language impairments. To do so, the committee examined trends in initial allowances and trends in the overall number of SSI child recipients for speech and language disorders, and examined these trends in the context of the cumulative effect of new children being entered into the program after establishment of this diagnostic eligibility in 1994 and the relatively few departures from the program. These findings are presented below.

The numbers of initial determinations, denials, and initial allowances for speech and language disorders are shown in Figure 5-11. An initial determination refers to a decision made by Disability Determination Services as to whether a child is allowed or denied SSI benefits based on disability.

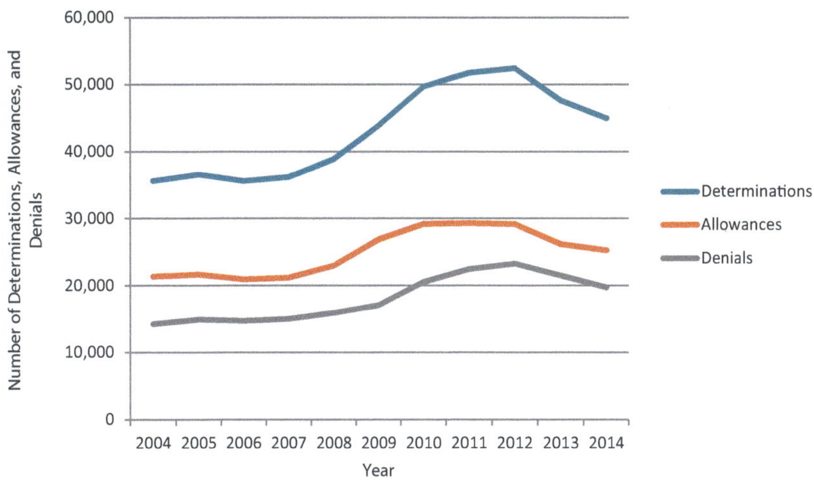

FIGURE 5-11 Number of determinations, allowances, and denials for speech and language disorders (includes primary impairment codes 3153 and 7840) at the initial level, fiscal years 2004-2014.
SOURCE: Unpublished dataset provided by the Social Security Administration.

Therefore, determinations equal the sum of initial allowances and denials. The committee's analysis showed that initial allowances for children with speech and language disorders exceed the number of denials. The data suggest that more children who meet the requirements for SSI disability benefits than children who do not meet the requirements are applying for benefits and being allowed into the SSI program.

The numbers of allowances for primary speech and language impairment over an 11-year period are shown in Figure 5-12. The figure also shows increases in allowances within the SSI program during years that correspond to the years of administration of the National Survey of Children with Special Health Care Needs and the National Survey of Children's Health.

The number of children who met the eligibility criteria each year for a marked or extreme speech or language impairment increased from 18,299 in 2004 to 22,727 in 2014. During that same period, the population of children aged 0-17 in the United States increased by just 0.39 percent (U.S. Census Bureau, 2015c). It is noteworthy that during the economic recession that began in 2007, the number of initial allowances increased sharply, and the number then decreased in 2013 and 2014 as the economy improved.

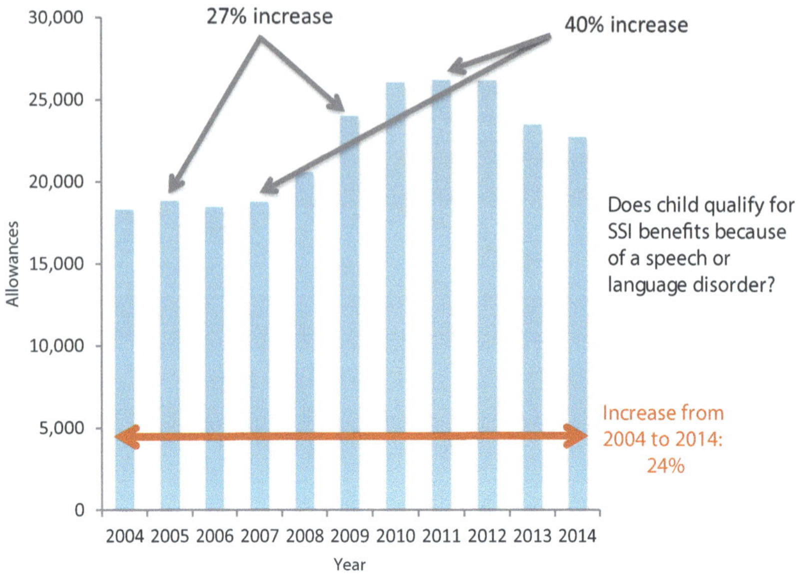

FIGURE 5-12 Initial allowances for speech and language impairment as a primary condition, fiscal years 2004-2014.
SOURCE: Unpublished dataset provided by the Social Security Administration.

The 27 percent increase in SSI allowances for children with speech and language impairments is markedly lower than the 56 percent increase in prevalence of these disorders reported by the National Survey of Children with Special Health Care Needs between 2005-2006 and 2009-2010. On the other hand, the 40 percent increase in SSI allowances is larger than the 26 percent increase in prevalence reported by the National Survey of Children's Health between 2007 and 2011 (compare Figures 5-2 [presented earlier] and 5-12).

Figure 5-13 illustrates the total number of children receiving SSI benefits for speech and language impairment over the period 2004 to 2014, showing a 171 percent increase from 78,827 to 213,688. However, the number of initial allowances per year (i.e., newly eligible beneficiaries) increased by only 24.2 percent during this same period.

Figure 5-14 illustrates why the annual number of initial allowances increased by 24.2 percent during this 11-year period, while the total number of recipients increased by 171 percent. As elaborated below, because the impairment code for speech and language impairment (3153) was not

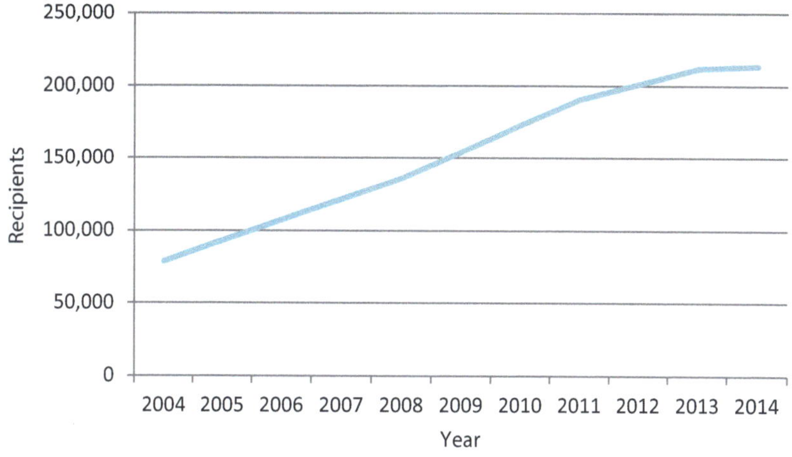

FIGURE 5-13 Numbers of child recipients of SSI benefits for speech and language impairment, fiscal years 2004-2014.
SOURCE: Unpublished dataset provided by the Social Security Administration.

established until 1994, and children qualifying for SSI benefits have severe disorders that are unlikely to remit, the growth in the number of overall recipients reflects the aggregation of new allowances over the 18 preceding years. In other words, the total number of participants in a particular year is an *accumulation* of new cases added in that year plus all of those deemed eligible in prior years (less those who age out or are otherwise no longer eligible). In most cases, children who are deemed eligible will continue to have a severe speech or language disorder, and unless their eligibility changes for some other reason, they will not exit the program until they reach 18 years of age. Thus, a 24.2 percent increase in the number of annual initial *allowances* leads to a much larger 171 percent increase in the total number of *beneficiaries* over time because once qualified for SSI, few children with severe speech and language disorders subsequently become ineligible for the program.

In 1994, the first year in which the new impairment code (3153) for speech and language impairment existed, only 1,585 children met the eligibility criteria for this new code. In 1995, an additional 4,109 children were allowed benefits under this new code; in 1996, an additional 4,119 children were allowed; and so forth for each subsequent year. Given that children with severe speech and language impairments are likely to continue

1993	1994	1995	1996	1997	1998	1999	2000	2001	2002	2003	2004	2005	2006	2007	2008	2009	2010	2011	2012	2013	2014	Total Recipients	Year	Increase
0	1,585	4,109	4,119	2,904	3,829	6,017	8,299	10,500	13,676	16,944	18,299	18,829	18,445	18,761	20,572	24,000	26,050	26,188	26,177	23,493	22,727	305,710	2014	18,608
0	1,585	4,109	4,119	2,904	3,829	6,017	8,299	10,500	13,676	16,944	18,299	18,829	18,445	18,761	20,572	24,000	26,050	26,188	26,177	23,493		287,102	2013	19,384
0	1,585	4,109	4,119	2,904	3,829	6,017	8,299	10,500	13,676	16,944	18,299	18,829	18,445	18,761	20,572	24,000	26,050	26,188	26,177			267,718	2012	24,592
0	1,585	4,109	4,119	2,904	3,829	6,017	8,299	10,500	13,676	16,944	18,299	18,829	18,445	18,761	20,572	24,000	26,050	26,188				243,126	2011	26,188
0	1,585	4,109	4,119	2,904	3,829	6,017	8,299	10,500	13,676	16,944	18,299	18,829	18,445	18,761	20,572	24,000	26,050					216,938	2010	26,050
0	1,585	4,109	4,119	2,904	3,829	6,017	8,299	10,500	13,676	16,944	18,299	18,829	18,445	18,761	20,572	24,000						190,888	2009	24,000
0	1,585	4,109	4,119	2,904	3,829	6,017	8,299	10,500	13,676	16,944	18,299	18,829	18,445	18,761	20,572							166,888	2008	20,572
0	1,585	4,109	4,119	2,904	3,829	6,017	8,299	10,500	13,676	16,944	18,299	18,829	18,445	18,761								146,316	2007	18,761
0	1,585	4,109	4,119	2,904	3,829	6,017	8,299	10,500	13,676	16,944	18,299	18,829	18,445									127,555	2006	18,445
0	1,585	4,109	4,119	2,904	3,829	6,017	8,299	10,500	13,676	16,944	18,299	18,829										109,110	2005	18,829
0	1,585	4,109	4,119	2,904	3,829	6,017	8,299	10,500	13,676	16,944	18,299											90,281	2004	18,299
0	1,585	4,109	4,119	2,904	3,829	6,017	8,299	10,500	13,676	16,944												71,982	2003	16,944
0	1,585	4,109	4,119	2,904	3,829	6,017	8,299	10,500	13,676													55,038	2002	13,676
0	1,585	4,109	4,119	2,904	3,829	6,017	8,299	10,500														41,362	2001	10,500
0	1,585	4,109	4,119	2,904	3,829	6,017	8,299															30,862	2000	8,299
0	1,585	4,109	4,119	2,904	3,829	6,017																22,563	1999	6,017
0	1,585	4,109	4,119	2,904	3,829																	16,546	1998	3,829
0	1,585	4,109	4,119	2,904																		12,717	1997	2,904
0	1,585	4,109	4,119																			9,813	1996	4,119
0	1,585	4,109																				5,694	1995	4,109
0	1,585																					1,585	1994	1,585

Terminations at 4% of recipients each year = 96,108

509	662	903	1,234	1,654	2,202	2,879	3,611	4,364	5,102	5,853	6,676	7,636	8,678	9,725	10,709	11,484	12,228

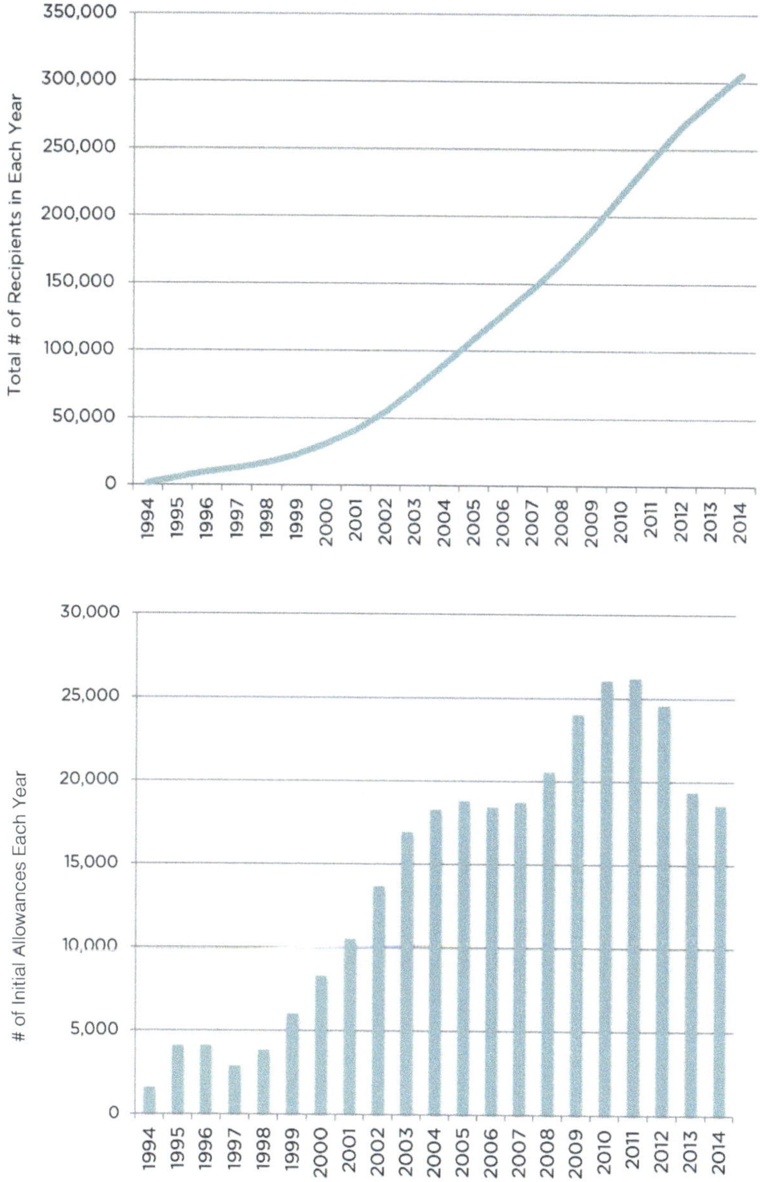

FIGURE 5-14 Illustration of how the total number of children receiving SSI benefits grew over time as a result of the addition of a new category, fiscal years 1994-2014.
SOURCE: Unpublished dataset provided by the Social Security Administration.

to have severe impairments throughout adolescence and into adulthood, the total number of children (aged 0-18) who received benefits under this new code in any given year approaches the total number of children who became eligible in each of the preceding 18 years (those years are shaded in Figure 5-14). Thus, the total number of children receiving SSI benefits for speech and language impairments in 2013 will include almost all of the children who became eligible in the years from 1996 through 2013, but will not include children who became eligible in 1994 or 1995. In fact, when the numbers in Figure 5-14 are adjusted for the approximately 4 percent[4] of children whose benefits are terminated each year (see the later discussion of suspensions and terminations), the graph of the number of recipients each year in Figure 5-14 is similar to the graph in Figure 5-13. In other words, the increase in the number of recipients is almost completely explained by the fact that a new category for speech and language impairment was created in 1994; that virtually all children in this category have marked or extreme forms of impairment (as required by the SSA eligibility criteria); and that very few of these children will cease to have marked or extreme impairments as a result of receiving the available treatments.

Comorbidities Among Allowances for Primary Speech and Language Disorders

Figure 5-15 shows the number of allowances for children with primary speech and language impairments who also had secondary impairments (comorbidities). The top two secondary impairment categories are none established, no medical evidence in file, and none/no secondary impairment for children with primary speech and language impairments. However, these data should be viewed with caution. In its review, the U.S. Government Accountability Office (GAO, 2012) found "significant inconsistencies" in how secondary impairments were coded nationwide. Furthermore, the absence of a *recorded* secondary impairment does not mean that the child did not actually have another impairment, only that it was not recorded as part of the eligibility determination process.

Only about one-third of children with speech and language impairments had a secondary impairment recorded. Among these children, autistic disorder and other developmental disorders was the secondary impairment category most commonly listed. The number of children with secondary autism spectrum disorder increased between 2004 and 2014 from 643 to 2,488. The second most commonly occurring secondary impairment, especially between 2007 and 2010, was attention deficit hyperactivity disorder.

[4] Based on unpublished data provided by the SSA, the 4 percent figure was calculated by dividing total child terminations by total child SSI recipients in 2008.

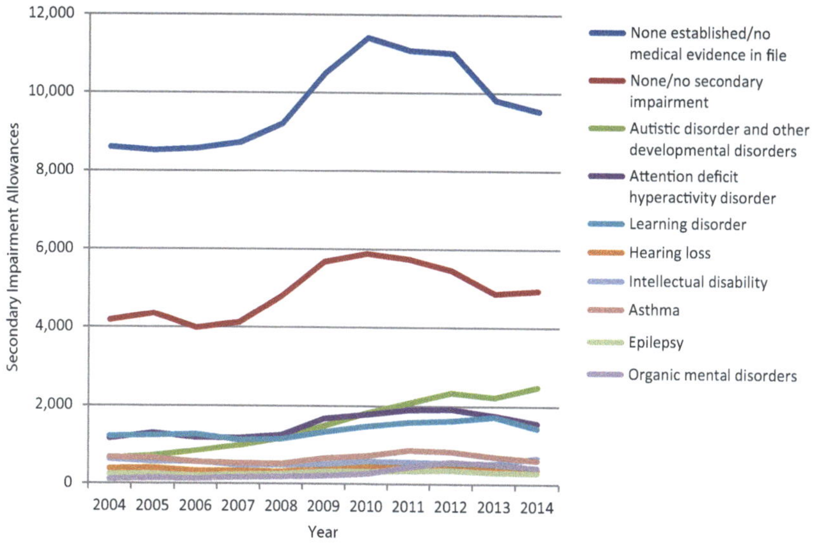

FIGURE 5-15 Top secondary impairments for initial allowances for primary speech and language disorder (includes impairment codes 3153 and 7840), fiscal years 2004-2014.
SOURCE: Unpublished dataset provided by the Social Security Administration.

Between 2008 and 2014, autism spectrum disorder, attention deficit hyperactivity disorder, and learning disability were the most frequent comorbid conditions associated with an allowance based on a primary speech or language impairment.

Primary Impairments for Which Speech and Language Impairments Were Secondary Impairments

Figure 5-16 shows the most frequent primary impairments among children for whom speech and language impairments were reported as a secondary condition. The most commonly occurring of these primary impairments was autism spectrum disorder, for which allowances ranged from 2,402 to 6,238 between 2008 and 2014. Between 2004 and 2007, the most commonly occurring primary impairment was intellectual disability. Commonly occurring in addition to autism spectrum disorder and intellectual disability were attention deficit hyperactivity disorder and learning disabilities.

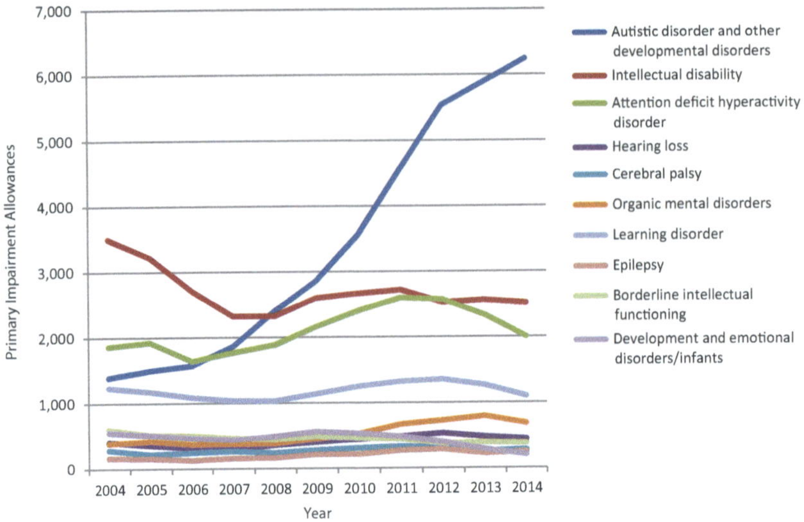

FIGURE 5-16 Top primary impairments for which speech and language disorders were secondary impairments (includes impairment codes 3153 and 7840), fiscal years 2004-2014.
SOURCE: Unpublished dataset provided by the Social Security Administration.

Exits from the Supplemental Security Income Program

Recipients may exit from the SSI program because of suspension, termination, age-18 transitions, or death. A suspension occurs when a recipient's payments are stopped because of ineligibility. Suspensions cannot last longer than 1 year. If a recipient does not become eligible again within 12 months, benefits are terminated. A termination is a permanent loss of SSI eligibility. A terminated recipient must file a new application to reinstate his or her benefits. (See also the discussion of the SSI program in Chapter 4.)

Figure 5-17 shows suspensions from the SSI program from 2004 through 2013. Notably, these data are for all children receiving SSI benefits, not just those with speech and language disorders as has been the case previously in this section. Depending on the year, suspensions represent 12-15 percent of the total number of SSI recipients under 18 years of age.

Most suspensions occurred because the child recipient's family income or assets exceeded SSI program limits. The number of such income-related suspensions increased from 84,900 in 2004 to 95,138 in 2013. Approximately 3.7 to 18.3 percent of the suspensions occurred because the child no longer qualified as having a marked or extreme impairment.

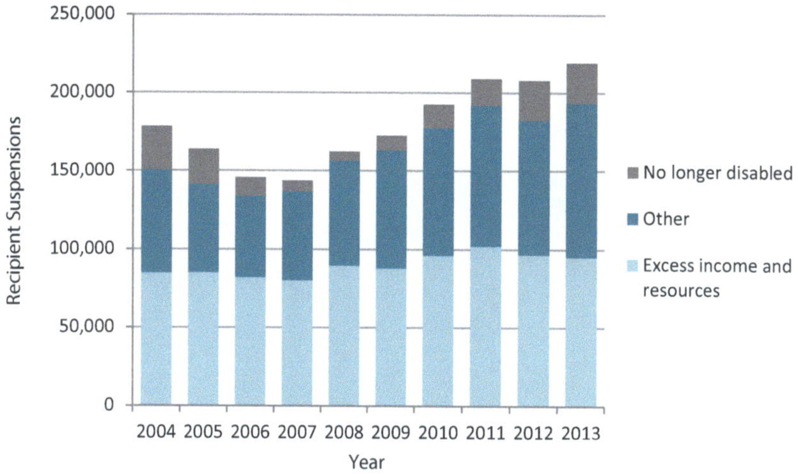

FIGURE 5-17 Number of all child SSI recipients suspended, fiscal years 2004-2013.
SOURCE: Unpublished dataset provided by the Social Security Administration.

This trend is consistent with information presented in Chapter 3 indicating that the severity of speech and language disorders required for SSI eligibility is unlikely to resolve over time, even when treatment is provided. Some children were suspended for "other" reasons, which include admission into a residential facility, whereabouts unknown, no representative payee, in public institution, failed to furnish report, moved outside United States, in transition, and other or unknown reasons.

Figure 5-18 shows the number of children (again not limited to those with speech and language disorders) whose SSI benefits were terminated between 2004 and 2013. As in Figure 5-17, the largest number of terminations occurred when recipients' families had income and/or resources that exceeded program limits—28,270 terminations in 2004, rising to 32,825 in 2013 (which represents 48.9 percent of all terminations in that year). Terminations due to no longer being disabled decreased by more than 70 percent between 2004 and 2008 before increasing to 27.5 percent in 2013—approximately the same level as in 2004.

Concentration of Lowest-Income Children Within the Supplemental Security Income Program Resulting from Suspensions and Terminations

The net result of suspending and terminating higher-income children from the SSI program is the concentration of children from the poorest

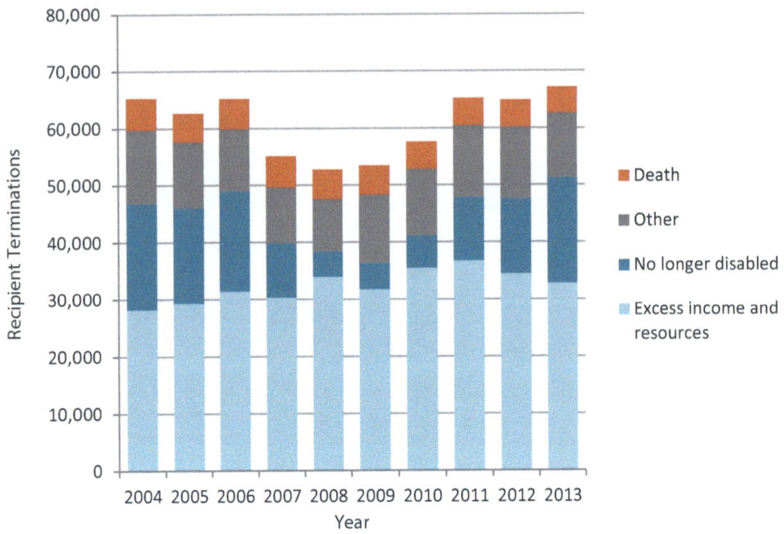

FIGURE 5-18 Number of SSI child recipients terminated, fiscal years 2004-2013.
SOURCE: Unpublished dataset provided by the Social Security Administration.

families remaining in the program (see Figure 5-19). The largest number of child SSI recipients are those with the lowest family incomes (at or below 100 percent of the FPL). Over time, a larger proportion of the lowest-income children thus are retained within the SSI program.

TRENDS IN CHILDHOOD SPEECH AND LANGUAGE DISORDERS AMONG MEDICAID BENEFICIARIES

Medicaid data are administrative and can be used to examine comorbid conditions and services among children receiving treatment for a medical diagnosis. As described below, entry into the SSI program establishes eligibility for Medicaid in most states. Consequently, most children eligible for SSI are also eligible for Medicaid. The Medicaid data on such children can then be tracked over time to examine trends in the number of Medicaid enrollees who are diagnosed with a speech or language disorder and their resulting utilization of treatment services, if any. This section first describes the relationship of children with speech and language disorders enrolled in SSI to the Medicaid program, with specific reference to their eligibility for, and entry into, Medicaid. It then illustrates the prevalence of speech and language disorders among a sample of Medicaid enrollees. The section ends by describing some of the limitations in the use of Medicaid data to

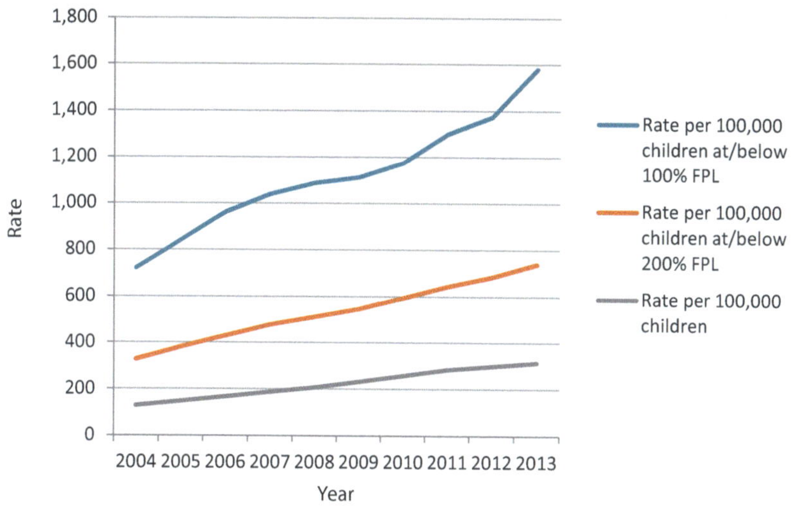

FIGURE 5-19 Rate of children receiving SSI benefits on the basis of speech and language disorders (includes impairment codes 3153 and 7840) by the federal poverty level (FPL), fiscal years 2004-2013.
NOTE: The Current Population Survey table creator was used to generate numbers of children below 200 percent of the FPL. Parameters used to generate the numbers include get count of: persons in poverty universe (everyone except unrelated individuals under 15); years: 2004 to 2013; Census 2010 weights; row variable: age; column variable: income-to-poverty ratio; and customized formatting: income-to-poverty ratio cutoff of 200 percent.
SOURCES: U.S. Census Bureau, 2015a,c, and unpublished dataset provided by the Social Security Administration.

establish trends in the prevalence of speech and language disorders among children with these disorders enrolled in the SSI program.

Established in July 1965 as Title 19 of the Social Security Act, Medicaid is the dominant insurer of low-income adults and children in the United States today. Jointly funded by the federal and state governments, Medicaid is administered by the states, which have latitude in determining program eligibility, available benefits, health care provider payment rates, drug formularies, and a range of program characteristics, within federal parameters. As a result, there is wide variability among states in program characteristics and beneficiary populations. (Detailed discussion of the origins and structure of Medicaid is available elsewhere [see, e.g., Engel, 2006, and Olson, 2010].)

As the description above implies, most children are eligible for Medicaid because their families have low incomes. However, states determine income limits for their Medicaid programs, as long as those limits meet or exceed federal minimums. The family income above which an infant below 1 year of age is no longer eligible for Medicaid, for example, varies from 139 percent of the FPL in Utah to 375 percent of the FPL in Iowa (HHS, 2015b).

Income is not the sole criterion by which children qualify for Medicaid. Children who are in certain highly vulnerable categories (e.g., disability status) and meet citizenship and state residency criteria are eligible for Medicaid in certain states under several other eligibility categories; being a recipient of SSI is one such category.

In 33 so-called 1634 states and the District of Columbia, SSI eligibility automatically qualifies an individual for Medicaid coverage (SSA, 2014). There are 10 "209(b) states" that use criteria more restrictive than those of the SSI program to determine Medicaid eligibility for their residents; in these states, meeting SSI eligibility criteria does not guarantee Medicaid eligibility (SSA, 2014). Additionally, there are 7 "SSI criteria states" that make their own determinations regarding Medicaid eligibility once an individual has met SSI eligibility criteria (SSA, 2014). The net result of all this variation is that the Medicaid and SSI beneficiary populations display substantial overlaps but are by no means identical.

Once a child SSI recipient is eligible for Medicaid, the child's parent or guardian must successfully seek services from a provider who bills Medicaid for those services. A diagnosis is necessary for such a bill (a "claim") to be paid. Medicaid claims are generated as a result of such a billing process, and represent units of services that are paid for by state Medicaid agencies. Medicaid data, therefore, reflect the receipt of health care services or treatment. These are data of a particular type: they reflect those services received by a child who is eligible for Medicaid, whose provider accepts Medicaid reimbursement, and whose treatment was paid for by the Medicaid agency in the state in which the child lives. Children who are unable to access services—for example, because no providers in their region will accept Medicaid reimbursement—will not appear on Medicaid rolls even if they are Medicaid beneficiaries or otherwise eligible for Medicaid. Furthermore, Medicaid claims data do not include claims of children who are in Medicaid managed care. This exclusion is substantial, as up to half of all children reflected in Medicaid data are in managed care and thus are not reported to state Medicaid agencies in most states. Hence their diagnoses or use of services cannot be established. Consequently, Medicaid data cannot be used to determine the prevalence of speech and language disorders in the general population—that is, they are not population data. They can be used only to quantify the rate of diagnoses of these disorders occurring among a treated population whose care was paid for by Medicaid under certain payment arrangements—that is, they are a type of service data. These data cannot be interpreted to include all low-income children with speech and language disorders, or even all children who receive Medicaid funding for their health insurance.

An analysis of Medicaid claims data from 20 states conducted by a team at Rutgers University sheds light on speech and language disorders among participants in the SSI and Medicaid programs. The Rutgers team examined claims data for children aged 3-17 with 11+ months of continuous Medicaid eligibility and no dual eligibility in a given year. Data were obtained for 2001-2010 from Alabama, Alaska, Arkansas, California, Florida, Idaho, Illinois, Indiana, Louisiana, Michigan, Mississippi, Montana, North Carolina, North Dakota, New Hampshire, New Mexico, South Dakota, Vermont, Virginia, and Wyoming.[5] Importantly, these are not longitudinal or panel data, as discussed earlier. Hence, these data should be interpreted as comparing diagnostic codes for speech and language disorders observed over time among correlated but possibly independent groups of children receiving services paid for by Medicaid.

Figure 5-20 displays the proportion of children in these 20 states whose Medicaid claims indicate a diagnosis of speech and language disorders (blue bars). It also shows the proportion of children who were eligible for Medicaid during 2001-2010 because they were SSI beneficiaries whose claims had the same diagnosis during the same time period (gray bars). As seen in the figure, a greater proportion of those children who were eligible for Medicaid because of participation in the SSI program had observed diagnoses of speech and language disorders compared with other children on Medicaid.

In calendar year 2010, for example, 11.9 percent of the children on Medicaid because of SSI program participation (n = 56,980) were diagnosed as having speech and language disorders, compared with 2.7 percent of all children on Medicaid (n = 221,630) diagnosed as having these disorders. This pattern reveals that, compared with non-SSI children on Medicaid, more children with speech and language disorders are concentrated within the SSI/Medicaid population. This pattern may reflect increased entry into the SSI program of children with speech and language disorders over time, as discussed earlier in this chapter. Some of these children on SSI, then, may have found their way into the Medicaid program through the eligibility

[5] This subset of 20 states was selected because they (1) had predominantly fee-for-service youth Medicaid populations or (2) had been identified as having relatively complete and usable managed care encounter data for that population. See https://www.cms.gov/Research-Statistics-Data-and-Systems/Computer-Data-and-Systems/MedicaidDataSourcesGenInfo/Downloads/MAX_IB_15_AssessingUsability.pdf and http://mathematicampr.com/publications/pdfs/health/MAX_IB14.pdf (accessed September 30, 2015).

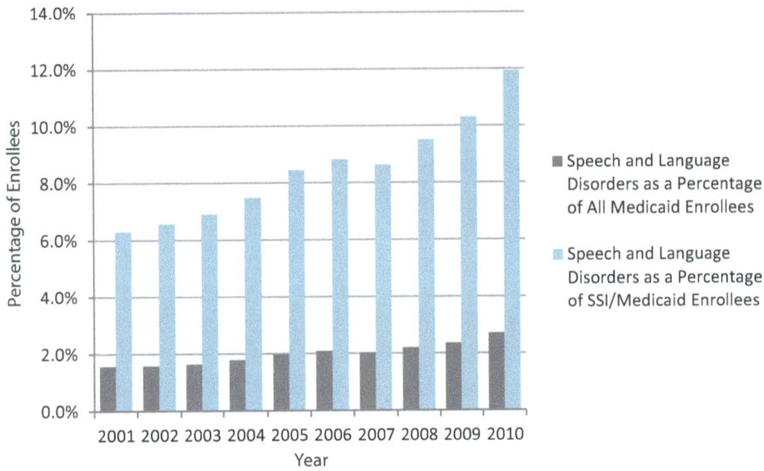

FIGURE 5-20 Speech and language disorders among Medicaid enrollees and SSI/Medicaid enrollees.
SOURCE: Medicaid Analytic eXtract [MAX] data.

mechanisms discussed earlier. The SSI program, therefore, may act as a gateway into Medicaid for some low-income children with severe speech and language disorders who do not already have Medicaid coverage. The alternative pathway may be equally operant, in which low-income children on Medicaid are diagnosed with speech and language disorders and then seek SSI program participation. Both of these trends support the increasing prevalence of speech and language disorders among children receiving SSI discussed earlier in this chapter. Irrespective of mode of entry, the two programs are highly complementary, with Medicaid resourcing the health care needs of children and SSI resourcing the added costs associated with raising children with speech and language disorders.

The concentration of children with speech and language disorders within the SSI program is also evident in the heights of the blue and red bars in Figure 5-20 over time. Between 2001 and 2010, the proportion of children in the SSI/Medicaid population with this diagnosis increased from 6.3 percent to nearly 12 percent; the rate of increase among the Medicaid population—from 1.6 percent to 2.7 percent—was far more moderate. The trends in the occurrence of speech and language disorder diagnoses over time within the SSI/Medicaid population, then, parallel the increase in the occurrence of these disorders over time among children receiving SSI benefits.

The increases in speech and language disorders in the SSI/Medicaid and Medicaid populations differ from the prevalence of speech and language disorders among children in the general U.S. population discussed in Chapter 2. The simplest explanation for this difference is that the estimated prevalence in the general population (up to 16 percent) includes children with conditions ranging from mild to severe. The 6.3-12 percent prevalence is for a treated (Medicaid) population, and children receiving SSI must have severe speech and language disorders to qualify for the program. Children receiving Medicaid-funded services by definition must have the condition for which services are necessary, and must also successfully procure the services. Even if children in the general population have speech and language disorders, they are not necessarily able to procure services successfully. Other explanations for this difference in percentages are cited in the discussion of data limitations below; they include such factors as ascertainment challenges inherent in speech and language disorders, differences in the severity of the ascertained disorders, and limitations in the nature of the data used to arrive at diagnoses of speech and language disorders.

Medicaid data can also be used to identify comorbid conditions. One approach is to examine additional diagnostic codes within the claims of children with a diagnosis of speech or language disorder. Using this strategy, the Rutgers University team determined that the most commonly occurring comorbid diagnosis in the claims of children with speech and language disorders is attention deficit hyperactivity disorder. Figure 5-21 displays the proportion of the SSI/Medicaid population with comorbid speech and language disorders and attention deficit hyperactivity disorder.

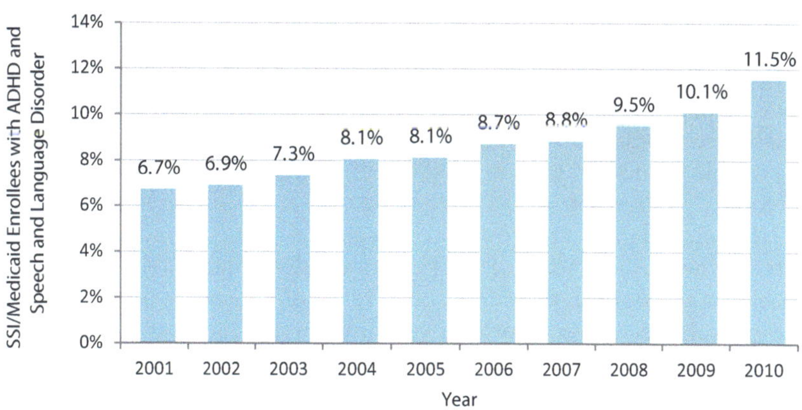

FIGURE 5-21 SSI/Medicaid enrollees with attention deficit hyperactivity disorder and a comorbid diagnosis of speech or language disorder.
NOTE: ADHD = attention deficit hyperactivity disorder.
SOURCE: MAX data.

Among children who were eligible for Medicaid because of SSI program participation, 6.7 percent (n = 38,466) had comorbid attention deficit hyperactivity disorder and speech or language disorder in calendar year 2001. This rate of comorbidity rose over time to reach 11.5 percent (n = 84,519) in calendar year 2010—roughly consonant with the 11.9 percent rate of speech and language disorders among the SSI/Medicaid population shown in Figure 5-20. These two rates differ because 11.5 percent is the rate of comorbidity, and not all children with speech and language disorders also have attention deficit hyperactivity disorder.

While the committee had access to Medicaid enrollment information, it lacked data on the number and nature of services received by Medicaid beneficiaries with speech and language disorders. Consequently, the committee was unable to answer questions related to treatment and service utilization among those eligible for Medicaid because of SSI program participation.

DATA STRENGTHS AND LIMITATIONS

This chapter has relied on three different types of data: clinical data drawn from small treatment studies; population data drawn from large national surveys; and service (administrative) data drawn from the SSA, IDEA, or Medicaid. Each of these three types of data has unique strengths and limitations, as described below.

The primary strength of clinical data is the high validity with which a diagnosis of speech and language disorders can be established. Because these clinical data often are derived from treatment studies, they typically yield high-quality and highly reliable information on the nature of a disorder; its antecedents, concomitants, and consequences; the nature of treatment received; and the outcomes resulting from treatment. Clinical data, however, cannot be used to establish the population prevalence of a disorder unless the study sample is nationally representative. These studies usually are conducted within a narrow geographic area and are, therefore, susceptible to local influences on the identification, treatment, course, and outcome of a disorder.

If clinical data are narrow and "deep dives" into a condition, population data are broad and shallow. The principal advantage of survey data is the ability to establish the rate of occurrence of a disorder in a population (the prevalence of the disorder). Because survey data cover broad geographic areas, even the entire United States, they are less susceptible than clinical data to local or regional variations in identification or treatment. This breadth comes with a few drawbacks, however. Because the surveys elicit information from large numbers of respondents and the time allotted for each respondent is very limited, they usually do not probe deeply into the condition a child may have. In many instances, the data are not specific enough to permit reliable ascertainment of speech and language disorders, and different surveys use different ways of identifying such disorders. In contrast with clinical studies, in which the investigators follow up with patients over time, surveys are difficult and expensive to implement on a larger scale. Consequently, most national health surveys obtain information at a single point in time, and cannot be used to monitor the evolution of a disorder within an individual over time. In addition, as noted previously, these data often are based on parent or guardian reports without clinical corroboration of a child's condition.

Administrative or service data capture the entire universe of children who receive services. Like clinical data, they are good sources of knowledge regarding the nature and types of services a child receives or consumes and the providers who treat them. Like survey data, they cover large geographic areas. But service data pose some unique problems. For IDEA data, many children who receive services for speech and language disorders do not have a primary speech or language category in special education. This situation creates problems in disaggregating which children are receiving treatment specifically for speech and language disorders. The diagnoses contained in Medicaid data may not be highly reliable, and data on services can be problematic as well (Bright et al., 1989). Moreover, all administrative data are sensitive to changes in rules, regulations, and funding, which may cause the number of children in the dataset to fluctuate even when there is no change in the population prevalence of the underlying disorder.

The three types of data also capture speech and language disorders very differently, as illustrated earlier in Table 5-1. The National Survey of Children with Special Health Care Needs elicits from respondents impressions of problems with speaking, communicating, and being understood, while the National Survey of Children's Health elicits whether a health care provider has diagnosed a fluency disorder. Other surveys focus on "speech problems" (e.g., National Health Interview Survey) without querying about language impairments. There is, consequently, great heterogeneity in the disorders that national surveys seek to identify and in the severity of conditions that are captured. These problems limit the extent to which national surveys can be used to answer questions about the prevalence of speech and language disorders at a national level. In addition, the questions used to ascertain speech and language disorders in these national surveys result in the identification and inclusion of children with relatively milder forms of the disorders. In contrast, children who are eligible for Medicaid because of SSI program participation are likely to have the most severe limitations. As discussed earlier, this is the case because the SSI program serves only children with "marked" and "extreme" disorders, and their Medicaid claims reflect this high level of impairment. Clinical data offer the greatest leeway in ascertaining levels of impairment. Because clinician-investigators can choose to focus on the entire range of severity of speech and language disorders, these data reflect the greatest variations in how the disorders are manifested.

Given these limitations to existing data, the committee's task was to obtain and utilize the best available data for the intended purposes of this study—minimizing the constraints of particular types of data while maximizing their particular utility in answering specific questions. As a result, this chapter relies on a mix of data sources. The overall purpose was to use clinical, national survey, and administrative data in ways that would build a valid picture of what childhood speech and language disorders look like in the general population and in the SSI population.

FINDINGS AND CONCLUSIONS

The committee's review of clinical, national survey, and administrative data and careful consideration of expert testimony yielded a picture of what is known about past and current trends in the prevalence of speech and language disorders among children (under age 18) in the general U.S. population and in the SSI population. Based on its review of the best available evidence, the committee reached the following findings and conclusions.

Findings

- 5-1. Multiple data sources provide estimates of speech and language disorders in children (under age 18) in the general U.S. population.
- 5-2. Administrative and service data provide estimates of children who receive benefits or services for speech and language disorders through large federal programs. The SSA established the impairment code for speech and language disorders (3153) in 1994.
- 5-3. The overall prevalence of reported speech and language disorders of any severity ranges from 2 to 16 percent of the general population of children and young adults aged birth through 21 years.
- 5-4. Two national surveys show that boys manifest speech and language disorders approximately twice as frequently as girls.
- 5-5. Two national surveys show increases in the prevalence of speech and language disorders of between 26 and 56 percent over 4-year periods within the past decade.
- 5-6. The number of children receiving SSI benefits for a primary speech or language impairment increased by 171 percent between 2004 and 2014. However, the number of initial allowances per year (i.e., newly eligible beneficiaries) increased by only 24 percent during this time period, with the exception of a more significant

increase (28 percent) during the recession (December 2007 to June 2009).

5-7. More than 40 percent of children with speech and language disorders in the general U.S. population experience comorbidities such as neurodevelopmental conditions, autism spectrum disorder, and behavioral problems.

5-8. The most commonly occurring comorbid diagnosis in the Medicaid claims of children with speech and language disorders is attention deficit hyperactivity disorder, seen in between 6.7 and 11.5 percent of children on Medicaid.

5-9. Only about one-third of children with speech and language impairments in the SSI program have a secondary impairment recorded. Among these children, autistic disorder and other developmental disorders was the most commonly occurring secondary impairment category listed.

5-10. Between 8.3 and 57.1 percent of children with speech problems in the general U.S. population are reported to have unmet needs for at least one indicator of health care access or service utilization.

5-11. Administrative data from IDEA suggest that between 1.5 and 1.7 percent of all U.S. children receive special education services as a result of a primary condition of speech and/or language impairment.

5-12. Children with speech and language disorders in the general U.S. population are more likely than children without such disorders to live in poverty (26 versus 21 percent) or low-income households (28 versus 23 percent).

5-13. The greatest number of child SSI recipients are those with the lowest family incomes (at or below 100 percent of the FPL).

Conclusions

5-1. No single dataset or even a small set of data sources can provide definitive population estimates of the prevalence of speech and language disorders over time among U.S. children.

5-2. Children with speech and language disorders in the general U.S. population are not comparable to the population of children who receive SSI benefits for speech and language disorders.

5-3. Changes in the SSA's program procedures, changes in eligibility and determination guidelines, cohort composition, and macroeconomic conditions all influence changes in the rate of identification of speech and language disorders within a given cohort of children at any point in time.

5-4. The information available on national trends in speech and language disorders in children—especially those disorders that are severe—is extremely limited. Available data suggest an increase in the overall prevalence of speech and language disorders in the general child population over the past decade.

5-5. The sharp increase in the number of SSI recipients eligible because of speech and language disorders observed between 2004 and 2014 is explained almost entirely by (1) the introduction in 1994 of a new impairment code for speech and language impairment, and (2) the marked and extreme levels of impairment among children who receive SSI benefits for speech and language disorders that are unlikely to be resolved by the time a child reaches age 18.

5-6. Children with speech and language disorders have a high likelihood of experiencing other health conditions as well.

5-7. The modest rates of comorbidities in the SSI data are due to inconsistencies in how secondary impairments are coded; the absence of a *recorded* secondary impairment does not mean that the child did not actually have another impairment, only that such a secondary impairment was not recorded as part of the eligibility determination process.

5-8. Children with speech and language disorders experience significant barriers to receiving needed health care services.

5-9. The net result of suspending and terminating higher-income children from the SSI program is the concentration of children from the poorest and most vulnerable families remaining in the program.

5-10. Data from national surveys indicate that speech and language disorders are more common among children from families living in poverty than among children from families not living in poverty.

REFERENCES

Bainbridge, K. 2015. *Speech problems among US children (age 3-17 years)*. Workshop presentation to the Committee on the Evaluation of the Supplemental Security Income (SSI) Disability Program for Children with Speech Disorders and Language Disorders, May 18, Washington, DC.

Black, L. I., A. Vahratian, and H. J. Hoffman. 2015. *Communication disorders and use of intervention services among children aged 3-17 years: United States, 2012*. NCHS data brief, no. 205. Hyattsville, MD: National Center for Health Statistics.

Blumberg, S. J. 2015. *Understanding speech and language data in the National Survey of Children with Special Health Care Needs*. Workshop presentation to the Committee on the Evaluation of the Supplemental Security Income (SSI) Disability Program for Children with Speech Disorders and Language Disorders, May 18, Washington, DC.

Boushey, H., C. Brocht, J. Bernstein, and B. Gundersen. 2001. *Hardships in America: The real story of working families*. Washington, DC: Economic Policy Institute.

Bright, R. A., J. Avorn, and D. E. Everitt. 1989. Medicaid data as a resource for epidemiologic studies: Strengths and limitations. *Journal of Clinical Epidemiology* 42(10):937-945.

CDC (Centers for Disease Control and Prevention). 2007. *2005-2006 National Survey of Children with Special Health Care Needs Datasets*. http://www.cdc.gov/nchs/slaits/cshcn.htm (accessed September 30, 2015).

CDC. 2012a. *About the National Health Interview Survey.* www.cdc.gov/nchs/nhis/about_nhis.htm (accessed August 18, 2015).

CDC. 2012b. *2009-2010 National Survey of Children with Special Health Care Needs Datasets.* http://www.cdc.gov/nchs/slaits/cshcn.htm (accessed September 30, 2015).

CDC. 2013a. *National Survey of Children's Health.* www.cdc.gov/nchs/slaits/nsch.htm (accessed August 18, 2015).

CDC. 2013b. *2007 National Survey of Children's Health.* http://www.cdc.gov/nchs/slaits/nsch.htm#nsch2007 (accessed September 30, 2015).

CDC. 2013c. *2011-2012 National Survey of Children's Health.* http://www.cdc.gov/nchs/slaits/nsch.htm#nsch2011 (accessed September 30, 2015).

CDC. 2014a. *National Survey of Children with Special Health Care Needs.* www.cdc.gov/nchs/slaits/cshcn.htm (accessed August 18, 2015).

CDC. 2014b. *2005-2006 National Survey of Children with Special Health Care Needs.* http://www.cdc.gov/nchs/slaits/cshcn.htm#2005CSHCN (accessed September 30, 2015).

CDC. 2014c. *2009-2010 National Survey of Children with Special Health Care Needs.* http://www.cdc.gov/nchs/slaits/cshcn.htm#09-10 (accessed September 30, 2015).

CDC. 2015. *Questionnaires, datasets, and related documentation 1997 to the present.* http://www.cdc.gov/nchs/nhis/quest_data_related_1997_forward.htm (September 17, 2015).

Coleman-Jensen, A., M. Nord, and A. Singh. 2013. *Household food security in the United States in 2012.* Washington, DC: U.S. Department of Agriculture, Economic Research Service. www.ers.usda.gov/media/1183208/err-155.pdf (accessed July 13, 2015).

DRC (Data Resource Center for Child and Adolescent Health). 2012a. *Frequently asked questions.* http://www.childhealthdata.org/learn/faq#what is NSCH (accessed April 1, 2015).

DRC. 2012b. *Guide to topics and questions asked: National Survey of Children's Health 2011/12.* http://www.childhealthdata.org/learn/topics_questions/2011-12-nsch (accessed September 17, 2015).

DRC. 2012c. *Guide to topics and questions asked: National Survey of Children with Special Health Care Needs, 2009/10.* http://www.childhealthdata.org/learn/topics_questions/3.3.0-2009-10-national-survey-of-cshcn--topics-questions (accessed September 17, 2015).

Engel, J. 2006. *Poor people's medicine: Medicaid and American charity care since 1965.* Durham, NC: Duke University Press.

GAO (U.S. Government Accountability Office). 2012. *Supplemental Security Income: Better management oversight needed for children's benefits.* GAO-12-497. http://purl.fdlp.gov/GPO/gpo25551 (accessed July 7, 2015).

HHS (U.S. Department of Health and Human Services). 2013. *Child Health USA 2012.* http://mchb.hrsa.gov/publications/pdfs/childhealth2012.pdf (accessed September 2, 2015).

HHS. 2015a. Annual update of the HHS poverty guidelines. *Federal Register* 80(14):3236-3237.

HHS. 2015b. *State Medicaid and CHIP income eligibility standards.* www.medicaid.gov/medicaid-chip-program-information/program-information/downloads/medicaid-and-chip-eligibility-levels-table.pdf (accessed September 2, 2015).

HHS. n.d. *Access to health services.* www.healthypeople.gov/2020/topics-objectives/topic/Access-to-Health-Services (accessed on September 2, 2015).

HHS, HRSA (Health Resources and Services Administration), and MCHB (Maternal and Child Health Bureau). 2008. *The National Survey of Children with Special Health Care Needs chartbook 2005-2006.* Rockville, MD: HHS.

Hoffman, H. 2015. *Speech and language impairments in the U.S. pediatric population: Findings from the National Health Interview Survey (NHIS) voice, speech, and language supplement.* Workshop presentation to the Committee on the Evaluation of the Supplemental Security Income (SSI) Disability Program for Children with Speech Disorders and Language Disorders, May 18, Washington, DC.

Ireys, H., D. Kasprzyk, A. Takyi, and J. Gillcrist. 2004. *Estimating the size and characteristics of the SSI child population: A comparison between the NSCF and three national surveys.* www.ssa.gov/disabilityresearch/documents/nscf/finalcomparison/nscf-comparison-final.pdf (accessed September 2, 2015).

NASEM (National Academies of Sciences, Engineering, and Medicine). 2015. *Mental disorders and disabilities among low-income children.* Washington, DC: The National Academies Press.

National Center for Children in Poverty. 2013. *Demographics of low-income children: United States.* New York: Columbia University, Mailman School of Public Health. www.nccp.org/profiles/US_profile_6.html (accessed September 1, 2015).

NBER (National Bureau of Economic Research). 2015. *SIPP data—reading Survey of Income and Program Participation (SIPP) data, using SAS, SPSS, or Stata.* http://www.nber.org/data/survey-of-income-and-program-participation-sipp-data.html (accessed September 30, 2015).

Newschaffer, C. J., M. D. Falb, and J. G. Gurney. 2005. National autism prevalence trends from United States special education data. *Pediatrics* 115(3):e277-e282.

Olson, L. K. 2010. *The politics of Medicaid.* New York: Columbia University Press.

SSA (Social Security Administration). 2014. *Program operations manual system: Medicaid and the Supplemental Security Income (SSI) program.* https://secure.ssa.gov/poms.nsf/lnx/0501715010 (accessed July 6, 2015).

U.S. Census Bureau. 2015a. *CPS table creator.* www.census.gov/cps/data/cpstablecrea tor.html (accessed July 13, 2015).

U.S. Census Bureau. 2015b. *Survey of income and program participation.* http://www.census.gov/programs-surveys/sipp/about/sipp-introduction-history.html (accessed September 30, 2015).

U.S. Census Bureau. 2015c. *Total population by child and adult populations.* http://datacenter.kidscount.org/data/tables/99-total-population-by-child-and-adult#detailed/1/any/false/869,15/39/416,417 (accessed September 23, 2015).

U.S. Department of Education. 2014. *36th annual report to congress on the implementation of the Individuals with Disabilities Education Act, 2014.* http://www2.ed.gov/about/reports/annual/osep/2014/parts-b-c/36th-idea-arc.pdf (accessed June 12, 2015).

U.S. Department of Education. 2015. *Children and youth with disabilities.* http://nces.ed.gov/programs/coe/indicator_cgg.asp (accessed September 2, 2015).

Visser, S. N., R. H. Bitsko, M. L. Danielson, R. Perou, and S. J. Blumberg. 2010. Increasing prevalence of parent-reported attention-deficit/hyperactivity disorder among children—United States, 2003 and 2007. *Morbidity and Mortality Weekly Report* 59(44):1439-1443.

6

Overall Conclusions

This report has two ultimate goals: (1) to synthesize what is known about trends in speech and language disorders in children in the general population and in the Supplemental Security Income (SSI) child disability population, and (2) to document the current state of knowledge regarding identification and treatment of speech and language disorders in children and levels of impairment associated with these conditions. As noted in each of the preceding chapters, the committee drew upon the existing literature and other relevant sources of information to formulate its findings and conclusions. The committee was not tasked with providing recommendations to the Social Security Administration (SSA). At the same time, the committee's findings and conclusions underscore potential directions and opportunities—for policy makers, and professionals in relevant fields of research and practice—related to the identification and treatment of speech and language disorders in children. In addition, the committee's findings and conclusions could be used to inform eligibility criteria and ongoing monitoring of children with speech and language disorders within the SSI program. Finally, the committee's review of the literature and multiple sources of data provides insight into current data collection efforts related to children with speech and language disorders. The committee's findings and conclusions in this area, in particular, offer significant opportunities for the SSA, for researchers, and for individuals who provide care for children with these disorders.

OVERALL CONCLUSIONS

Chapters 2 through 5 of this report each end with a list of findings and conclusions related to the topics examined within the respective chapters. Collectively, these findings and conclusions address the objectives, goals, and activities specified in the committee's statement of task (see Box 1-1 in Chapter 1). The findings are statements of the evidence; the conclusions are inferences, interpretations, or generalizations drawn from the evidence and supported by the committee's findings. (A complete list of the committee's findings and conclusions, by chapter, is presented later in this chapter.) From this more extensive set of findings and conclusions, the committee drew seven overall conclusions. This final chapter highlights supporting evidence and examples included in the report for each of these overall conclusions. The chapter ends with the committee's reflections on how its work can contribute to advancing understanding of and improving outcomes for children with severe speech and language disorders.

Impact of Severe Speech and Language Disorders

As noted in Chapter 2, severe speech and language disorders in children are associated with significant impairment in functioning. Children with severe speech and language disorders—those whose functioning is considered two to three standard deviations from the norm—may lack the ability to communicate effectively. The committee found that these disorders can have a lasting and profound impact on the children and families they affect. Specifically, the committee concluded that

1. **Severe speech and language disorders in children are conditions that interfere with communication and learning and represent serious lifelong threats to social, emotional, educational, and employment outcomes.**

Severe disruptions in speech or language acquisition have both direct and indirect consequences for child and adolescent development, not only in communication but also in associated abilities such as reading and academic achievement that depend on speech and language skills. In a 15-year follow-up study of children with speech and language disorders, for example, more than half (52 percent) of the children initially identified with speech and language disorders had residual learning disabilities and poor academic achievement later in life (King, 1982). Research has shown that the consequences of speech and language disorders extend beyond communication and learning. For example, a longitudinal study of children with severe language disorders found that in their mid-30s, these individuals experienced poor social adaptation, prolonged unemployment, and few close social relationships (Clegg et al., 2005).

Finally, as noted in Chapter 3, the functional requirements for language and communication increase continually throughout childhood. For children with moderate to severe speech and language disorders, these requirements often outpace their development. Thus, even if children with such disorders make some progress from growth and with treatment, the gap between their abilities and functional expectations widens.

Prevalence and Comorbidity

The committee was asked to identify past and current trends in the prevalence of speech and language disorders in the general U.S. population under age 18. As a first step to this end, the committee sought to arrive at a current estimate of the overall prevalence of speech and language disorders among children in the United States. In addition, the committee was asked to identify common comorbidities (or co-occurring conditions) of childhood speech and language disorders. To do so, the committee consulted numerous sources of data, including clinical data from small treatment studies, population-based data from large national surveys, and administrative data from large federal programs. (See Chapter 5 and Appendix B for detailed descriptions of these data sources.) From this review, the committee concluded that

2. **Speech and language disorders affect between 3 and 16 percent of U.S. children. Approximately 40 percent of children with speech and language disorders in nationally representative studies have serious comorbidities such as intellectual disabilities, autism spectrum disorder, and other neurodevelopmental and behavioral disorders.**

This range is based on prevalence estimates of speech and language disorders from peer-reviewed studies of U.S. children (between 3.8 and 15.6 percent) and from three national surveys (between 3.2 percent and 7.7 percent). As noted in Chapter 5, the data available regarding the prevalence of childhood speech and language disorders within the general population are limited in several ways. In particular, the sources of data considered by the committee vary markedly in how speech and language impairments are identified, the level of severity documented, the reporting sources, and the populations within the dataset. For example, many of the sources of data include information reported by a parent or caregiver but include no corroborating information from clinical assessment.

The few but varied data collection strategies used to estimate the prevalence of speech and language disorders in children leave room for both undercounts and overcounts. For example, conditions that commonly co-occur with speech and language disorders, such as autism spectrum disorder and attention deficit hyperactivity disorder, may initially be identified as speech and language disorders, thereby inflating the number of speech and language disorders reported. Conversely, speech and language disorders may be included in other reported categories, such as "development delays" or "multiple disabilities," or reported as secondary impairments, thereby effectively deflating the number of speech and language disorders reported.

Although the committee encountered challenges, it found sufficient evidence to estimate that 3 to 16 percent of the general population of children from birth to through age 21 experience problems with speech or language.[1] Specifically, studies on childhood *speech sound disorders* show overall prevalence rates ranging from 2 to 13 percent (Campbell et al., 2003; Eadie et al., 2015; Shriberg et al., 1999). Research on childhood *language disorders* shows overall prevalence rates between 6 and 15 percent, depending on age (Law et al., 2000; McLeod and Harrison, 2009). And one population-based study of *specific language impairment* found a prevalence rate of 7.4 percent among children in kindergarten (Tomblin et al., 1997).

Given the complex, multidimensional nature of language acquisition and the integral role of speech and language across multiple domains of child development, speech and language disorders occur at relatively high rates (Kena et al., 2014) and, as noted in Chapter 2, are frequently identified in association with (i.e., comorbid with) a wide range of other neurodevelopmental disorders. For example,

- in clinical practice, when children present with significant delays in the development of communication skills, autism spectrum disorder is one of the primary diagnostic considerations (Myers and Johnson, 2007);
- all children and adolescents with intellectual disability have varying degrees of impairment in communication skills (American Psychiatric Association, 2013); and
- multiple studies have demonstrated a strong association between attention deficit hyperactivity disorder and speech and language disorders (Pennington and Bishop, 2009; Tomblin and Nippold, 2014).

National Health Interview Survey data from 2000 to 2012 indicate that more than 40 percent of children with speech and language problems

[1] While the primary population of focus for this study is children under age 18, the committee reviewed and has included here relevant Individuals with Disabilities Education Act (IDEA) data (which include children from birth to age 21).

experienced comorbidities such as developmental delay (estimated at 32 percent), autism (estimated at 12 percent), and intellectual disability (estimated at 10 percent) (Bainbridge, 2015). Finally, young children with language impairments are at high risk for later manifestation of learning and mental health disorders.

Thus, it is important both to carefully examine the speech and language skills of children with other developmental disorders and to identify other neurodevelopmental disorders among children presenting with speech and language impairments. Among populations of children with conditions as diverse as autism spectrum disorder, attention deficit hyperactivity disorder, traumatic brain injury, and genetic disorders, speech and language disorders may be the most easily identified area of impairment because of the central role of language and communication in the functional capacity of children and adolescents.

Supplemental Security Income

Research shows that children living in poverty are at greater risk for a disability relative to those not living in poverty (Emerson and Hatton, 2005; Farran, 2000; Fujiura and Yamaki, 2000; Msall et al., 2006; Parish and Cloud, 2006), as well as that childhood disability increases the risk of a family's living in poverty (Lustig and Strauser, 2007; NASEM, 2015). Data from the U.S. Census 2010 showed that families raising children with a disability experienced poverty at higher rates than families raising children without a disability (21.8 and 12.6 percent, respectively) (Wang, 2005). At the same time, childhood poverty and the accompanying deprivations have significant adverse implications for children with disabilities and their families. Research has established that childhood poverty can exacerbate disabilities and their effects and lead to deleterious outcomes across a range of indicators, including emotional, social, and mental development; academic achievement; and employment during adulthood (Fujiura and Yamaki, 2000; Kuhlthau and Perrin, 2001; Kuhlthau et al., 2005; Parish et al., 2008). The converse is true as well: the consequences of poverty are likely to be especially serious for children with disabilities because of their heightened vulnerabilities, elevated needs for health care, and overall poor health (Kuhlthau et al., 2005; Newacheck and Kim, 2005).

As described in Chapter 4, the SSI program for children was established to address the needs of children with disabilities living in low-income households because they were determined to be "among the most disadvantaged of all Americans and are deserving of special assistance" (U.S. House of Representatives, 1971). SSI recipients include children whose health conditions or disabilities are severe enough to meet the program's disability eligibility criteria and whose family income and assets are within limits specified by the Social Security Administration. The committee concluded that

> 3. **Children of families with low incomes are more likely than the general population to have disabilities, including speech and language disorders. The Supplemental Security Income (SSI) program is designed to award benefits to the most severely impaired children from low-income, resource-limited families. Currently, 0.31 percent of U.S. children receive SSI benefits for speech and language disorders.**

An analysis of the impact of SSI revealed that the receipt of children's SSI benefits reduced the percentage of families with incomes below the federal poverty level from 58 percent to 32 percent. Still, economic vulnerability remains notable for these families. Bailey and Hemmeter (2014) found that approximately 58 percent of families receiving children's SSI benefits continued to have incomes below 150 percent of the federal poverty level,[2] even after accounting for receipt of the benefit.

To qualify for SSI benefits, children must meet a complex and detailed set of eligibility criteria that are income- and asset-related, work-related, and disability-related. The evidence required to document severity of disability is extensive and includes both medical evidence—such as formal testing to provide developmental and functional information, signs, symptoms, and laboratory findings—and parental and teacher reports. Under the SSA's standards, observations and information from a single source—such as a parent or caregiver—are an insufficient basis for a finding of disability.

Assessment, Evaluation, and Standards of Care

In accordance with its charge, the committee reviewed standards of care, including diagnostic evaluation and assessment, treatments and protocols, and educational interventions for children with speech and language disorders. The committee reviewed the literature and invited speech, language, and special education experts to provide additional insights into current standards of care and practices for children with these disorders. Chapters 2 and 3 provide an overview of this review and, when available, include evidence on the efficacy of treatments and interventions.

In addition, the committee was asked to identify the kinds of care documented or reported to be received by children in the SSI disability program. As described in Chapter 4, the committee requested a review of a

---

[2] Poverty researchers typically identify 200 percent of the federal poverty level as the income threshold for adequate subsistence (Boushey et al., 2001).

random sample of case files of children who receive SSI benefits for speech and language disorders. The results of this review helped demonstrate the kinds of evidence the SSA considers when making a disability determination for a child. Based on its review of professional standards of care and the documentation included in a random sample of case files, the committee concluded that

> 4. **To determine the severity of speech and language disorders in children, the Social Security Administration employs the results of professionally administered assessments and also takes into account other clinical evidence that would be consistent with severe speech and language disorders.**

As described in Chapter 4, the evidence in the sample of case files reviewed by the committee was derived overwhelmingly from diagnostic, evaluation, and treatment information. This evidence helped the committee understand the types of treatment the children in the sample were documented or reported to have received and the extent to which such diagnostic and evaluation services reflect the professional standards described in Chapters 2 and 3. For example, Chapter 2 describes the standardized tests typically used to diagnose speech and language disorders in children. Of the 152 cases included in the committee's review, 143 included evidence of standardized testing. Three case files that lacked information regarding standardized testing included diagnostic evidence derived from nonstandardized ratings and measurements as well as spontaneous language samples, evidence that is often used to make diagnoses of speech and language disorders in children. Finally, nearly all of the case files in the sample included information from speech-language pathologists regarding the child's speech and language status, and more than half contained developmental screening reports from a pediatrician. In all, only two of all of the cases reviewed lacked the type of specialized, objective clinical and evaluative data one would expect to find in a case based on functional equivalency. As noted in Chapter 4, while these findings cannot be considered representative of the entire SSI child population with speech and language disorders, the committee's review yielded valuable information that is consistent with other sources of evidence considered for this study.

In addition, as noted in Chapter 4, the process for identifying children with speech and language disorders who are eligible for SSI benefits is consistent with the multidimensional, multimethod, and multisource perspective that is evident in current professional practice. This process includes the assessment of children across multiple domains to determine the presence and severity of impairments in any individual areas, as well as their combined and interacting effects on day-to-day functioning. Likewise, children's case records include multiple forms of evidence concerning impairment and functioning (e.g., test scores, classroom records, progress in intervention), with no single piece of evidence being considered in isolation. Finally, information from parents, caregivers, and others with direct knowledge of children's daily functioning in age-appropriate environments and activities (e.g., Child Function Report Forms [SSA 3375-3379], Teacher Questionnaire Form [SSA 5565]) also is used to ensure that formal and criterion-referenced scores in the case record are consistent with levels of functioning in typical settings.

The descriptions of "marked" and "extreme" limitations that are used to identify impairments sufficiently severe to functionally equal the SSA's Listing of Impairments ("Listings") also are consistent with professional practice in interpreting norm- and criterion-referenced tests of speech and language. For example, meeting the functional equivalence standard requires marked limitations in at least two of the six domains of function or an extreme limitation in one domain (C.F.R. 416.926a). Marked and extreme limitations are defined, respectively, as levels of impairment that "seriously" or "very seriously" interfere with the ability "to independently initiate, sustain or complete activities" in a domain. On norm-referenced tests, marked limitations correspond to the level of functioning that would be expected of children whose scores are at least two but less than three standard deviations below the mean. As noted in Chapter 2, in a sample of 100 children, only 2 would be expected to have scores sufficiently low to meet this standard. Even fewer children—only about 1 of every 1,000—would be expected to have scores more than three standard deviations below the mean, the standard for extreme limitation.

In children younger than 3 years of age, for whom norm-referenced testing is generally infeasible, chronological age is used as the reference standard for defining limitations sufficiently severe to functionally equal the Listings. Such children have a marked limitation if their functioning in a domain is comparable to that of children who are more than one-half but less than two-thirds of their chronological age; they have an extreme limitation if their functioning is typical of children one-half their chronological age or younger. This means that a 24-month-old child functioning at a level consistent with that of typical children between 13 and 18 months of age would have a marked limitation; a 24-month-old functioning at the level of a typical child 12 months of age or younger would have an extreme limitation. These definitions of marked and extreme limitations are comparable to and in some cases more stringent than standards for identifying children (aged birth to 3 years) eligible for early intervention under the Individuals with Disabilities Education Act (IDEA) Part C based on developmental delays (U.S. Department of Education, 2011; see also Rosenberg et al., 2013).

Trends in Prevalence of the General U.S. Population Compared with Trends in the Supplemental Security Income Population

One of the committee's primary objectives was to consider past and current trends in the prevalence of speech and language disorders among the general U.S. population under age 18 and to compare those trends with trends observed among participants in the SSI childhood disability program. To do so, the committee analyzed clinical studies, nationally representative survey data, and administrative or service data from a range of sources. These data, however, are primarily serial cross-sections as opposed to longitudinal—that is, they do not follow individual children over time. Instead, these data reflect changes in the prevalence of speech and language disorders observed within populations of respondents (in the case of survey data) or beneficiaries (in the case of SSI data) over successive years. Because children observed in one year may not be the same as children observed in another, the composition of these populations will change over time; consequently, these data cannot be used to describe the natural history of speech and language disorders over time. Not only may changes in population composition over time affect rates of observed occurrence; changes in programs for children with severe disabilities also will affect the size and characteristics of the population of children who receive benefits based on a severe disability in any given year. Thus, over time, SSI eligibility standards and the eligibility determination process itself, along with broader economic factors such as the Great Recession (from December 2007 to June 2009), also may influence the rate at which speech and language disorders are observed among any given population of children at any given point in time.

Despite these data limitations, the committee was able to draw certain conclusions from the evidence regarding the extent to which speech and language disorders are documented in specific populations of children over time.

Trends in the General U.S. Population

The committee used the best available evidence to assess trends in the prevalence of speech and language disorders in the general U.S. child population. Several sources that collect data on these disorders in children suggest that over the past decade their prevalence has increased. The two nationally representative surveys that include measures of speech and language disorders in children at multiple points in time are the National Survey of Children's Health and the National Survey of Children with Special Health Care Needs. The National Survey of Children's Health showed an increase in prevalence of speech and language disorders from

3.8 percent (n = 2,697) in 2007 to 4.8 percent (n = 3,916) in 2011, a 26 percent increase. The National Survey of Children with Special Health Care Needs showed an increase in prevalence from 3.2 percent (n = 8,435) in 2005-2006 to 5.0 percent (n = 11,936) in 2009-2010, an increase of 56 percent. Although not directly comparable, the committee reviewed SSI data on initial allowances for speech and language disorders for two points in time to determine the percent increase in those initial allowances. The number of initial allowances for speech and language disorders in 2007 (n = 21,135) and the number in 2011 (n = 29,309) show a 40 percent increase. Therefore, the committee concluded that

5. **The best available evidence shows an increase in the prevalence of speech and language disorders over the past decade in the U.S. child population. Trends in annual Supplemental Security Income initial allowances parallel this overall increase.**

Causes, Treatment, and Persistence

The committee was asked to identify causes of speech and language disorders and to determine how often these impairments are the result of known causes. Chapter 2 notes that a variety of congenital and acquired conditions may result in abnormal speech and/or language development. These conditions include primary disorders of hearing, as well as specific genetic diseases, brain malformation syndromes, toxic exposures, nutritional deficiencies, injuries, and epilepsy. (Box 2-3 in Chapter 2 includes examples of speech and language disorders with known causes.) In some cases, the cause of speech and language disorders in children may not be known. In these cases, research points to an array of possible risk factors for these disorders in children. To date, the evidence best supports a cumulative risk model in which increases in risk are greater for combinations of risk factors than for individual factors (Harrison and McLeod, 2010; Lewis et al., 2015; Pennington and Bishop, 2009; Reilly et al., 2010; Whitehouse et al., 2014). For example, one study of speech sound disorders found that three variables—male sex, low maternal education, and positive family history of developmental communication disorders—were individually associated with increased odds of speech sound disorder, but the odds of such a disorder were nearly eight times greater in a child with all three risk factors than in a child with none of them (Campbell et al., 2003).

As detailed in Chapter 3, a range of different strategies are used to treat mild, moderate, and severe speech and language disorders in children. These strategies vary based on the particular needs and circumstances of the child. Several important factors shape the intervention program for any given child. These factors include treatment objectives (e.g., conventional or compensatory communication goals), the nature of the disorder, the developmental level of the child, the individuals involved in the intervention (or "agents of change"), and the settings in which treatment is provided (e.g., school-based, home-based, or clinic-based). In reviewing the evidence, the committee found that, with treatment, mild speech and language disorders may completely resolve or be limited to relatively minor impairments; moderate speech and language disorders may substantially diminish, with residual impairments in an associated domain, such as reading and literacy. In the most severe cases, however, even with treatment, core speech and language deficits will likely continue into adolescence and may be lifelong. Therefore, committee concluded that

6. **Children with mild to moderate speech and language disorders will benefit from a variety of treatments. For children with severe speech and language disorders, treatment improves function; with few exceptions, however, substantial functional limitations will persist.**

An implication of this conclusion is that a severe disorder will persist over time, thereby necessitating ongoing educational, social, and health supports and, in the case of children from low-income families, continuing eligibility for financial assistance through the SSI program.

Trends Among Supplemental Security Income Program Participants

To identify trends among participants in the SSI program, the committee reviewed administrative data collected by the SSA on initial allowances and recipients based on primary speech and language impairments. Between 2004 and 2014, the number of children receiving SSI benefits for speech and language disorders increased from 90,281 to 315,523, a 249 percent increase. Given the substantial increase in the total number of recipients, the committee reviewed older data to help explain this growth. At the committee's request, the SSA provided supplemental data for review beginning in 1994, the year in which the impairment code for speech and language impairment (3153) was introduced. From its review of the data, the committee concluded that

7. **The total number of children receiving Supplemental Security Income for speech and language disorders more than tripled in the past decade. In addition to an increase in prevalence of these disorders in the general U.S. child population, this growth is explained primarily by two factors:**

- **the introduction of a new impairment code for speech and language disorders in 1994, and**
- **the continuing eligibility of children whose severe speech and language disorders persist throughout childhood.**

Prior to 1994, there were zero initial allowances for the impairment code for speech and language impairment in children (3153). The current total number of recipients reflects both the accumulation over time of new individuals in this impairment category and the very low attrition from the program due to the above-noted persistence of severe speech and language disorders throughout childhood and adolescence.

As described in Chapter 5, in 1994, the first year that the new impairment code existed, only 1,585 children met the eligibility criteria under this new code. In 1995, an additional 4,109 children began receiving benefits under this new code; in 1996, an additional 4,119 children were allowed benefits, and so forth for each subsequent year. Given that children with severe speech and language impairments are likely to continue to have those severe impairments throughout adolescence and into adulthood, the total number of SSI recipients who received benefits under this new code in any given year approaches the total number of children who became eligible in each of the preceding 18 years. As a result, the total number of children receiving SSI benefits for speech and language impairments in 2013 will include almost all of the children who became eligible in the years from 1996 through 2013.

Several additional factors contribute to the changes observed in the number of children who receive SSI benefits for speech and language disorders. For example, the total number of child SSI recipients fluctuates depending on the number of initial allowances, terminations, suspensions, and suspension reentries. When the number of allowances exceeds the number of terminations and suspensions in a year, the total number of recipients increases for that year. Overall growth in the population of children would be expected to contribute some growth to the program as well. Consequently, the number of children who are allowed (found eligible for the program) in a given year can be expected to exceed the number who exit the program. Finally, allowances are affected by macroeconomic conditions. During a period of economic expansion, as family income increases and joblessness decreases, fewer children are likely to meet the SSA's financial eligibility criteria. By contrast, during periods of economic downturn, such as the Great Recession (from December 2007 to June 2009), more children will meet the program's financial eligibility criteria as a result of relatively higher unemployment.

Supporting Evidence for the Committee's Overall Conclusions

Box 6-1 shows the connections between each of the committee's overall conclusions and its chapter-specific findings and conclusions. Box 6-2 collects all of the committee's chapter-specific findings and conclusions organized by chapter.

BOX 6-1
Overall Conclusions and Supporting Evidence*

1. **Severe speech and language disorders in children are conditions that interfere with communication and learning and represent serious lifelong threats to social, emotional, educational, and employment outcomes.**

   Findings

   1-3. In a 15-year follow-up study of children with speech and language disorders, 52 percent of the children initially identified with such disorders had residual learning disabilities and poor academic achievement later in life.

   2-6. Children with severe speech and language disorders have an increased risk of a variety of adverse outcomes, including mental health and behavior disorders, learning disabilities, poor academic achievement, and limited employment and social participation.

   Conclusions

   1-2. Mild speech and language impairments in preschool will sometimes be transient; severe forms of these disorders have a high probability of being long-term disabilities.

   2-1. Severe speech and language disorders represent serious threats to children's social, emotional, educational, and employment outcomes.

   2-2. Severe speech and language disorders are debilitating at any age, but their impacts on children are particularly serious because of their widespread adverse effects on development and the fact that these negative consequences cascade and build on one another over time.

2. **Speech and language disorders affect between 3 and 16 percent of U.S. children. Approximately 40 percent of children with speech and language disorders in nationally representative studies have serious comorbidities such as intellectual disabilities, autism spectrum disorder, and other neurodevelopmental and behavioral disorders.**

   Findings

   1-4. Twenty-one percent of all special education eligibility in the United States is for speech and language impairments—three times greater than eligibility for autism or intellectual disability.

continued

BOX 6-1 Continued

2-1. Speech and language disorders are prevalent, affecting between 3 and 16 percent of U.S. children. Prevalence estimates vary according to age and the diagnostic criteria employed, but best evidence suggests that approximately 2 percent of children have speech and/or language disorders that are severe according to clinical standards.

2-5. Speech and language disorders frequently co-occur with other neurodevelopmental disorders and may be among the earliest symptoms of serious neurodevelopmental conditions.

5-3. The overall prevalence of reported speech and language disorders of any severity ranges from 2 to 16 percent of the general population of children and young adults aged birth through 21 years.

5-4. Two national surveys show that boys manifest speech and language disorders approximately twice as frequently as girls.

5-8. The most commonly occurring comorbid diagnosis in the Medicaid claims of children with speech and language disorders is attention deficit hyperactivity disorder, seen in between 6.7 and 11.5 percent of children on Medicaid.

5-9. Only about one-third of children with speech and language impairments in the SSI program have a secondary impairment recorded. Among these children, autistic disorder and other developmental disorders was the most commonly occurring secondary impairment category listed.

3. Children of families with low incomes are more likely than the general population to have disabilities, including speech and language disorders. The Supplemental Security Income (SSI) program is designed to award benefits to the most severely impaired children from low-income, resource-limited families. Currently, 0.31 percent of U.S. children receive SSI benefits for speech and language disorders.

Findings

4-1. To qualify for the SSI program, children and their families must meet a number of eligibility standards that are designed to restrict the program to children with severe conditions and those whose families have low incomes and very limited resources.

4-2. The SSI program is designed to assist the families of children whose conditions are severe and for whom the persistence of severity is expected, as measured by duration over time.

5-12. Children with speech and language disorders in the general U.S. population are more likely than children without such disorders to live in poverty (26 versus 21 percent) or low-income households (28 versus 23 percent).

5-13. The greatest number of child SSI recipients are those with the lowest family incomes (at or below 100 percent of the federal poverty level).

Conclusions

5-8. Children with speech and language disorders experience significant barriers to receiving needed health care services.

5-9. The net result of suspending and terminating higher-income children from the SSI program is the concentration of children from the poorest and most vulnerable families remaining in the program.

5-10. Data from national surveys indicate that speech and language disorders are more common among children from families living in poverty than among children from families not living in poverty.

4. To determine the severity of speech and language disorders in children, the Social Security Administration employs the results of professionally administered assessments and also takes into account other clinical evidence that would be consistent with severe speech and language disorders.

Findings

5-5. Two national surveys show increases in the prevalence of speech and language disorders of between 26 and 56 percent over 4-year periods within the past decade.

5-6. The number of children receiving SSI benefits for a primary speech or language impairment increased by 171 percent between 2004 and 2014. However, the number of initial allowances per year (i.e., newly eligible beneficiaries) increased by only 24 percent during this time period, with the exception of a more significant increase (28 percent) during the recession (December 2007 to June 2009).

5. The best available evidence shows an increase in the prevalence of speech and language disorders over the past decade in the U.S. child population. Trends in annual Supplemental Security Income initial allowances parallel this overall increase.

Findings

4-5. To qualify for SSI benefits, children must meet a complex and detailed set of financial-related, work-related, and disability-related eligibility criteria. The evidence required to document severity of disability is extensive and rests on clinical and educational data and information, as well as information gleaned from professionals and standardized testing. Parental observations and reports alone are an insufficient basis for a finding of disability.

4-6. The SSA's standard for marked or extreme impairment requires that children display a degree of disability that places them at least two and three standard deviations, respectively, below normal age-appropriate functional levels.

4-7. To determine the severity of speech and language disorders in children, the SSA employs the results of professionally administered assessments and also takes into account other clinical evidence that would be consistent with severe speech and language disorders.

continued

BOX 6-1 Continued

6. Children with mild to moderate speech and language disorders will benefit from a variety of treatments. For children with severe speech and language disorders, treatment improves function; with few exceptions, however, substantial functional limitations will persist.

Findings

3-1. Few treatments exist that can alter the underlying cause of a speech or language disorder.

3-5. Evidence indicates that speech and language therapy results in gains in the skills and behaviors targeted by the therapy.

3-6. Toddlers who are late talkers often make developmental gains; however, these gains may be less likely in children whose condition is severe and who have other neurodevelopmental and socioeconomic risk factors.

3-7. Children with language disorders at the age of 5 or 6 are likely to have persistent language problems throughout childhood.

Conclusions

3-1. Severe speech and language disorders are likely to persist throughout childhood.

3-2. Speech and language therapy does not substantially alter the course of these disorders and thus is not curative; however, it provides improved function in those areas that are targeted.

7. The total number of children receiving Supplemental Security Income for speech and language disorders more than tripled in the past decade. In addition to an increase in prevalence of these disorders in the general U.S. child population, this growth is explained primarily by two factors:

- **the introduction of a new impairment code for speech and language disorders in 1994, and**
- **the continuing eligibility of children whose severe speech and language disorders persist throughout childhood.**

Findings

5-2. Administrative and service data provide estimates of children who receive benefits or services for speech and language disorders through large federal programs. The SSA established the impairment code for speech and language disorders (3153) in 1994.

5-6. The number of children receiving SSI benefits for a primary speech or language impairment increased by 171 percent between 2004 and 2014. However, the number of initial allowances per year (i.e., newly eligible beneficiaries) increased by only 24 percent during this time period, with the exception of a more significant increase (28 percent) during the recession (December 2007 to June 2009).

Conclusion

5-5. The sharp increase in the number of SSI recipients eligible because of speech and language disorders observed between 2004 and 2014 is explained almost entirely by (1) the introduction in 1994 of a new impairment code for speech and language impairment, and (2) the marked and extreme levels of impairment among children who receive SSI benefits for speech and language disorders that are unlikely to be resolved by the time a child reaches age 18.

---

* This committee was not charged with making recommendations to the Social Security Administration.

BOX 6-2
Chapter-Specific Findings and Conclusions

Chapter 1: Introduction

Findings

1-1. Developmental disorders are identified when expected functional skills in children fail to emerge.

1-2. Underlying factors that contribute to developmental disorders are likely to have been present well before the signs are manifest in the child's development.

1-3. In a 15-year follow-up study of children with speech and language disorders, 52 percent of the children initially identified with such disorders had residual learning disabilities and poor academic achievement later in life.

1-4. Twenty-one percent of all special education eligibility in the United States is for speech and language impairments—three times greater than eligibility for autism or intellectual disability.

Conclusions

1-1. It is generally more accurate to describe the "age of identification" of a speech or language disorder than to focus on the "age of onset."

1-2. Mild speech and language impairments in preschool will sometimes be transient; severe forms of these disorders have a high probability of being long-term disabilities.

Chapter 2: Childhood Speech and Language Disorders in the General U.S. Population

Findings

2-1. Speech and language disorders are prevalent, affecting between 3 and 16 percent of U.S. children. Prevalence estimates vary according to age and the diagnostic criteria employed, but best evidence suggests that approximately 2 percent of children have speech and/or language disorders that are severe according to clinical standards.

2-2. Some speech and language disorders result from known biological causes.

2-3. In many cases, these disorders have no identifiable cause, but factors including male sex and reduced socioeconomic and educational resources have been associated with an increased risk of the disorders.

2-4. Diagnosing speech and language disorders in children is a complex process that requires integrating information on speech and language with information on biological and medical factors, environmental circumstances, and other areas of development.

2-5. Speech and language disorders frequently co-occur with other neurodevelopmental disorders and may be among the earliest symptoms of serious neurodevelopmental conditions.

2-6. Children with severe speech and language disorders have an increased risk of a variety of adverse outcomes, including mental health and behavior disorders, learning disabilities, poor academic achievement, and limited employment and social participation.

Conclusions

2-1. Severe speech and language disorders represent serious threats to children's social, emotional, educational, and employment outcomes.

2-2. Severe speech and language disorders are debilitating at any age, but their impacts on children are particularly serious because of their widespread adverse effects on development and the fact that these negative consequences cascade and build on one another over time.

2-3. Severe speech and language disorders may be one of the earliest detectable symptoms of other serious neurodevelopmental conditions; for this reason, they represent an important point of entry to early intervention and other services.

2-4. It is critically important to identify such disorders for two reasons: first, because they may be an early symptom of other serious neurodevelopmental disorders, and second, so that interventions aimed at forestalling or minimizing their adverse consequences can be undertaken.

Chapter 3: Treatment and Persistence of Speech and Language Disorders in Children

Findings

3-1. Few treatments exist that can alter the underlying cause of a speech or language disorder.

3-2. Alternative and augmentative communication treatment can provide nonspeech alternatives to speech that lead to functional gains in communication.

3-3. Speech and language therapy during the preschool years focuses on the promotion of implicit learning of an abstract system of principles and symbols.

3-4. In accordance with policies and practice guidelines, speech-language intervention often is conducted in the home and/or classroom and incorporates communication needs within the family and the educational curriculum.

3-5. Evidence indicates that speech and language therapy results in gains in the skills and behaviors targeted by the therapy.

3-6. Toddlers who are late talkers often make developmental gains; however, these gains may be less likely in children whose condition is severe and who have other neurodevelopmental and socioeconomic risk factors.

3-7. Children with language disorders at the age of 5 or 6 are likely to have persistent language problems throughout childhood.

continued

BOX 6-2 Continued

Conclusions

3-1. Severe speech and language disorders are likely to persist throughout childhood.

3-2. Speech and language therapy does not substantially alter the course of these disorders and thus is not curative; however, it provides improved function in those areas that are targeted.

3-3. Although there is a large literature on treatment effects, data are lacking on the effect of treatment on more general quality-of-life outcomes, particularly among children with severe disorders and those living in poverty.

Chapter 4: Supplemental Security Income for Children with Speech and Language Disorders

Findings

4-1. To qualify for the SSI program, children and their families must meet a number of eligibility standards that are designed to restrict the program to children with severe conditions and those whose families have low incomes and very limited resources.

4-2. The SSI program is designed to assist the families of children whose conditions are severe and for whom the persistence of severity is expected, as measured by duration over time.

4-3. An analysis of the impact of SSI revealed that children's SSI benefits raised family income above the federal poverty level by 26.4 percent for families with child SSI beneficiaries. However, 58.0 percent of families receiving children's SSI benefits continued to have income below 150 percent of the federal poverty level, even after accounting for receipt of the benefit.

4-4. More children receive services under the Individuals with Disabilities Education Act (IDEA) and the Title V Program for Children with Special Health Care Needs—which are designed to identify children with substantial disability-related needs for health and educational services—than receive SSI. Neither of these programs uses a "marked or extreme" standard for disability, and neither has financial eligibility regulations.

4-5. To qualify for SSI benefits, children must meet a complex and detailed set of financial-related, work-related, and disability-related eligibility criteria. The evidence required to document severity of disability is extensive and rests on clinical and educational data and information, as well as information gleaned from professionals and standardized testing. Parental observations and reports alone are an insufficient basis for a finding of disability.

4-6. The SSA's standard for marked or extreme impairment requires that children display a degree of disability that places them at least two and three standard deviations, respectively, below normal age-appropriate functional levels.

4-7. To determine the severity of speech and language disorders in children, the SSA employs the results of professionally administered assessments and also takes into account other clinical evidence that would be consistent with severe speech and language disorders.

Conclusions

4-1. SSI is a safety net for severely disabled children whose conditions are expected to persist over time and who live in low-income, resource-limited families.

4-2. Children of families with low incomes are more likely than the general population to have disabilities, including speech and language disorders. The SSI program is designed to award benefits to the most severely impaired children from low-income, resource-limited families. Currently, 0.31 percent of U.S. children receive SSI benefits for speech and language disorders.

4-3. The disability standard for SSI (at least two to three standard deviations below normal age-appropriate functional levels) places a child far below his or her same-age peers in function and is well beyond the severity of a clinical diagnosis for speech and language disorders.

4-4. SSI benefits have the effect of lifting some children and their families out of poverty.

Chapter 5: Comparison of Trends in Childhood Speech and Language Disorders in the General Population and the SSI Program Population

Findings

5-1. Multiple data sources provide estimates of speech and language disorders in children (under age 18) in the general U.S. population.

5-2. Administrative and service data provide estimates of children who receive benefits or services for speech and language disorders through large federal programs. The SSA established the impairment code for speech and language disorders (3153) in 1994.

5-3. The overall prevalence of reported speech and language disorders of any severity ranges from 2 to 16 percent of the general population of children and young adults aged birth through 21 years.

5-4. Two national surveys show that boys manifest speech and language disorders approximately twice as frequently as girls.

5-5. Two national surveys show increases in the prevalence of speech and language disorders of between 26 and 56 percent over 4-year periods within the past decade.

continued

BOX 6-1 Continued

5-6. The number of children receiving SSI benefits for a primary speech or language impairment increased by 171 percent between 2004 and 2014. However, the number of initial allowances per year (i.e., newly eligible beneficiaries) increased by only 24 percent during this time period, with the exception of a more significant increase (28 percent) during the recession (December 2007 to June 2009).

5-7. More than 40 percent of children with speech and language disorders in the general U.S. population experience comorbidities such as neurodevelopmental conditions, autism spectrum disorder, and behavioral problems.

5-8. The most commonly occurring comorbid diagnosis in the Medicaid claims of children with speech and language disorders is attention deficit hyperactivity disorder, seen in between 6.7 and 11.5 percent of children on Medicaid.

5-9. Only about one-third of children with speech and language impairments in the SSI program have a secondary impairment recorded. Among these children, autistic disorder and other developmental disorders was the most commonly occurring secondary impairment category listed.

5-10. Between 8.3 and 57.1 percent of children with speech problems in the general U.S. population are reported to have unmet needs for at least one indicator of health care access or service utilization.

5-11. Administrative data from IDEA suggest that between 1.5 and 1.7 percent of all U.S. children receive special education services as a result of a primary condition of speech and/or language impairment.

5-12. Children with speech and language disorders in the general U.S. population are more likely than children without such disorders to live in poverty (26 versus 21 percent) or low-income households (28 versus 23 percent).

5-13. The greatest number of child SSI recipients are those with the lowest family incomes (at or below 100 percent of the federal poverty level).

Conclusions

5-1. No single dataset or even a small set of data sources can provide definitive population estimates of the prevalence of speech and language disorders over time among U.S. children.

5-2. Children with speech and language disorders in the general U.S. population are not comparable to the population of children who receive SSI benefits for speech and language disorders.

5-3. Changes in the SSA's program procedures, changes in eligibility and determination guidelines, cohort composition, and macroeconomic conditions all influence changes in the rate of identification of speech and language disorders within a given cohort of children at any point in time.

5-4. The information available on national trends in speech and language disorders in children—especially those disorders that are severe—is extremely limited. Available data suggest an increase in the overall prevalence of speech and language disorders in the general child population over the past decade.

5-5. The sharp increase in the number of SSI recipients eligible because of speech and language disorders observed between 2004 and 2014 is explained almost entirely by (1) the introduction in 1994 of a new impairment code for speech and language impairment, and (2) the marked and extreme levels of impairment among children who receive SSI benefits for speech and language disorders that are unlikely to be resolved by the time a child reaches age 18.

5-6. Children with speech and language disorders have a high likelihood of experiencing other health conditions as well.

5-7. The modest rates of comorbidities in the SSI data are due to inconsistencies in how secondary impairments are coded; the absence of a recorded secondary impairment does not mean that the child did not actually have another impairment, only that such a secondary impairment was not recorded as part of the eligibility determination process.

5-8. Children with speech and language disorders experience significant barriers to receiving needed health care services.

5-9. The net result of suspending and terminating higher-income children from the SSI program is the concentration of children from the poorest and most vulnerable families remaining in the program.

5-10. Data from national surveys indicate that speech and language disorders are more common among children from families living in poverty than among children from families not living in poverty.

FINAL THOUGHTS

This report represents the National Academies of Sciences, Engineering, and Medicine's first comprehensive study of speech and language disorders in children. Using available data drawn from various sources, the committee carried out the study called for in its statement of task. First, this report presents an overview of the current status of diagnosis and treatment of speech and language disorders and the level of impairment these disorders cause among children. Second, the report identifies past and current trends in the prevalence and persistence of speech and language disorders among the general population of U.S. children and compares these trends with those found in the SSI childhood disability population. The evidence presented in this report underscores the long-term and profound impact of severe speech and language disorders on children and their families, as well as the degree to which children with such disorders can be expected to be a significant presence in a program such as SSI, whose purpose is to provide basic financial assistance to families of children with the severest disabilities. It is the committee's hope that this report will make a substantial contribution to understanding the nature of severe speech and language disorders in children and will provide a strong foundation for future efforts in policy, practice, and research.

The committee's findings and conclusions characterize the current state of knowledge. Its findings also highlight the challenges that arise in undertaking a close examination of children's health status in the area of speech and language because of deficiencies in the evidence across both the general population and, in this case, the specific population of children enrolled in the SSI program. In particular, the committee notes that its ability to address salient questions more thoroughly was limited by the absence of two basic types of information: (1) longitudinal data on children who receive SSI benefits on the basis of speech and language disorders, and (2) comprehensive information on the prevalence of these disorders among the general U.S. child population that captures a range of health, demographic, and socioeconomic characteristics such as gender, income, race/ethnicity, and condition severity. Longitudinal data on children who receive SSI benefits on the basis of speech and language disorders would provide insight into these children's status over time, as well as the types and range of treatments and their impact on health and functioning. This information would be useful in assessing the impact of treatment on continuing eligibility and would significantly enhance the SSA's ability to shape its continuing disability review process for children. More complete information on the prevalence of speech and language disorders in the general U.S. child population would enable the SSA to better determine the extent to which its initial SSI eligibility determination rates align with the prevalence of these disorders within both the general child population and the population of low-income children. It is this latter group of children who are most likely to qualify for SSI benefits if they experience speech and language disorders that reach the degree of severity required to satisfy the SSI program's rigorous eligibility standard.

Despite its limitations, the evidence presented in this report offers valuable insight into the relationship between the general population of children with speech and language disorders on the one hand and the presence of children with these disorders in the SSI program on the other. Furthermore, the evidence presented here can assist policy makers, health and education professionals, and SSI program administrators in understanding the extent to which the program's basic design and administrative process operate together to connect the nation's most severely impaired and disadvantaged children with speech and language disorders to the benefits the program offers.

REFERENCES

American Psychiatric Association. 2013. *Diagnostic and statistical manual of mental disorders: DSM-5* (5th ed.). Washington, DC: American Psychiatric Association.

Bailey, M. S., and J. Hemmeter. 2014. *Characteristics of noninstitutionalized DI and SSI program participants, 2010 update.* http://www.ssa.gov/policy/docs/rsnotes/rsn2014-02.html (accessed July 10, 2015).

Bainbridge, K. 2015. *Speech problems among US children (age 3-17 years).* Workshop presentation to the Committee on the Evaluation of the Supplemental Security Income (SSI) Disability Program for Children with Speech Disorders and Language Disorders, May 18, Washington, DC.

Boushey, H., C. Brocht, B. Gundersen, and J. Bernstein. 2001. *Hardships in America: The real story of working families.* Washington, DC: Economic Policy Institute.

Campbell, T. F., C. A. Dollaghan, H. E. Rockette, J. L. Paradise, H. M. Feldman, L. D. Shriberg, D. L. Sabo, and M. Kurs-Lasky. 2003. Risk factors for speech delay of unknown origin in 3-year-old children. *Child Development* 74(2):346-357.

Clegg, J., C. Hollis, L. Mawhood, and M. Rutter. 2005. Developmental language disorders—A follow-up in later adult life. Cognitive, language and psychosocial outcomes. *Journal of Child Psychology and Psychiatry and Allied Disciplines* 46(2):128-149.

Eadie, P., A. Morgan, O. C. Okoumunne, K. T. Eecen, M. Wake, and S. Reilly. 2015. Speech sound disorder at 4 years: Prevalence, comorbidities, and predictors in a community cohort of children. *Developmental Medicine & Child Neurology* 57(6):578-584.

Emerson, E., and C. Hatton. 2005. The socio-economic circumstances of families with disabled children. *Disability and Society* 22(6):563-580.

Farran, D. 2000. Another decade of intervention for children who are low-income or disabled: What do we know now? In *Handbook of early childhood intervention* (2nd ed.), edited by J. P. Shonkoff and S. J. Meisels. Cambridge, England: Cambridge University Press. Pp. 510-548.

Fujiura, G. T., and K. Yamaki. 2000. Trends in demography of childhood poverty and disability. *Exceptional Children* 66:187-199.

Harrison, L. J., and S. McLeod. 2010. Risk and protective factors associated with speech and language impairment in a nationally representative sample of 4- to 5-year-old children. *Journal of Speech, Language, and Hearing Research* 53(2):508-529.

Kena, G., S. Aud, F. Johnson, X. Wang, J. Zhang, A. Rathbun, S. Wilkinson-Flicker, and P. Kristapovich. 2014. *The condition of education 2014*. NCES 2014-083. Washington, DC: U.S. Department of Education, National Center for Education Statistics.

King, R. R. 1982. In retrospect: A fifteen-year follow-up report of speech-language-disordered children. *Language, Speech, and Hearing Services in Schools* 13(1):24-32.

Kuhlthau, K. A., and J. M. Perrin. 2001. Child health status and parental employment. *Archives of Pediatric and Adolescent Medicine* 155(12):1346-1350.

Kuhlthau, K. A., K. Hill, R. Yucel, and J. Perrin. 2005. Financial burden for families of children with special health care needs. *Maternal and Child Health Journal* 9(2):207-218.

Law, J., J. Boyle, F. Harris, A. Harkness, and C. Nye. 2000. Prevalence and natural history of primary speech and language delay: Findings from a systematic review of the literature. *International Journal of Language & Communication Disorders* 35(2):165-188.

Lewis, B. A., L. Freebairn, J. Tag, A. A. Ciesla, S. K. Iyengar, C. M. Stein, and H. G. Taylor. 2015. Adolescent outcomes of children with early speech sound disorders with and without language impairment. *American Journal of Speech-Language Pathology* 24(2):150-163.

Lustig, D. C., and D. R. Strauser. 2007. Causal relationships between poverty and disability. *Rehabilitation Counseling Bulletin* 50(4):194-202.

McLeod, S., and L. J. Harrison. 2009. Epidemiology of speech and language impairment in a nationally representative sample of 4- to 5-year-old children. *Journal of Speech, Language, and Hearing Research* 52(5):1213-1229.

Msall, M. E., F. Bobis, and S. Field. 2006. Children with disabilities and supplemental security income. Guidelines for appropriate access in early childhood. *Infants & Young Children* 19(1):2-15.

Myers, S. M., and C. P. Johnson. 2007. Management of children with autism spectrum disorders. *Pediatrics* 120(5):1162-1182.

NASEM (National Academies of Sciences, Engineering, and Medicine). 2015. *Mental disorders and disabilities among low-income children*. Washington, DC: The National Academies Press.

Newacheck, P. W., and S. E. Kim. 2005. A national profile of health care utilization and expenditures for children with special health care needs. *Archives of Pediatric and Adolescent Medicine* 159(1):10-17.

Parish, S. L., and J. M. Cloud. 2006. Financial well-being of young children with disabilities and their families. *Social Work* 51(3):223-232.

Parish, S. L., R. A. Rose, M. Grinstein-Weiss, E. L. Richman, and M. E. Andrews. 2008. Material hardship in US families raising children with disabilities. *Exceptional Children* 75(1):71-92.

Pennington, B. F., and D. V. M. Bishop. 2009. Relations among speech, language, and reading disorders. *Annual Review of Psychology* 60:283-306.

Reilly, S., M. Wake, O. C. Ukoumunne, E. Bavin, M. Prior, E. Cini, L. Conway, P. Eadie, and L. Bretherton. 2010. Predicting language outcomes at 4 years of age: Findings from Early Language in Victoria study. *Pediatrics* 126:e1530-e1537.

Rosenberg, S. A., C. C. Robinson, E. F. Shaw, and M. C. Ellison. 2013. Part C early intervention for infants and toddlers: Percentage eligible versus served. *Pediatrics* 131(1):38-46.

Shriberg, L. D., J. B. Tomblin, and J. L. McSweeny. 1999. Prevalence of speech delay in 6-year-old children and comorbidity with language impairment. *Journal of Speech, Language, and Hearing Research* 42(6):1461-1481.

Tomblin, J. B., and M. A. Nippold. 2014. *Understanding individual differences in language development across the school years.* New York: Psychology Press.

Tomblin, J. B., N. L. Records, P. Buckwalter, X. Xhang, E. Smith, and M. O'Brien. 1997. Prevalence of specific language impairment in kindergarten children. *Journal of Speech, Language, and Hearing Research* 40(6):1245-1260.

U.S. Department of Education. 2011. Early intervention program for infants and toddlers with disabilities; assistance to states for the education of children with disabilities. Final Rule and Proposed Rule 34 CFR Part 303. *Federal Register* 76(188)60140-60283.

U.S. House of Representatives. 1971. *Social Security Amendments of 1971: Report of the Ways and Means Committee on H.R. 1.* H. Report No. 92-251, pp. 146-148.

Wang, Q. 2005. Disability and American families: 2000. *Bulletin* 62(4):21-30.

Whitehouse A. J. O., W. M. R. Shelton, C. Ing, and J. P. Newnham. 2014. Prenatal, perinatal, and neonatal risk factors for specific language impairment: A prospective pregnancy cohort study. *Journal of Speech, Language, and Hearing Research* 57(4):1418-1427.

Appendix A

Glossary of Key Terms

Award: An administrative determination that an individual is eligible for a Supplemental Security Income benefit (SSA, 2014).

Child: A blind or disabled individual who is neither married nor the head of household and who is (1) under age 18, or (2) under the age of 22 and a student regularly attending a school, college, or university or a course of vocational or technical training designed to prepare him or her for gainful employment. A child 18 or older is subject to the adult definition of disability and is not subject to parental deeming (SSA, 2014).

Continuing disability review (CDR): A review of the beneficiary's medical condition to determine whether there has been sufficient medical improvement so that the individual is no longer disabled or whether the individual has demonstrated the ability to engage in substantial gainful activity (SSA, 2006).

Deeming: The process by which the Social Security Administration considers the income and resources of an ineligible individual to be available to a recipient when determining eligibility or payment amount. Deeming applies only between

- the living-with ineligible spouse and the eligible spouse;
- the living-with ineligible parent(s) and eligible child(ren) under age 18; and
- the immigration sponsors of some noncitizens and the noncitizen(s) (SSA, 2014).

Disability: For individuals aged 18 or older, the inability to engage in any substantial gainful activity by reason of any medically determinable physical or mental impairment that can be expected to result in death or that has lasted or can be expected to last for a continuous period of at least 12 months. An individual under age 18 must have a medically determinable physical or mental impairment that results in marked and severe functional limitations and that can be expected to result in death or that has lasted or can be expected to last for a continuous period of at least 12 months (SSA, 2014).

Disability Determination Services (DDS): The state agency responsible for developing medical evidence and rendering the initial determination and reconsideration as to whether a claimant is disabled or a beneficiary continues to be disabled within the meaning of the law (SSA, 2006).

Listing of Impairments: Issued by the Social Security Administration and used to identify medical conditions for purposes of determining disability. Also referred to as the Medical Listings (SSA, 2006).

Recipient: A person who is receiving Supplemental Security Income payments based on an evaluation of his or her countable income and resources, age, and disability status (SSA, 2014).

Substantial gainful activity (SGA): The level of work activity used to establish disability. A finding of disability requires that a person be unable to engage in SGA. A person who is not statutorily blind and is earning above the SGA level in 1 month (net of impairment-related work expenses) is ordinarily considered to be engaging in SGA. According to regulation, the Social Security Administration bases yearly increases in the SGA level on increases in the national average wage base (SSA, 2014).

Suspension: Benefits are suspended for various reasons, including excess income for Supplemental Security Income recipients and work above the substantial gainful activity level for Social Security Disability Insurance beneficiaries, among others. Under benefit suspension, the individual remains eligible for the program but does not collect a cash benefit (SSA, 2006).

Termination: For an individual, cessation of benefits, which can occur for a number of reasons, including death, medical improvement, or a period of suspension lasting longer than 12 months (SSA, 2014).

REFERENCES

SSA (Social Security Administration). 2006. *Trends in the Social Security and Supplemental Security Income disability programs*. http://www.ssa.gov/policy/docs/chartbooks/disability_trends/trends.pdf (accessed June 10, 2015).

SSA. 2014. *Annual report of the Supplemental Security Income Program*. http://ssa.gov/oact/ssir/SSI14/ssi2014.pdf (accessed June 10, 2015).

Appendix B

Descriptions of Data Sources

ADMINISTRATIVE OR SERVICE DATA

Individuals with Disabilities Education Act Data

Since 1975, the U.S. Department of Education has collected data on early intervention and special education services provided to children with disabilities as required by the Individuals with Disabilities Education Act (IDEA). The U.S. Department of Education maintains and provides public access to state-supplied administrative records about children and young adults with disabilities until the age of 21 (U.S. Department of Education, 1995). The act requires each state that receives assistance to report annually the number and percentage of children with disabilities who are receiving educational services, by race, ethnicity, limited English proficiency status, gender, and disability category (Wexler and Miceli, 2015). IDEA data include annual counts of services provided to children ages birth-2 (Part C) and ages 3-21 (Part B).

Part B data are collected from 60 reporting entities and provide information on the number of children with disabilities, ages 3-21, who received special education and related services under IDEA between October 1 and December 1 each year (based on the state-designated child count date). The data are collected by disability category, race/ethnicity, gender, and discrete age (Wexler and Miceli, 2015). The Part B data are reported by primary disability category. As a result, these data may be artificially deflated when speech and language impairments are reported as "developmental delay" or "multiple disabilities." On the other hand, there is potential for inflation in the speech or language impairment category when autism, for example, is reported in this category (Wexler and Miceli, 2015). The Part C data reflect the number of infants and toddlers, ages birth-2, who received early intervention services under IDEA as of the annual state-designated child count date (October 1-December 1). The data are collected from 56 Part C reporting entities by race/ethnicity, gender, and discrete age. The data provide information on service utilization and the number and distribution of students served under the law. They also provide information on such topics as the site of service (e.g., regular classroom, special education classroom, community-based setting); service providers (e.g., speech and language pathologist, special education teacher, special education paraprofessional); graduation rates for students, broken out by disability category; and the prevalence of the disability categories (e.g., autism, emotional disturbance, specific learning disabilities, speech or language impairments, visual impairments, intellectual disabilities) (U.S. Department of Education, 2014). The Part C data are not reported by disability category.

Medicaid Analytic eXtract (MAX) Data

An analysis of MAX data, commissioned for this study, was conducted by a team at Rutgers University. The study population included all Medicaid-eligible youth ages 3 to 17 years in a subset of 20 states for the years 2001-2010 (the most recent year for which MAX data are publicly available). For purposes of inclusion in this analysis, enrollee age was computed as of July 1 each year, and 11 consecutive or nonconsecutive months of Medicaid eligibility in a single year was required. The 20 states selected were those found to provide relatively complete diagnosis and treatment detail (Byrd and Dodd, 2012; Nysenbaum et al., 2012).[1] The analysis was based primarily on Medicaid enrollment, claims, and prescription drug-fill data from the MAX. These data provided a set of research files constructed from mandated periodic data submissions by the state Medicaid programs; these submissions had been compiled and processed by the Centers for Medicare & Medicaid Services (CMS). Enrollment data include information on such beneficiary characteristics as age, sex, and race/ethnicity; Medicaid eligibility class; diagnoses recorded; services received; and prescriptions filled. Claims data are provided separately for inpatient, long-term care, and other (primarily outpatient) services and include details

[1] The preliminary MAX data analysis included 44 states and the District of Columbia. A subset of 20 states was identified that in 2009 either (1) had predominantly fee-for-service youth Medicaid populations or (2) had been identified as having relatively complete and usable managed care encounter data for that population (Byrd and Dodd, 2012; Nysenbaum et al., 2012).

on diagnoses received and services delivered. The few youth with dual Medicaid/Medicare eligibility were excluded from the analysis because records from Medicare, which is the first payer for many services, were not observable for this population.

Enrollees were assigned to one of three basis-of-eligibility (BoE) groups following examination of their eligibility records: Supplemental Security Income (SSI)/Medicaid, foster care, and other (including a large group eligible solely because of household income). In general, households eligible for Medicaid on the basis of income are poor or near-poor (living below 200 percent of the federal poverty level [FPL]). Analyses were stratified by this grouping variable. Each enrollee's last observed BoE category in each year was used to assign her or him an overall status for the year, in order to establish mutually exclusive categories. Preliminary analysis revealed 96 percent consistency throughout the year for the focal SSI/Medicaid group, suggesting that this method of assigning BoE categories on the basis of the last observation of the year did not distort these enrollees' eligibility histories. A threshold of either one or more inpatient claims or two or more outpatient claims on different dates was used to establish the presence of speech and language disorders and nine other conditions for each enrollee for each year of analysis (using codes from the *International Classification of Diseases, Ninth Revision, Clinical Modification* [ICD-9-CM]). Once enrollees' eligibility, sociodemographic characteristics, diagnoses, prescriptions, and services had been identified, analyses were performed to track diagnosis and treatment trends between 2001 and 2010.

Supplemental Security Income Data

Allowance and recipient data are collected and maintained by two different divisions within the Social Security Administration (SSA): (1) the Office of Disability Program Management Information (ODPMI) for allowances, and (2) the Office of Research, Evaluation, and Statistics (ORES) for recipients.

Office of Disability Program Management Information

The ODPMI tracks information on the outcomes of the SSI adjudication process. Specifically, the ODPMI records information on whether an applicant is eligible according to the SSI work, income, and resource criteria (Step 1) and the disability criteria (Steps 2 and 3). Administrative information regarding the outcome of a determination of disability is recorded on a standard form called the SSA-831 "Disability Determination and Transmittal" form. Data collected from the SSA-831 form are maintained in a database known as the Disability Research File (DRF). Data on determinations collected by the SSA also include information on three aspects of every determination: (1) a medical diagnosis associated with the determination, (2) the level of adjudication at which the allowance was made, and (3) the regulation basis for the allowance. These three key data elements are discussed in the following subsections.

Diagnostic categories for determinations of SSI benefits The SSA's Program Operations Manual requires that the diagnosis or medical basis for an applicant's disability most pertinent to the determination of eligibility be recorded. The SSA collects information on a primary diagnosis and an optional secondary diagnosis for each determination. According to the Program Operations Manual, "The primary diagnosis for an allowance refers to the basic condition that rendered the individual disabled, or in (the case of) a denial, the one which the evidence shows to have the most significant effect on the individual's ability to work." A secondary diagnosis is defined as the "most significant diagnosis following the primary diagnosis in severity" (SSA, 2014).

The SSA disability examiners are required to record an "impairment code" for every disability determination. The SSA's impairment codes are a list of numeric codes loosely informed by ICD-9, used to classify medical diagnoses that are the basis for disability claims. Each impairment code is linked to a diagnostic category within the SSA's "Listing of Impairments" based in part on the *Diagnostic and Statistical Manual of Mental Disorders, Third Edition, Revised* (DSM-III-R) (SSA, 2010). For each allowance that meets or equals a listing, the examiner is required to record the correlated impairment code. For every allowance that functionally equals a Listing, the examiner must record the impairment code that most closely matches the diagnosis in the applicant's case file and is the basis of his or her disability. For denials, examiners are instructed to record an impairment code for the diagnosis that has the most effect on the claimant's function, or a code for "none established" if there is no diagnosis.

Level of adjudication The ODPMI also collects information on the level of adjudication at which a determination is made.

Regulation basis of determinations Finally, the ODPMI keeps records on whether allowances are for disabilities that meet, medically equal, or functionally equal the listings.

Office of Research, Evaluation, and Statistics

The ORES collects and maintains data on the number of individuals who receive SSI benefit payments. These data are known as the Supplemental

Security Record (SSR). The SSR is a record of the number of individuals who apply for SSI disability benefits; the number of applicants who become eligible for benefits under both the nondisability (work, income, and resource) and disability criteria (awards[2]); and the number of individuals who are currently recipients of SSI disability benefit payments. The recipient data in the SSR refer to the number of recipients within a time period—specifically, within December of the year.

POPULATION DATA

National Health Interview Survey

The National Health Interview Survey (NHIS), conducted by the Centers for Disease Control and Prevention's National Center for Health Statistics (NCHS), is a cross-sectional household interview survey that collects data annually to monitor the health of the U.S. population. The sample consists of the civilian noninstitutionalized population residing in the United States, and the sample size is approximately 35,000 households with 87,500 persons (CDC, 2012). The survey's core questions include four major components: Household, Family, Sample Adult, and Sample Child. Major health topics addressed include physical and mental health status; chronic conditions, including asthma and diabetes; access to and use of health care services; health insurance coverage and type of coverage; health-related behaviors; measures of functioning and activity limitations; immunizations; and injuries and poisonings (CDC, 2014a).

National Health Interview Survey—Voice, Speech, and Language Supplement

In 2012, the NHIS included a Voice, Speech, and Language Supplement with Child Communication Disorders (CCD) being added to the Sample Child section of the survey. The CCD Supplement sampled children ages 3 to 17 with difficulties in voice, swallowing, speech, and language lasting for 1 week or longer in the past 12 months (CDC and HHS, 2013). The supplement also included questions related to diagnosis, age of onset, severity, and receipt of speech-language therapy or other intervention services (Hoffman, 2015).

[2] An award is an administrative status indicating that an applicant has met both disability and nondisability (work, income, and resource) eligibility criteria.

National Survey of Children's Health

The NSCH is a national survey sponsored by the Maternal and Child Health Bureau of the Health Resources and Services Administration. Data are collected using a State and Local Area Integrated Telephone Survey (SLAITS) (Data Resource Center for Child and Adolescent Health, 2012). Conducted in years 2003-2004, 2007-2008, and 2011-2012, the NSCH provides parent-reported information on children's health and well-being at the national and state levels for a representative sample of noninstitutionalized children in the United States aged 0-17 years (Data Resource Center for Child and Adolescent Health, 2012). The number of interviews for the 2003-2004 survey was 102,353, for the 2007-2008 survey 91,642 (CDC, 2013), and for the 2011-2012 survey 95,677 (CDC, 2013). Topics covered in the NSCH include child and family demographics, children's physical and mental health status, early childhood-specific information (ages 0-5 years), middle-childhood- and adolescent-specific information (ages 6-17 years), family health and activities, parental health status, and parents' perceptions of neighborhood characteristics (Data Resource Center for Child and Adolescent Health, 2012), as well as access to and use of health care services, access to medical homes, and health insurance status and type of coverage (Data Resource Center for Child and Adolescent Health, 2012).

National Survey of Children with Special Health Care Needs

Sponsored by the Maternal and Child Health Bureau of the Health Resources and Services Administration, the National Survey of Children with Special Health Care Needs (NS-CSHCN) is a national survey that was conducted using SLAITS in years 2001, 2005-2006, and 2009-2010 (Data Resource Center for Child and Adolescent Health, 2012). The NS-CSHCN provides parent-reported information on the health and functional status of children with special health care needs at the national and state levels; the survey sample consists of the noninstitutionalized population of children in the United States with special health care needs aged 0-17 years (Data Resource Center for Child and Adolescent Health, 2012). The survey included 38,866 interviews in 2001 and 40,840 interviews in 2005-2006 (CDC, 2014b). The 2009-2010 survey consisted of 40,242 detailed interviews (CDC, 2014b). Topics covered in the NS-CSHCN include child's health and functional status (expanded to include current conditions and functional limitations beginning in 2005-2006), child's health insurance status, adequacy of coverage, and the impact of the child's health on the family. The survey also covers access to health care, including types of health care services required by a child, any unmet health care needs, care coordination, and the family-centeredness of the child's health care (Data Resource Center for Child and Adolescent Health, 2012).

Survey of Income and Program Participation

The Survey of Income and Program Participation (SIPP) is a national household-based survey administered by the U.S. Census Bureau that collects information on income, labor force participation, social program participation and eligibility, and general demographic characteristics (U.S. Census Bureau, 2013). The survey design consists of a continuous series of national panels ranging in duration from 2.5 to 4 years, with interviews conducted every 4 months (U.S. Census Bureau, 2013). Each panel consists of a nationally representative sample of noninstitutionalized individuals and households, with sample sizes ranging from 14,000 to 52,000 interviewed households (U.S. Census Bureau, 2013). Interviews to collect parent-reported information for children are performed in person and by telephone. The focus is on documenting the economic well-being of respondents by focusing on labor force participation, program participation (e.g., Temporary Assistance for Needy Families [TANF], SSI, Supplemental Nutrition Assistance Program [SNAP], and income) (U.S. Census Bureau, 2013). Additional SIPP topics include personal history, child care, wealth, program eligibility, child support, utilization and cost of health care, disability, school enrollment, taxes, and annual income (U.S. Census Bureau, 2013).

REFERENCES

Byrd, V. L. H., and A. H. Dodd. 2012. *Accessing the usability of encounter data for enrollees in comprehensive managed care across MAX 2007-2009*. Mathematica Policy Research Medicaid Policy Brief No. 15. www.cms.gov/Research-Statistics-Data-and-Systems/Computer-Data-and-Systems/MedicaidDataSourcesGenInfo/Downloads/MAX_IB_15_AssessingUsability.pdf (accessed July 18, 2015).

CDC (Centers for Disease Control and Prevention). 2012. *National Health Interview Survey*. http://www.cdc.gov/nchs/nhis/about_nhis.htm (accessed June 12, 2015).

CDC. 2013. *State and Local Area Integrated Telephone Survey*. http://www.cdc.gov/nchs/slaits/nsch.htm (accessed April 15, 2015).

CDC. 2014a. *NCHS fact sheet*. http://www.cdc.gov/nchs/data/factsheets/factsheet_nhis.htm (accessed June 12, 2015).

CDC. 2014b. *State and local area integrated telephone survey*. http://www.cdc.gov/nchs/slaits/cshcn.htm (accessed April 15, 2015).

CDC and HHS (U.S. Department of Health and Human Services). 2013. *2012 National Health Interview Survey (NHIS) public use data release*. http://ftp.cdc.gov/pub/health_statistics/nchs/Dataset_Documentation/NHIS/2012/srvydesc.pdf (accessed June 12, 2015).

Data Resource Center for Child and Adolescent Health. 2012. *Frequently asked questions*. http://www.childhealthdata.org/learn/faq#whatisNSCH (accessed April 1, 2015).

Hoffman, H. J. 2015. *Speech and language impairments in the US pediatric population: Findings from the National Health Interview Survey (NHIS) voice, speech, and language supplement*. PowerPoint presentation.

Nysenbaum, J., E. Bouchery, and R. Malsberger. 2012. *The availability and usability of behavioral health organization encounter data in MAX 2009*. Mathematica Policy Research Medicaid Policy Brief No. 14. www.mathematica-mpr.com/~/media/publications/PDFs/health/MAX_IB14.pdf (accessed July 18, 2015).

SSA (Social Security Administration). 2010. *20 CFR parts 404 and 416 revised medical criteria for evaluating mental disorders; proposed rule*. http://www.gpo.gov/fdsys/pkg/FR-2010-08-19/pdf/2010-20247.pdf (accessed August 10, 2015).

SSA. 2014. *DI 26510.015 completing item 16a and 16b on the SSA-831 disability determination and transmittal*. https://secure.ssa.gov/poms.nsf/lnx/0426510015 (accessed April 23, 2015).

U.S. Census Bureau. 2013. *Survey of income and program participation*. http://www.census.gov/programs-surveys/sipp/about/sipp-introduction-history.html (accessed April 1, 2015).

U.S. Department of Education. 1995. *Individuals with Disabilities Education Act amendments of 1995: Reauthorization of the Individuals with Disabilities Education Act (IDEA)*. Washington, DC: U.S. Department of Education.

U.S. Department of Education. 2014. *36th annual report to Congress on the implementation of the Individuals with Disabilities Education Act, 2014*. http://www2.ed.gov/about/reports/annual/osep/2014/parts-b-c/36th-idea-arc.pdf (accessed June 12, 2015).

Wexler, L., and M. Miceli. 2015. *Using IDEA section 618 data to explore prevalence of students with speech and language impairments*. PowerPoint presentation.

Appendix C

Population and Administrative/Service Data for Speech and Language Disorders

TABLE C-1 Number of Children Aged 3-21 Served Under the Individuals with Disabilities Education Act (IDEA) Part B, by Disability Type: School Year 2011-2012 (refers to Figure 1-3 in Chapter 1)

Disability Type	Ages 3-21
Specific learning disabilities	2,363,890
Speech or language impairments	1,413,289
Other health impairments	754,527
Autism	458,209
Intellectual disabilities	443,054
Developmental delay	393,138
Emotional disturbance	374,552
Multiple disabilities	132,986
Hearing impairments	78,545
Orthopedic impairments	61,763

NOTE: The sample size of children aged 3-21 served under IDEA Part B for all disabilities is 6,530,552.
SOURCES: Kena et al., 2014; U.S. Department of Education, 2012.

TABLE C-2 Number of Child SSI Recipients, by Family Income Relative to the Federal Poverty Level, with and Without SSI Payments, September-December 2010 (refers to Figure 4-1 in Chapter 4)

Federal Poverty Level	Without SSI Payments	With SSI Payments
Under 100% FPL	692,696	377,256
100-150% FPL	187,481	309,207
150% or more FPL	313,670	507,385

NOTES: Totals do not necessarily equal the sum of rounded components. The sample size is 1,193,848. FPL = federal poverty level; SSI = Supplemental Security Income.
SOURCE: Bailey and Hemmeter, 2014.

TABLE C-3 Number of Children with Speech and Language Disorders in the General U.S. Population Based on the 2005-2006 and 2009-2010 National Survey of Children with Special Health Care Needs (refers to Figure 5-1 in Chapter 5)

Years	Number	Sample Size of Children with Special Health Care Needs	Weighted Percentage of Children with Special Health Care Needs	Percentage of U.S. Children with Special Health Care Needs
2005/6	8,435	38,296	23.00%	13.90%
2009/10	11,936	39,747	30.00%	15.10%

SOURCES: CDC, 2007, 2014; HHS, 2013; HHS et al., 2008.

TABLE C-4 Number of Children with Speech and Language Disorders in the General U.S. Population Based on the 2007 and 2011 National Survey of Children's Health (refers to Figure 5-2 in Chapter 5)

Years	Number	Sample size
2007	2,697	81,955
2011	3,916	85,581

SOURCES: CDC 2013a,b.

TABLE C-5 Number of Children in the General U.S. Population of Children Aged 6-21 Years Served Under IDEA Part B, by Year and Disability Category, Fall 2003 Through Fall 2012 (refers to Figure 5-3 in Chapter 5)

Disability Type	2003	2004	2005	2006	2007	2008	2009	2010	2011	2012
Learning disabilities	2,866,908	2,789,895	2,727,802	2,654,668	2,559,722	2,522,735	2,483,391	2,412,801	2,354,790	2,338,273
Other health impairments	452,442	508,085	557,121	595,073	624,688	648,112	678,640	703,912	733,960	770,648
Speech or language impairments	1,129,260	1,137,692	1,143,195	1,144,277	1,135,638	1,121,496	1,107,029	1,089,976	1,071,200	1,061,762
Intellectual disabilities	582,663	555,524	533,426	511,041	487,175	475,713	460,964	444,894	430,819	424,530

SOURCES: U.S. Department of Education, 2014a,b.

TABLE C-6 Prevalence of Speech and Language Disorders by Race/Ethnicity Among Children Aged 0-17 Years Based on the 2007 and 2011 National Survey of Children's Health (refers to Figure 5-5 in Chapter 5)

Race/Ethnicity	2007	2011
Non-Hispanic White	1,697	2,449
Non-Hispanic Black	313	403
Other Non-Hispanic	261	447
Hispanic	373	529

NOTE: The sample size is 81,955 in 2007 and 85,581 in 2011.
SOURCES: CDC, 2013a,b.

TABLE C-7 Children Aged 6-17 with Speech and Language Disorders, by Family Income Relative to the Federal Poverty Level Based on the 2010 Survey of Income and Program Participation (refers to Figure 5-7 in Chapter 5)

Federal Poverty Level	Number
Under 100% FPL	75
100-150% FPL	78
150% or more FPL	124

NOTES: The sample size is 277. FPL = federal poverty level.
SOURCE: NBER, 2015.

TABLE C-8 Children Aged 6-17 Without Speech and Language Disorders, by Family Income Relative to the Federal Poverty Level Based on the 2010 Survey of Income and Program Participation (refers to Figure 5-8 in Chapter 5)

Federal Poverty Level	Number
Under 100% FPL	3,150
100-150% FPL	3,493
150% or more FPL	7,864

NOTES: The sample size is 14,507. FPL = federal poverty level.
SOURCE: NBER, 2015.

TABLE C-9 Material Hardship Among Families with and Without Children with Speech and Language Disorders Based on the 2010 Survey of Income and Program Participation (refers to Figure 5-9 in Chapter 5)

Types of Hardship	Households with 6- to 17-Year-Olds with Speech and Language Disorders	Households with 6- to 17-Year-Olds Without Speech Problems
Unmet essential expenses	99	3,397
Low food security	65	2,122
Child food insecurity	22	961

NOTE: The sample size of children with speech and language disorders is 277 and without speech and language disorders is 14,507.
SOURCE: NBER, 2015.

TABLE C-10 Unmet Health Care Needs for Children with Speech Problems (refers to Figure 5-10 in Chapter 5) Based on the 2007 and 2011 National Survey of Children's Health

Indicators of Receiving Health Care	2007	2011
No preventive care in past year	218	367
≥ 1 unmet health need	397	519
No help with care coordination	598	624

NOTE: In 2007, the sample sizes for no preventive care in past year, ≥ 1 unmet health need, and no help with care coordination are 2,469, 2,487, and 980, respectively. In 2011, the respective sample sizes are 3,529, 3,548, and 1,410.
SOURCES: CDC, 2013a,b.

TABLE C-11 Number of Determinations, Allowances, and Denials for Speech and Language Disorders (includes primary impairment codes 3153 and 7840) at the Initial Level Based on Fiscal Year 2004-2014 SSI Data (refers to Figure 5-11 in Chapter 5)

Year	Determinations	Allowances	Denials
2004	35,588	21,337	14,251
2005	36,507	21,610	14,897
2006	35,613	20,904	14,709
2007	36,153	21,135	15,018
2008	38,858	22,944	15,914
2009	43,889	26,839	17,050
2010	49,661	29,144	20,517
2011	51,740	29,309	22,431
2012	52,403	29,165	23,238
2013	47,604	26,142	21,462
2014	44,985	25,244	19,741

SOURCE: Unpublished dataset provided by the Social Security Administration.

TABLE C-12 Initial Allowances for Speech and Language Disorders Based on Fiscal Year 1994-2014 SSI Data (refers to Figures 5-12 and 5-14a in Chapter 5)

Year	3153—Speech and Language Impairment Allowances	7840—Loss of Voice Allowances	Speech/Language Impairment and Loss of Voice Allowances
1994	1,585	2,108	3,693
1995	4,109	1,969	6,078
1996	4,119	1,893	6,012
1997	2,904	1,965	4,869
1998	3,829	2,055	5,884
1999	6,017	2,810	8,827
2000	8,299	3,266	11,565
2001	10,500	2,858	13,358
2002	13,676	2,730	16,406
2003	16,944	2,866	19,810
2004	18,299	3,038	21,337
2005	18,829	2,781	21,610
2006	18,445	2,459	20,904
2007	18,761	2,374	21,135
2008	20,572	2,372	22,944
2009	24,000	2,839	26,839
2010	26,050	3,094	29,144
2011	26,188	3,121	29,309
2012	26,177	2,988	29,165
2013	23,493	2,649	26,142
2014	22,727	2,517	25,244

SOURCE: Unpublished dataset provided by the Social Security Administration.

TABLE C-13 Numbers of Recipients for Speech and Language Disorders Based on Fiscal Year 2004-2014 SSI Data (refers to Figure 5-13 in Chapter 5)

Year	3153—Speech and Language Impairment	7840—Loss of Voice	Speech/Language Impairment and Loss of Voice Recipients
2004	78,827	15,201	94,028
2005	93,162	15,462	108,624
2006	107,318	16,009	123,327
2007	121,771	16,577	138,348
2008	135,990	17,018	153,008
2009	154,229	17,716	171,945
2010	173,102	18,285	191,387
2011	190,714	19,011	209,725
2012	201,044	19,788	220,832
2013	211,865	19,721	231,586
2014	213,688	18,635	232,323

SOURCE: Unpublished dataset provided by the Social Security Administration.

TABLE C-14 Top Secondary Impairments for Initial Allowances for Primary Speech and Language Disorders (includes impairment codes 3153 and 7840) Based on Fiscal Year 2004-2014 SSI Data (refers to Figure 5-15 in Chapter 5)

	2004	2005	2006	2007
0000—Unknown, No Medical Evidence	8,610	8,523	8,574	8,724
None—Secondary Code Blank	4,180	4,352	3,985	4,120
2990—Autistic Disorder and Developmental Disorders	643	714	839	978
3140—Attention Deficit Hyperactivity Disorder	1,159	1,304	1,183	1,178
3152—Learning Disorder	1,222	1,244	1,263	1,128
3890—Hearing Loss	388	397	330	323
3180—Intellectual Disability	624	570	571	478
4930—Asthma	668	657	557	522
3450—Epilepsy	243	244	209	240
2940—Organic Mental Disorders	118	143	135	165

SOURCE: Unpublished dataset provided by the Social Security Administration.

TABLE C-15 Top Primary Impairments for Secondary Speech and Language Disorders (includes impairment codes 3153 and 7840) Based on Fiscal Year 2004-2014 SSI Data (refers to Figure 5-16 in Chapter 5)

	2004	2005	2006	2007
2990—Autistic Disorder and Developmental Disorders	1,392	1,494	1,571	1,864
3180—Intellectual Disability	3,500	3,222	2,710	2,322
3140—Attention Deficit Hyperactivity Disorder	1,859	1,922	1,638	1,766
3890—Hearing Loss	402	353	311	291
3430—Cerebral Palsy	283	219	242	263
2940—Organic Mental Disorders	383	417	370	376
3152—Learning Disorder	1,235	1,174	1,086	1,036
3450—Epilepsy	160	157	125	154
3195—Borderline Intellectual Functioning	596	514	500	465
3150—Development and Emotional Disorders/Infants	549	511	465	438

SOURCE: Unpublished dataset provided by the Social Security Administration.

2008	2009	2010	2011	2012	2013	2014
9,220	10,497	11,408	11,076	11,007	9,815	9,537
4,808	5,682	5,891	5,746	5,462	4,878	4,952
1,177	1,486	1,814	2,077	2,337	2,226	2,488
1,249	1,675	1,784	1,902	1,920	1,759	1,564
1,155	1,332	1,485	1,583	1,624	1,722	1,438
315	394	470	478	484	410	371
483	502	587	565	543	521	676
517	654	716	857	824	696	605
257	320	319	334	353	293	288
180	202	265	430	572	502	418

2008	2009	2010	2011	2012	2013	2014
2,402	2,855	3,558	4,568	5,535	5,889	6,238
2,326	2,596	2,665	2,720	2,526	2,561	2,517
1,884	2,155	2,402	2,598	2,575	2,330	2,002
353	399	442	488	533	476	439
238	278	304	329	318	256	277
382	452	526	666	728	786	682
1,032	1,134	1,245	1,321	1,349	1,265	1,099
160	209	207	268	281	219	241
439	488	461	443	376	386	378
490	560	529	481	400	280	197

TABLE C-16 Number of all SSI Child Recipients Suspended Based on Fiscal Year 2004-2013 SSI Data (refers to Figure 5-17 in Chapter 5)

Year	Excess Income and Resources	Other	No Longer Disabled	Total
2004	84,900	65,800	27,600	150,700
2005	85,180	56,270	22,400	141,450
2006	82,062	51,817	11,845	133,879
2007	80,409	56,591	6,588	137,000
2008	89,563	67,079	5,800	156,642
2009	88,031	75,578	9,073	163,609
2010	96,165	81,721	14,721	177,886
2011	102,161	90,184	16,572	192,345
2012	96,647	85,949	25,353	182,596
2013	95,138	98,485	25,484	193,623

SOURCE: Unpublished dataset provided by the Social Security Administration.

TABLE C-17 Number of SSI Child Recipients Terminated Based on Fiscal Year 2004-2013 SSI Data (refers to Figure 5-18 in Chapter 5)

Year	Excess Income and Resources	No Longer Disabled	Other	Death	Total
2004	28,270	18,550	12,950	5,500	65,270
2005	29,347	16,747	11,531	5,051	62,676
2006	31,498	17,536	10,862	5,236	65,132
2007	30,384	9,516	9,759	5,488	55,147
2008	34,045	4,478	8,986	5,194	52,703
2009	31,858	4,528	11,940	5,041	53,367
2010	35,528	5,720	11,543	4,824	57,615
2011	36,772	11,152	12,507	4,805	65,236
2012	34,522	13,103	12,575	4,686	64,886
2013	32,825	18,432	11,341	4,484	67,082

SOURCE: Unpublished dataset provided by the Social Security Administration.

TABLE C-18 Rate of SSI Child Speech and Language Impairment Recipients by the Federal Poverty Level Based on Fiscal Year 2004-2013 SSI Data (refers to Figure 5-19 in Chapter 5)

Speech Year	Speech and Language Impairment and Loss of Voice Recipients	No. of Children Under 200% FPL (CPS)	No. of Children Under 100% FPL (CPS)	U.S. Under 18 Population	Rate per 100,000 Children At/Below 100% FPL	Rate per 100,000 Children At/Below 200% FPL	Rate per 100,000 Children
2004	94,028	28,753,000	13,041,000	73,297,735	721	327	128
2005	108,624	28,539,000	12,896,000	73,523,669	842	381	148
2006	123,327	28,757,000	12,827,000	73,757,714	961	429	167
2007	138,348	28,999,000	13,324,000	74,019,405	1,038	477	187
2008	153,008	30,064,000	14,068,000	74,104,602	1,088	509	206
2009	171,945	31,505,000	15,451,000	74,134,167	1,113	546	232
2010	191,387	32,254,000	16,286,000	74,119,556	1,175	593	258
2011	209,725	32,678,000	16,134,000	73,902,222	1,300	642	284
2012	220,832	32,269,000	16,073,000	73,708,179	1,374	684	300
2013	231,586	31,364,000	14,659,000	73,585,872	1,580	738	315

NOTES: The Current Population Survey table creator was used to generate numbers of children below 100 percent and 200 percent of the federal poverty level. Parameters used to generate the numbers include get count of: persons in poverty universe (everyone except unrelated individuals under 15); years: 2004 to 2013; Census 2010 weights; row variable: age; column variable: income-to-poverty ratio; and customized formatting: income-to-poverty ratio cutoff of 100 percent and 200 percent. CPS = Current Population Survey; FPL = federal poverty level.
SOURCES: U.S. Census Bureau, 2015a,b; unpublished dataset provided by the Social Security Administration.

TABLE C-19 Speech and Language Disorders Among Medicaid Enrollees and SSI/Medicaid Enrollees Based on Fiscal Year 2001-2010 Medicaid Analytic eXtract (MAX) Data (refers to Figure 5-20 in Chapter 5)

	2001	2002	2003	2004	2005	2006	2007	2008	2009	2010
Speech and Language Disorders Among Medicaid Enrollees	83,713	91,997	98,317	114,415	133,167	139,239	131,870	151,794	181,082	221,630
Speech and Language Disorders Among SSI/Medicaid Enrollees	22,750	24,829	27,305	30,578	34,975	37,528	37,143	41,813	48,280	56,980

SOURCE: MAX data.

TABLE C-20 SSI/Medicaid Enrollees with Attention Deficit Hyperactivity Disorder (ADHD) and a Comorbid Diagnosis of Speech or Language Disorder Based on Fiscal Year 2001-2010 MAX Data (refers to Figure 5-21 in Chapter 5)

	2001	2002	2003	2004	2005	2006	2007	2008	2009	2010
SSI/Medicaid Enrollees with ADHD and a Comorbid Diagnosis of Speech or Language Disorder	38,466	42,603	48,485	53,357	59,756	60,492	62,787	69,149	81,051	84,519

SOURCE: MAX data.

REFERENCES

Bailey, M. S., and J. Hemmeter. 2014. *Characteristics of noninstitutionalized DI and SSI program participants, 2010 update.* www.ssa.gov/policy/docs/rsnotes/rsn2014-02.html (accessed July 10, 2015).

CDC (Centers for Disease Control and Prevention). 2007. *2005-2006 National Survey of Children with Special Health Care Needs Datasets.* http://www.cdc.gov/nchs/slaits/cshcn.htm (accessed September 30, 2015).

CDC. 2013a. *2007 National Survey of Children's Health.* http://www.cdc.gov/nchs/slaits/nsch.htm#nsch2007 (accessed September 30, 2015).

CDC. 2013b. *2011-2012 National Survey of Children's Health.* http://www.cdc.gov/nchs/slaits/nsch.htm#nsch2011 (accessed September 30, 2015).

CDC. 2014. 2005-2006 *National Survey of Children with Special Health Care Needs.* http://www.cdc.gov/nchs/slaits/cshcn.htm#2005CSHCN (accessed September 30, 2015).

HHS (U.S. Department of Health and Human Services). 2013. *Child Health USA 2012.* http://mchb.hrsa.gov/publications/pdfs/childhealth2012.pdf (accessed September 2, 2015).

HHS, HRSA (Health Resources and Services Administration), and MCHB (Maternal and Child Health Bureau). 2008. *The National Survey of Children with Special Health Care Needs chartbook 2005-2006.* Rockville, MD: HHS.

Kena, G., S. Aud, F. Johnson, X. Wang, J. Zhang, A. Rathbun, S. Wilkinson-Flicker, and P. Kristapovich. 2014. *The condition of education 2014.* NCES 2014-083. Washington, DC: U.S. Department of Education, National Center for Education Statistics.

NBER (National Bureau of Economic Research). 2015. *SIPP data—reading Survey of Income and Program Participation (SIPP) data, using SAS, SPSS, or Stata.* http://www.nber.org/data/survey-of-income-and-program-participation-sipp-data.html (accessed September 30, 2015).

U.S. Census Bureau. 2015a. *CPS table creator.* www.census.gov/cps/data/cpstablecrea tor.html (accessed July 13, 2015).

U.S. Census Bureau. 2015b. *Total population by child and adult populations.* http://datacenter.kidscount.org/data/tables/99-total-population-by-child-and-adult#detailed/1/any/false/869,15/39/416,417 (accessed September 23, 2015).

U.S. Department of Education. 2012. *Historical state-level IDEA data files.* http://tadnet.public.tadnet.org/pages/712 (accessed November 9, 2015).

U.S. Department of Education. 2014a. *36th annual report to Congress on the implementation of the Individuals with Disabilities Education Act, 2014.* http://www2.ed.gov/about/reports/annual/osep/2014/parts-b-c/36th-idea-arc.pdf (accessed June 12, 2015).

U.S. Department of Education, 2014b. *OSEP's annual reports to Congress on implementation of the Individuals with Disabilities Education Act (IDEA).* http://www2.ed.gov/about/reports/annual/osep/index.html (accessed November 9, 2015).

Appendix D

Description of Methods Used to Calculate Trends in National Survey Data

METHODS

This report includes analyses of three datasets: (1) the 2008 panel of the Survey of Income and Program Participation (SIPP), (2) the 2007 and 2011-2012 iterations of the National Survey of Children's Health (NSCH), and (3) the 2005-2006 and 2009-2010 iterations of the National Survey of Children with Special Health Care Needs (NS-CSHCN).

Survey of Income and Program Participation

The SIPP is a nationally representative survey of the noninstitutionalized population of the United States. The 2008 panel was administered to household units over 16 waves occurring every 4 months. In addition to core questions asked at each wave, additional sets of questions referred to as topic modules were asked at 12 of the waves. The Wave 6 topic module was administered from May to August 2010, and it contained questions about the functional limitations and disabilities of adults (defined by the SIPP as those aged 15 years or older) and children aged 6-14 in the surveyed families. Wave 6 of the 2008 SIPP included 88,164 people in 34,850 households. Of these, there were 14,784 children aged 6-17 in 8,836 families.

Children aged 6-17 were identified as having a speech disorder if a positive response was recorded for the question asking whether he or she had "any difficulty having [his or her] speech understood" or if "speech problems" was identified as a condition underlying any difficulty with activities of daily living. In addition, because those aged 15-17 were treated as adults in the SIPP and additional questions were asked of them, children of these ages were identified as having a speech disorder if "speech problems" was identified as a condition underlying difficulty that they had with working or as a reason for their having fair or poor health.

The SIPP provides various weighting variables that take into account its complex design (including clustering) and the probability of someone being in the sample. These allow for relatively direct estimates of how many people and households across the Unites States each surveyed person and household represents. Person-weights were used to calculate descriptive statistics for individual-level variables, such as race and gender. For household-level variables, such as the percentage of households experiencing low food security, household-weights were used. Because child Supplemental Security Income (SSI) receipt was recorded at the household level in the SIPP, it was treated as a household-level variable. Child SSI receipt for those aged 15-17 was sometimes labeled in the survey as individual adult SSI receipt given the SIPP's treatment of this age group as adults. These were counted as instances of child SSI and added to household-level calculations.

For variance estimations, the committee used Fay's modified balanced repeat replication method. To prevent respondents from small geographic areas from being identifiable, the SIPP alters its primary sample units (PSUs) by combining them into larger variance strata and then splitting each stratum into two variance units. Fay's method is recommended by the SIPP for variance estimation because it is able to account for both halves of the strata that are generated. Resulting variance estimates are nominally conservative. STATA (version 13.0) was used to calculate point and variance estimates using the weight and variance estimation variables in the SIPP.

National Survey of Children's Health

The NSCH is nationally representative of noninstitutionalized children aged 0-17 in the United States. The survey is administered through dialing of random telephone numbers. One child in each household including children is then selected at random, and the survey is administered to the adult in the household who is most knowledgeable about the child's health and health care. The 2007 NSCH included data on 91,642 children with completed surveys, and the 2011-2012 NSCH included 95,677.

Children with speech disorders were identified in the survey through a series of questions. Respondents were first asked general questions about whether the child had any functional limitations or if he or she needed or received any medicines, services, therapies, or treatments. Those with positive responses to any of these questions were then asked about a series of diagnoses and whether the child had received any of them. Included in this list for those aged 2-17 was the diagnosis of any speech or other language problem. Finally, for each diagnosis with an affirmative response, it was determined whether the child currently had the diagnosis. The committee used this final step to determine whether an individual child currently had a speech disorder.

The NSCH provided one weight for each child in the survey based on the probability of being sampled. Numerous adjustments were then made, including adjustments for nonresponse bias, multiple land and/or cell phone lines, and subsampling of children within the household. This allowed for weighted point estimates. For weighted variance estimates, the NSCH directly provided stratum and PSU variables. These were applied using STATA for the analysis.

National Survey of Children with Special Health Care Needs

The NS-CSHCN is nationally representative of noninstitutionalized children aged 0-17 with one or more special health care needs in the United States. It was administered by the same organization (the Data Resource Center for Child and Adolescent Health, or DRC) as the NSCH and used similar procedures. Respondents were selected using the same methods outlined above, with the added step of having interviewers assess whether there were children in the household with special health care needs. This allowed for an estimate of the proportion of children in the country with special health care needs, in addition to detailed information about this population. The 2005-2006 NS-CSHCN included data on 40,804 children with special health care needs with completed surveys, and the 2009-2010 NS-CSHCN included 40,242 children.

Regarding speech disorders in children aged 1-17, respondents were asked whether the child, compared with others his or her age, experienced "a lot, a little, or no difficulty with . . . speaking, communicating, or being understood." Children who had either a little or a great deal of difficulty in this area were identified as having a speech disorder.

Weights for point and variance estimates were constructed and provided similarly to those for the NSCH, although the NS-CSHCN provided additional weights related to estimating the proportion of children nationally who had special health care needs. To develop estimates of the proportion of children in the United States with speech disorders, the proportion of children with special health care needs who had a speech disorder was multiplied by the proportion of children in the general population who had special health care needs.

Appendix E

Review of Social Security Administration Case Files

To help carry out its task, as set forth by the Social Security Administration (SSA), the National Academies of Sciences, Engineering, and Medicine Committee on the Evaluation of the Supplemental Security Income (SSI) Disability Program for Children with Speech Disorders and Language Disorders requested that the SSA conduct a review of case files to address two primary objectives.

Objective 1:
Describe the characteristics of the SSI child recipient population that has speech and language delays as the primary impairment code.

This objective will help the committee address items 1-5 in the task order as they relate to the SSI childhood disability population.

Objective 2:
Determine whether professional standards of pediatric and adolescent health care are received by children alleging a speech or a language disorder who apply for SSI and whose cases are allowed.

This objective will help the committee "identify the kinds of care documented or reported to be received by children in the SSI program."

CASE FILE CHARACTERISTICS

The committee requested that the SSA review a **random sample of 152 case files** from **fiscal year (FY) 2014** that meet the following criteria:

- Type of claim—**Initial Determinations**
  - — Eighty percent "functionally equal" the Listings
  - — Twenty percent "meet or medically equal" the Listings
- Primary impairment code on Form SSA-831—**3153 Speech and Language Delays**
- Secondary impairment code on Form SSA-831—**Any**
- Regulation basis code—**All allowances (meets, medically equals, and functionally equals)**

CASE FILE EXCLUSION CRITERION

The primary impairment code identified by Disability Determination Services (DDS) on Form SSA-831 does not correspond to the child's primary impairment based on the medical evidence of record.

SPECIFIC QUESTIONS AND VARIABLES

The committee developed a list of variables and questions derived from SSA Forms 3375-BK, 3376-BK, 3377-BK, 3378-BK, 3379-BK, and 3820-BK (see below). The committee requested that the random sample of 150 case files be reviewed for these variables and to answer these questions (to the extent to which this information is documented).

RESULTS

The SSA's Office of Disability Policy used SurveyMonkey® to conduct internal case reviews and exported the results to an Excel file for the committee to analyze. The following results were reported:

A. **About the Child**
   1. Date of birth
   2. Age at date of filing
   3. Age at date of determination
   4. Gender
   5. Can the child speak and understand English?
   6. Age of onset of speech or language impairment?
   7. Countable income

B. Identification of Speech/Language Disorders

1. Disabling illnesses, injuries, or conditions (from the child's file)
2. Do the child's illnesses, injuries, or conditions cause pain or other symptoms?
3. Does the child have problems seeing?
4. Does the child have problems hearing?
5. Is the child totally unable to talk?
6. Are the child's physical abilities limited?
7. Does the child display any behavioral problems?

B.1 Medical Assessment

1. Has the child been tested for behavioral or learning problems?
   - If "yes" list the tests administered.
2. Has the child had, or will he/she have, any medical tests for illnesses, injuries, or conditions?
   - If "yes" list the tests administered.

B.2 Disability Assessment

1. Has the child been tested or examined by Head Start (Title V)?
2. Has the child been tested or examined by a public or community health department?
3. Has the child been tested or examined by a child welfare or social service agency or Special Supplemental Nutrition Program for Women, Infants, and Children (WIC)?
4. Has the child been tested or examined by an early intervention service?
5. Has the child been tested or examined by a program for children with special health care needs?
6. Has the child been tested or examined by a mental health/mental retardation center?

C. Receipt of Treatment/Evolution of Treatment

1. Has the child received one or more interventions for speech disorder (as applicable)?
2. Has the child received one or more interventions for language disorder (as applicable)?
3. Has the child received one or more interventions for hearing disorder (as applicable)?
   - If "yes" list the services received.
4. As of the date of filing, does the child take any medications?
   - If "yes" give name of medicine.
   - If "yes" give reason for medicine.
5. Does the child have autism?

D. Disability Evaluation

1. Does the child's impairment meet a listing?
2. Does the child's impairment medically equal a listing?
3. If the impairment does not meet or medically equal a listing, note "marked" or "extreme" for each of the domains of functional equivalence:
   - Acquiring and using information
   - Attending to and completing tasks
   - Interacting and relating with others
   - Moving about and manipulating objects
   - Caring for yourself
   - Health and physical well-being

E. Types of Evidence in File

1. What information does this file contain with regard to the child's speech and language status?
2. Are there scores or summary information from standardized speech and language measures?
3. Is there information from systematic nonstandardized speech and language observations (observational rating forms, speech-language samples)?
4. Is there information regarding speech and language based on informal observation?
5. Was information provided regarding the child's hearing?
6. Which of the following documentation does the file include
   - Speech and language records
   - Occupational therapy records
   - Physical therapy records
   - Child health records
   - Child Find, Early Intervention (Individual Family Service Plan or Individualized Education Program)
   - Psychological consultative exam
   - Speech and language consultative exam
   - Forms SSA-3375, SSA-3376, SSA-3377, SSA-3378, SSA-3379, or 3820-BK

Appendix F

Workshop Agendas

March 9, 2015
National Academy of Sciences Building
2101 Constitution Ave., NW, Room 125
Washington, DC 20418

AGENDA

Meeting Objectives

1. Discuss the significance and impact of severe speech and language disorders in the lives of children and their families.
2. Discuss the Supplemental Security Income (SSI) childhood disability program and determination process to gain a better understanding of the child disability population with speech and language disorders.
3. Discuss the identification of and treatment for speech and language disorders in children.
4. Discuss the stakeholders' perspectives.

8:30-9:00 a.m. **REGISTRATION**

9:00 a.m. **Welcome, Introductions, and Opening Remarks**
Sara Rosenbaum, Committee Chair

9:15 a.m.	**The Significance and Impact of Severe Speech and Language Disorders in the Lives of Children and Their Families** **Rhea Paul, Ph.D., CCC-SLP,** Professor of Speech Language Pathology, Sacred Heart University Q&A and Discussion
10:00 a.m.	**Understanding the SSI Disability Determination Process for Children with Speech Disorders and Language Disorders** **Joanna Firmin,** Office of Disability Policy, Social Security Administration Q&A and Discussion
11:00 a.m.	**Panel 1: Identification of and Treatment for Speech and Language Disorders** *Moderator: Stephen Camarata, Committee Member* **Ann P. Kaiser, Ph.D.,** Susan Gray Chair in Education and Human Development and Professor of Special Education and Psychology, Peabody College at Vanderbilt University **Cheryl K. Messick, Ph.D., CCC-SLP,** Associate Professor and Director of Clinical Education Communication Science and Disorders Department, University of Pittsburgh **Steven F. Warren, Ph.D.,** Professor of Speech-Language-Hearing, Department of Hearing and Speech, University of Kansas Q&A and Discussion
12:15 p.m.	**LUNCH BREAK**
1:15 p.m.	**Panel 2: Stakeholder Panel** *Moderator: William Barbaresi, Committee Member* **Lemmietta G. McNeilly, Ph.D., CCC-SLP, CAE,** Chief Staff Officer, Speech-Language Pathology, American Speech-Language-Hearing Association

	Michelle M. Macias, M.D., FAAP, American Academy of Pediatrics, Council on Children with Disabilities **Nora Wells, M.S.Ed.,** Executive Director, Family Voices
	Q&A and Discussion
2:30 p.m.	**Open Comment Period**
3:00 p.m.	**Closing Remarks and Adjourn Public Session**

May 18-19, 2015
Keck Center of the National Academies of
Sciences, Engineering, and Medicine
500 Fifth Street, NW
Washington, DC 20001

AGENDA

Meeting Objectives

1. Discuss data collection efforts by a range of sources related to childhood disability with an emphasis on speech and language disorders.
2. Highlight what is known from such efforts, including
   - identification and treatment;
   - service needs and utilization;
   - co-occurring conditions; and
   - child and family characteristics.

8:00-8:30 a.m.	**REGISTRATION**
8:30 a.m.	**Welcome, Introductions, and Opening Remarks** *Sara Rosenbaum, Committee Chair*
8:45 a.m.	**Findings from the National Survey of SSI Children and Families** *Moderator: Ramesh Raghavan, Committee Member* **Kalman Rupp, Ph.D.,** Office of Policy, Office of Research, Evaluation, and Statistics, Social Security Administration

	Paul S. Davies, Ph.D., Office of Data Exchange and Policy Publications, Social Security Administration **Jeffrey Hemmeter, Ph.D.,** Office of Program Development, Social Security Administration Q&A with Committee
9:45 a.m.	**Speech and Language Impairments in the U.S. Pediatric Population: Findings from the National Health Interview Survey—Voice, Speech, and Language Supplement** *Moderator: J. Bruce Tomblin, Committee Member* **Howard J. Hoffman, M.A.,** National Institute on Deafness and Other Communication Disorders, National Institutes of Health **Kathy Bainbridge, Ph.D., M.P.H.,** National Institute on Deafness and Other Communication Disorders, National Institutes of Health Q&A with Committee
10:45 a.m.	BREAK
11:00 a.m.	**Understanding Speech and Language Data in the National Survey of Children with Special Health Care Needs** *Moderator: Susan Parish, Committee Member* **Stephen J. Blumberg, Ph.D.,** Division of Health Interview Statistics, National Center for Health Statistics, Centers for Disease Control and Prevention Q&A with Committee
12:00 p.m.	LUNCH BREAK
1:00 p.m.	**Surveillance of Speech and Language Impairments in Special Education** *Moderator: Audrey Sorrells, Committee Member* **Larry Wexler, Ed.D.,** Office of Special Education Programs, U.S. Department of Education **Meredith Miceli, Ph.D.,** Office of Special Education Programs, U.S. Department of Education

	Q&A with Committee
2:00 p.m.	**Open Comment Period**
2:30 p.m.	**Closing Remarks and Adjourn Public Session**

Appendix G

Summary of *Mental Disorders and Disabilities Among Low-Income Children*

In 2013, the Social Security Administration's Office of Disability Policy requested that the Institute of Medicine (IOM) convene a consensus committee to identify past and current trends with the prevalence and persistence of mental disorders for the general U.S. population under age 18; compare those trends with trends in the Social Security Income (SSI) childhood disability population; and provide an overview of the current status of the diagnosis and treatment of mental disorders and the levels of impairment associated with these disorders in the U.S. population under age 18 (see Box G-1 for the committee's statement of task). This study was conducted at the same time that the study of the Committee on the Evaluation of the Supplemental Security Income (SSI) Disability Program for Children with Speech Disorders and Language Disorders was under way. While the two studies had related statements of task, they entailed separate committees, meetings, and report review processes.

The report of the Committee on the Evaluation of the Supplemental Security Income Disability Program for Children with Mental Disorders—*Mental Disorders and Disabilities Among Low-Income Children*—was released in September 2015. Box G-2 provides the report's key conclusions. The full text of the report can be found online at http://www.nap.edu/catalog/21780.

BOX G-1
Statement of Task

The task order objective is to:

- Identify past[a] and current trends[b] in the prevalence and persistence of mental disorders[c] for the general U.S. population under age 18, and compare those trends to trends in the SSI childhood disability population.
- Provide an overview of the current status of the diagnosis and treatment of mental disorders, and the levels of impairment, in the U.S. population under age 18.

To accomplish this objective, the committee shall:

1. Compare the national trends in the number of children with mental disorders under age 18 with the trends in the number of children receiving SSI on the basis of mental disorders, and describe the possible factors that may contribute to any differences between the two groups.
2. Identify current professional standards of pediatric and adolescent mental health care and identify the kinds of care documented or reported to be received by children in the SSI childhood disability population.

To perform the above activities, the committee shall do the following with respect to the two child populations:

1. Identify national trends in the prevalence of mental disorders in children; and assess factors that influence these trends (for example, increased awareness or improved diagnosis).
2. Identify the average age of onset and the gender distribution; and assess the levels of impairment within age groups.
3. Assess how age, development, and gender may play a role in the progression of some mental disorders.
4. Identify common comorbidities among pediatric mental disorders.
5. Identify which mental disorders are most amenable to treatment; and assess typical or average time required for improvement in mental disorder to manifest following diagnosis and treatment.
6. Identify professionally accepted standards of care (such as diagnostic evaluation and assessment, treatment planning and protocols, medication management,[d] and behavioral and educational interventions) for children with mental disorders.

---

[a] For at least the past 10 years.

[b] In context of current trends in child health and development, and in pediatric and adolescent medicine.

[c] Including disorders such as attention deficit hyperactivity disorder, autism and other developmental disorders, intellectual disability, learning disorders, and mood and conduct disorders.

[d] Including appropriateness of how medications are being prescribed.

BOX G-2
Key Conclusions

1. Information about trends in the rates of mental disorders, and the disability associated with mental disorders, among children in the United States is limited. In addition, it is difficult to directly compare these trends to trends in the number of allowances and recipients* of SSI benefits for child mental disorders. Information about the severity, comorbidities, treatment, outcomes, and other characteristics (including race and ethnicity) of children who are SSI recipients is also limited.
2. While the number of children allowed (that is new beneficiaries of) SSI benefits for mental disorders has fluctuated from year to year between 2004 to 2013, over the 10-year period, the percentage of poor children who are allowed SSI benefits for mental disorders has decreased.
3. After taking child poverty into account, the increase in the percentage of poor children receiving SSI benefits for mental disorders (from 1.88 percent in 2004 to 2.09 percent in 2013) is consistent with and proportionate to trends in prevalence of mental disorders among children in the general population.
4. The trend in child poverty was a major factor affecting trends observed in the SSI program for children with mental disorders during the study period. Increases in numbers of children applying for and receiving SSI benefits on the basis of mental health diagnoses are strongly tied to increasing rates of childhood poverty because more children with mental health disorders become financially eligible for the program when poverty rates increase.
5. Better data about diagnoses, comorbidities, severity of impairment, and treatment, with a focus on trends in these characteristics, is necessary to inform improvements to the SSI program for children. The expansion of data collection and analytical capacities to obtain critical information about SSI allowances for, and recipients with mental disorders should be given consideration by the SSA and related stakeholders.
6. Important policy issues identified during this study, but outside of the scope of this committee's statement of task, include improving methods for the evaluation of impairment and disability in children, effects of SSI benefits for children on family income and work, and state to state variation within the SSI program. Further investigation of these topics, building on the findings and conclusions of this report, could provide expert policy advice on how to improve the SSI program for children.

* An allowance is determination by the disability determination service, an administrative law judge, or the Appeals Council that an applicant meets the medical definition of disability under the law. A recipient is an individual who receives SSI benefits.

Appendix H

Committee Member Biographies

Sara Rosenbaum, J.D. (*Chair*), is Harold and Jane Hirsh professor of health law and policy and founding chair of the Department of Health Policy, Milken Institute School of Public Health, George Washington University. She also holds a professorship by courtesy in the George Washington Law School and is a member of the faculty of the School of Medicine and Health Sciences. A graduate of Wesleyan University and Boston University Law School, Ms. Rosenbaum has devoted her professional career to issues of health justice for populations who are medically underserved as a result of race, poverty, disability, or cultural exclusion. An honored teacher and scholar, a highly popular speaker, and a widely read writer on many aspects of health law and policy, she has emphasized public engagement as a core element of her professional life, providing public service to six presidential administrations and 15 Congresses since 1977. Ms. Rosenbaum is best known for her work on the expansion of Medicaid, the expansion of community health centers, patients' rights in managed care, civil rights and health care, and national health reform. Between 1993 and 1994, she worked for President Clinton, directing the drafting of the Health Security Act and designing the Vaccines for Children program, which offers near-universal coverage of vaccines for low-income and medically underserved children. She also regularly advises state governments on health policy matters and has served as a testifying expert in legal actions involving the rights of children under Medicaid. Professor Rosenbaum is the lead author of *Law and the American Health Care System*, 2nd edition (May 2012), a landmark textbook that provides an in-depth exploration of the interaction of American law and the U.S. health care system. She has received national awards for her work, serves on governmental advisory committees and private organizational and foundation boards, and is a past chair of AcademyHealth. She is a member of the Centers for Disease Control and Prevention (CDC) Director's Advisory Committee; has served as a member of CDC's Advisory Committee on Immunization Practice (ACIP); and is a commissioner on the Medicaid and Children's Health Insurance Program (CHIP) Payment and Access Commission (MACPAC), which advises Congress on federal Medicaid policy. Ms. Rosenbaum was elected to the National Academy of Medicine in 2012.

William J. Barbaresi, M.D., is director of the Developmental Medicine Center and associate chief, Division of Developmental Medicine, at Boston Children's Hospital, where he holds the Wade Family Foundation Chair in Developmental Medicine. He is associate professor of pediatrics at Harvard Medical School. Prior to his appointment at Boston Children's Hospital, Dr. Barbaresi was an associate professor in the division of developmental and behavioral pediatrics, Mayo Clinic College of Medicine. He earned his B.A. in psychology from Dartmouth College and his M.D. from the University at Buffalo School of Medicine and Biomedical Sciences. Dr. Barbaresi's research and clinical practice focus on childhood and adult attention deficit hyperactivity disorder (ADHD) and autism spectrum disorder and the co-occurrence of these conditions with other neurodevelopmental conditions and developmental disabilities. He serves as medical director for the University Centers for Excellence in Developmental Disabilities Education, Research, and Service, a collaborative effort of the Division of Developmental Medicine and the Institute for Community Inclusion at Boston Children's Hospital and the University of Massachusetts Boston to support training and education in the field of intellectual and developmental disabilities.

Stephen M. Camarata, Ph.D., is professor of hearing and speech sciences and former acting director of the Vanderbilt Kennedy Center for Research on Human Development, where he directed the research program on communication and learning in the Test and Technology Center. He is a nationally renowned researcher on speech and language development and intervention. Much of Dr. Camarata's work is focused on the Child Language Intervention Project (CLIP), which he also directs. CLIP provides individualized treatments for children with a variety of speech and language disorders, serving 200 children locally and more than 1,500 children in other states and countries. The National Institutes of Health (NIH) designated CLIP as a National Center for the Study of Language Intervention during 1998-2003. Dr. Camarata received B.A. and M.A. degrees in speech pathology and audiology from San Diego State University and a Ph.D. in 1984 from Purdue University. He was a postdoctoral fellow at the Early Childhood Language Laboratory in the Department of Hearing and Speech Sciences at the University of Arizona. He was a faculty member in special education and communication disorders at Pennsylvania State University from 1985 to 1988, and was on the faculty of Speech and Hearing Sciences at the University of California, Santa Barbara, from 1988 to 1990. He joined the Vanderbilt Hearing and Speech Sciences faculty in 1990. Dr. Camarata teaches graduate courses on how children acquire language, on child language and speech disorders, and on research design. Nationally, he is a member and fellow of the American Speech-Language-Hearing Association, and he previously chaired the association's Division on Treatment Efficacy. He also is active in the International Association for the Study of Child Language.

Christine Dollaghan, Ph.D., is an associate dean and professor in the School of Behavioral and Brain Sciences at the University of Texas at Dallas. Prior to joining the University of Texas at Dallas faculty in 2006, she was a professor of communicative disorders at the University of Pittsburgh. Her research focuses on diagnosis, treatment, and prediction in children with various speech and language disorders, including children with specific language impairment (SLI) and those recovering from severe traumatic brain injury. In addition to developing and exploring the validity of diagnostic measures for children of differing linguistic and demographic backgrounds, Dr. Dollaghan has reported on studies and meta-analyses concerning the accuracy of early language measures for predicting later outcomes. She is particularly interested in the quality of evidence available for clinical decision making, and authored a text on evidence-based practice in communication disorders in 2007. She has headed several research-related committees of the American Speech-Language-Hearing Association and received the Honors of the association in 2012.

Sidney M. Gospe, Jr., M.D., Ph.D., holds the Herman and Faye Sarkowsky Endowed Chair and is head of the Division of Pediatric Neurology at the University of Washington and Seattle Children's Hospital. Prior to joining the faculty of the University of Washington in 2000, he served on the faculty of the University of California, Davis, for 13 years. Dr. Gospe received his undergraduate education at Stanford University and earned his M.D. and Ph.D. degrees from Duke University. He completed his postgraduate medical education in both pediatrics and child neurology at Baylor College of Medicine in Houston. He has more than 25 years of experience in caring for infants, children, and adolescents with neurological and neuromuscular disorders. Dr. Gospe's laboratory research has focused on neurotoxicology, in particular on the neurodevelopmental effects of maternal exposure to certain toxicants during pregnancy. His clinical research concerns pyridoxine (vitamin B6)-dependent epilepsy (PDE), a rare familial cause of infantile seizures and associated developmental disability. He participates in biochemical, molecular, and radiological studies of patients with PDE and has established a national registry for patients with this uncommon inherited disorder.

Gloria L. Krahn, Ph.D., M.P.H., holds the Barbara Emily Knudson Endowed Chair in Family in the College of Public Health and Human Sciences at Oregon State University. Previously, she served for 5 years as division director of human development and disability at CDC, and for almost 25 years on the faculty of the Oregon Health & Science University (OHSU) in clinical practice, research, and training. Positions at OHSU in Portland included professor of pediatrics in public health and preventive medicine, director of the Oregon Institute on Disability & Development/University Center for Excellence in Developmental Disabilities, director of the Rehabilitation Research and Training Center on Health of People with Long Term Disabilities, and associate director of the Child Development and Rehabilitation Center. Dr. Krahn's areas of expertise relate to disability and public health. She has specific expertise in public health and disability across the life span, disability and health disparities, health policy, and human development. She has served in a number of national and international leadership roles, and has contributed to the growth of the field of disabilities and public health by co-editing the first textbook in the field (2009), supporting the development of the *Disability and Health Journal* and continuing to serve on its editorial board, providing oversight for Healthy People 2020 objectives on disability and health, and supporting the U.S. Department of Health and Human Services' (HHS's) cross-agency planning on disability-related health disparities. Dr. Krahn earned an M.A. and a Ph.D. in psychology from the University of Manitoba, Canada; received an M.P.H. from the University of California, Berkeley; and completed a postdoctoral residency at OHSU.

Elysa Marco, M.D., is a cognitive and behavioral child neurologist. She cares for children with all types of neurologic concerns; however, she specializes in the evaluation and treatment of children with cognitive, sensory, and behavioral challenges. Dr. Marco participates in the care of children at the University of California, San Francisco (UCSF), Medical Center Pediatric Neurology Clinic and the UCSF Marin-based practice in Greenbrae. In addition to her general child neurology and cognitive-behavioral focused clinics, she co-directs the monthly Autism NeuroGenetics Clinic, where children on the autism spectrum can receive coordinated evaluation and treatment from specialists in neurology and genetics. Dr. Marco also has an active neuroscience laboratory at UCSF that focuses on understanding and finding treatments for individuals with neurodevelopmental disorders. Her research is based on a thorough cognition and sensory evaluation of each child, combined with innovative functional imaging to better understand how children's brains process sound, touch, and visual information. Dr. Marco's current research involves individuals with autism disorders, sensory processing disorders, neuroanatomic disorders (such as agenesis of the corpus callosum), and specific genetic disorders (such as 16p11.2 copy number variations). In addition, she is an active collaborator with investigators studying the effects of autism on maternal health and the neural underpinnings of Tourette's syndrome. Her lab also is combining structural and functional brain imaging with computer-based training interventions to determine whether computer games can help children resist distracting information and improve visual motor planning. The overarching goal of her research is to use basic science findings to create beneficial treatments for children. Dr. Marco received her B.A. in psychology at the University of Pennsylvania and then obtained her M.D. at UCSF. She continued her residency training at UCSF in pediatrics, neurology, and child neurology. In addition, she completed a cognitive and behavioral fellowship with an emphasis on the genetics of cognitive impairment. She joined the faculty of UCSF in 2005 and is an active clinician, researcher, and educator.

Mary Pat Moeller, Ph.D., is director of the Center for Childhood Deafness and the Language Development Laboratory at Boys Town National Research Hospital in Omaha, Nebraska. Following many years of clinical practice, she obtained a Ph.D. in child language at the University of Nebraska–Lincoln. Her current research explores factors influencing the outcomes of children who are deaf or hard of hearing. She is co-principal investigator with J. Bruce Tomblin of an National Institutes of Health (NIH)-funded, prospective, multisite, longitudinal study of spoken language development in children who are hard of hearing. In addition to her longitudinal research efforts, Dr. Moeller conducted NIH-funded health communication research related to newborn hearing screening. She led a consensus conference in Austria in 2012 that resulted in a best practice statement on family-centered early intervention practices for children who are deaf or hard of hearing. Dr. Moeller has published and lectured internationally on topics related to developmental outcomes and early intervention practices for children who are deaf or hard of hearing. She received the Honors of the American Speech-Language-Hearing Association in 2013. She is the association's representative to the Joint Committee on Infant Hearing.

Susan L. Parish, Ph.D., is Nancy Lurie Marks professor of disability policy, director of the Lurie Institute for Disability Policy, and associate dean for research at the Heller School for Social Policy and Management, Brandeis University. Prior to joining Brandeis, she served on the faculty of the School of Social Work at the University of North Carolina at Chapel Hill. Dr. Parish's research examines the health and financial well-being of children and adults with disabilities and their caregiving families. She is particularly interested in the impact of health, income transfer, and poverty policies on these populations. Her research has been funded by federal, state, and foundation sources, including NIH, HHS (Health Resources and Services Administration), and the U.S. Department of Education (National Institute on Disability and Rehabilitation Research). Dr. Parish teaches classes in disability policy and both quantitative and qualitative research methods. She has won numerous awards for her teaching and her research, including the Padgett Early Career Achievement Award from the Society for Social Work and Research and the Research Matters! award from the Arc of the United States. She is a fellow of the American Association of Intellectual & Developmental Disabilities. Dr. Parish received a B.A. in English and an M.S.W. from Rutgers University and her Ph.D. in public health from the University of Illinois at Chicago. She completed a National Institute of Child Health and Human Development (NICHD)-funded post-doctoral research fellowship at the University of Wisconsin–Madison.

Ramesh Raghavan, M.D., Ph.D., is Professor and Associate Dean for Research in the School of Social Work at Rutgers, The State University of New Jersey. He focuses his research on access to and quality of mental health services for vulnerable children, especially those in the child welfare system. The instrumental focus of much of his work on access has been on Medicaid policy making, and he has examined the effects of Medicaid managed care on mental health service use, the longitudinal stability of health insurance coverage for child welfare-involved children, and insurance discontinuities for children leaving foster care. His work on quality has focused on receipt of mental health care consistent with national standards among children in the child welfare system, geographic variations in mental health services, and policy approaches to supporting implementation of mental health services. His current work focuses on developing better predictive models of the risk of mental health service use among child Medicaid beneficiaries and understanding the determinants of racial/ethnic disparities in Medicaid expenditures for child mental health services. A keen translator of research findings to policy making and vice versa, Dr. Raghavan has served on state and national commissions and advisory bodies, and conducts much of his research with active policy makers as co-investigators. In early 2015, he served as Senior Advisor in the Office of the Commissioner of the Administration on Children, Youth and

Families in Washington, DC. His work has received financial support from the Agency for Healthcare Research and Quality, the Administration for Children and Families, the National Institute of Mental Health (NIMH), and the State of Missouri. Dr. Raghavan is chair of NIMH's Mental Health Services Research review committee. He is a psychiatrist and health services researcher by training.

Audrey M. Sorrells, Ph.D., is associate dean of students for research in the Office of the Dean of Students, Division of Student Affairs, at the University of Texas at Austin. She is also associate professor of special education in the university's College of Education and past fellow in the Lee Hage Jamail Regents Chair in Education, as well as senior Ford fellow, National Research Council. Prior to her appointment in the Office of the Dean of Students, Dr. Sorrells served as undergraduate advisor and minority liaison officer in the Department of Special Education, as well as chair of several department, college, and university committees. She has 27 years of higher education teaching and research experience, from 1987 to 1997 at Southeastern Louisiana University and since 1997 at the University of Texas at Austin. Prior to her university appointments, Dr. Sorrells taught in K-12 settings, teaching students at risk and in high-poverty rural and urban schools, including students with learning and behavioral disabilities. Her research in higher education has focused on the first-year experience; first-generation students; veteran students with posttraumatic stress, mild traumatic brain injury (mTBI), and substance use disorders; and students with disabilities, as well as professional development and interdisciplinary partnerships in higher education. Other areas on which her research has focused include minority and disproportionate representation in K-12 schools for students with disabilities, reading instruction in middle and secondary schools, and college readiness. In addition to having authored and coauthored many refereed publications, Dr. Sorrells is a consultant and presenter at the local, state, and national levels, and currently serves as a principal investigator or co-investigator of several state and federally funded grants. She served as co-editor of the *Journal of Multiple Voices for Ethnically Diverse Exceptional Learners* and is co-author of the book *Critical Issues in Special Education: Access, Diversity and Accountability*. The recipient of many honors, including a doctoral leadership award from the University of Florida, Dr. Sorrells has also been a Ford Foundation postdoctoral fellow and a dean's fellow at the University of Texas at Austin and is listed in *Who's Who Among Educators in America*. She earned a B.A. in business administration and education and master of education degree in special education from Southeastern Louisiana University. She holds a Ph.D. in education from the University of Florida.

J. Bruce Tomblin, Ph.D., CCC-SP, is Child Language Research Center director and an emeritus professor at the University of Iowa. His research and teaching have long been in children's language development and disorders. In recent years, his research has been concerned with the development of and the genetic influence on the occurrence of certain forms of children's language problems. Much of this research has been supported by NIH research grants and contracts. Dr. Tomblin earned a B.A. in psychology from the University of La Verne, an M.A. in speech from the University of Redlands, and a Ph.D. in communicative disorders from the University of Wisconsin–Madison. He is a fellow of the American Speech-Language-Hearing Association and the Iowa Speech and Hearing Association. He holds a certificate of clinical competence in speech-language pathology from the American Speech-Language-Hearing Association.

Karl R. White, Ph.D., is a professor of psychology, holder of the Emma Eccles Jones Endowed Chair in Early Childhood Education, and founding director of the National Center for Hearing Assessment and Management. He has also held positions as a senior Fulbright scholar at Wilhelms Westfälische Universität in Germany, a congressional science fellow with the United States Senate, and chair of the Department of Research and Development at the National Technical Institute for the Deaf. Dr. White is recognized as one of the world's leading authorities on early identification and treatment of childhood hearing loss. His work has been recognized with awards from such diverse organizations as the Deafness Research Foundation, the American Speech-Language-Hearing Association, the Swedish Society of Medicine, the Alexander Graham Bell Association for the Deaf, and the Ali Yavar Jung National Institute for the Hearing Handicapped in India. He has produced hundreds of publications and made numerous presentations at scholarly meetings, and has been an invited speaker to more than 35 countries, where he has assisted in the implementation of newborn hearing screening and intervention programs. Dr. White has been the principal investigator or co–principal investigator for competitively funded grants and contracts at Utah State University totaling more than $60 million. He also serves on many national and international advisory groups for such organizations as HHS; the World Health Organization; the National Academies of Sciences, Engineering, and Medicine; the March of Dimes; and the American Academy of Pediatrics.

CONSULTANTS

Howard H. Goldman, M.D., Ph.D., is professor of psychiatry at the University of Maryland School of Medicine. He received joint M.D.-M.P.H.

degrees from Harvard University in 1974 and a Ph.D. in social policy research from the Heller School at Brandeis University in 1978. He is the author or coauthor of 325 publications in the professional literature. Dr. Goldman is the editor of *Psychiatric Services*, a mental health services research and policy journal published monthly by the American Psychiatric Association. He also has served on the editorial boards of several other journals, including the *American Journal of Psychiatry*, *Health Affairs*, and the *Journal of Mental Health Policy and Economics*. He served as senior scientific editor of the *Surgeon General's Report on Mental Health* from 1997 to 1999, for which he was awarded the Surgeon General's Medallion. During 2002 and 2003, Dr. Goldman was a consultant to the President's New Freedom Commission on Mental Health. In 1996 he was elected to membership in the National Academy of Social Insurance, and in 2002 he was elected to the National Academy of Medicine. He has chaired the National Academies of Sciences, Engineering, and Medicine's Standing Committee to Provide Medical Advice to the Disability Program of the Social Security Administration since 2009.

Barbara C. Sonies, Ph.D., formerly chief of the Speech-Language Pathology Section and chief of the Oral Motor Function Section, Department of Rehabilitation Medicine, NIH, is currently a research professor at the University of Maryland, Department of Hearing and Speech Sciences; she also is former adjunct professor at the George Washington University Speech and Hearing Department. She is currently a consultant to the Human Genome Research Institute at NIH on swallowing and oral motor function. Her clinical experience includes work with adults and children with a variety of cognitive, communicative, and developmental issues at the University of Minnesota Hospitals, where she was chief of speech-language pathology. She received the Honors of the American-Speech-Language Hearing Association, of which she is a fellow. Dr. Sonies founded the association's Dysphagia Special Interest Division and developed the original plan for board certification in swallowing and swallowing disorders. She holds a specialty certification in swallowing and swallowing disorders and was secretary of the Specialty Certification Board. Dr. Sonies has published many articles and presented hundreds of seminars and workshops on dysphagia and neurological disorders. She continues to mentor students and professionals in dysphagia practice. She originated the use of ultrasound to image the oral cavity for speech and swallowing and has conducted research on various conditions that impact swallowing function.